Anticancer Treatments and Cardiotoxicity

Anticancer Treatments and Cardiotoxicity

Mechanisms, Diagnostic, and Therapeutic Interventions

Edited by

Patrizio Lancellotti, PhD, MD
Professor of Cardiology, University of Liège, Liège, Belgium

Jose L. Zamorano Gómez, MD, FESC
Professor and Head of Cardiology, University Hospital Ramón y Cajal, Madrid, Spain

Maurizio Galderisi, MD, FESC
Associate Professor of Cardiology, Clinical Director, Federico II University Hospital, Naples, Italy

ELSEVIER

AMSTERDAM • BOSTON • HEIDELBERG • LONDON
NEW YORK • OXFORD • PARIS • SAN DIEGO
SAN FRANCISCO • SINGAPORE • SYDNEY • TOKYO
Academic Press is an imprint of Elsevier

Academic Press is an imprint of Elsevier
125 London Wall, London EC2Y 5AS, United Kingdom
525 B Street, Suite 1800, San Diego, CA 92101-4495, United States
50 Hampshire Street, 5th Floor, Cambridge, MA 02139, United States
The Boulevard, Langford Lane, Kidlington, Oxford OX5 1GB, United Kingdom

Notices

Knowledge and best practice in this field are constantly changing. As new research and experience broaden our understanding, changes in research methods, professional practices, or medical treatment may become necessary.

Practitioners and researchers must always rely on their own experience and knowledge in evaluating and using any information, methods, compounds, or experiments described herein. In using such information or methods they should be mindful of their own safety and the safety of others, including parties for whom they have a professional responsibility.

To the fullest extent of the law, neither the Publisher nor the authors, contributors, or editors, assume any liability for any injury and/or damage to persons or property as a matter of products liability, negligence or otherwise, or from any use or operation of any methods, products, instructions, or ideas contained in the material herein.

British Library Cataloguing-in-Publication Data
A catalogue record for this book is available from the British Library

Library of Congress Cataloging-in-Publication Data
A catalog record for this book is available from the Library of Congress

ISBN: 978-0-12-802509-3

For Information on all Academic Press publications
visit our website at https://www.elsevier.com

Publisher: Mica Haley
Acquisition Editor: Stacy Masucci
Editorial Project Manager: Sam W. Young
Production Project Manager: Lucía Pérez
Designer: Victoria Pearson

Typeset by MPS Limited, Chennai, India

Contents

Section V
Detection of Cardiac Dysfunction and Predictors of Cardiotoxicity

Section VI
Cardiotoxicity in Childhood

27. Cardiotoxicity of Childhood Cancer Treatments

J.L. Zamorano Gómez, J. Ramos, G. Alcidi and M. Galderisi

Section VII
Management of Anticancer Drugs Related Cardiotoxicity

28. Nonpharmacologic Therapy

G.L. Alonso Salinas and J.L. Zamorano Gómez

29. Beta-Blockers

G.L. Alonso Salinas and J.L. Zamorano Gómez

List of Contributors

R.A. Abellás-Sequeiros Complejo Hospitalario Universitario de Santiago de Compostela, Santiago de Compostela, Spain; University Clinical Hospital of Santiago de Compostela, Santiago de Compostela, Spain

G. Alcidi Federico II University, Naples, Italy

G.L. Alonso Salinas Hospital Ramón y Cajal, Madrid, Spain

G. Arpino AOU Federico II, Napoli, Italy

B. Ayach The University of Manitoba, Winnipeg, MB, Canada

R. Boni Regional Center of Nuclear Medicine, University of Pisa, Pisa, Italy

V. Bours University of Liège, Liège, Belgium; CHU Liège, Liège, Belgium

J. Brown The Methodist Hospital, Houston, TX, United States

C. Bucciarelli-Ducci University of Bristol, Bristol, United Kingdom; Imperial College London, London, United Kingdom

D. Cardinale European Institute of Oncology, Milan, Italy

C. Coppola Istituto Nazionale per lo Studio e la Cura dei Tumori "Fondazione Giovanni Pascale," IRCCS, Naples, Italy

B. Cosyns Centrum voor Hart en Vaatziekten, Jette, Belgium

R. Dulgheru University Hospital Sart Tilman, Liège, Belgium

T. Edvardsen Oslo University Hospital, Oslo, Norway

P.A. Erba Regional Center of Nuclear Medicine, University of Pisa, Pisa, Italy

P. Freres CHU Sart Tilman, Liège, Belgium

M. Galderisi Federico II University Hospital, Naples, Italy

J.R. González-Juanatey Complejo Hospitalario Universitario de Santiago de Compostela, Santiago de Compostela, Spain; University Clinical Hospital of Santiago de Compostela, Santiago de Compostela, Spain

R. Hinojar University Hospital Ramón y Cajal, Madrid, Spain

F. Ilardi Federico II University Hospital, Naples, Italy

G. Jerusalem CHU Sart Tilman, Liège, Belgium; E.S. Health Science Foundation, Lugo, Italy

D. Kerkhove Center voor Hart- en Vaatziekten, UZ Brussel, Jette, Brussels, Belgium

P. Lancellotti University of Liège, Liège, Belgium

T. López Fernández IdiPaz Research Institute, Madrid, Spain

A. López López University Clinical Hospital of Santiago de Compostela, Santiago de Compostela, Spain

J. López Sendón IdiPaz Research Institute, Madrid, Spain

C.R. Manrique Montefiore-Einstein Center for Heart and Vascular Care, Bronx, NY, United States

N. Maurea Istituto Nazionale per lo Studio e la Cura dei Tumori "Fondazione Giovanni Pascale," IRCCS, Naples, Italy

M.J. Monagham King's College Hospital, London, United Kingdom

M. Moonen University of Liège, Liège, Belgium; CHU Sart Tilman, Liège, Belgium

C. Oury University of Liège, Liège, Belgium

I. Paciolla AOU Federico II, Napoli, Italy

J.C. Plana Baylor College of Medicine, Houston, TX, United States; Texas Heart Institute, Houston, TX, United States

J. Ramos University of Alcalá, Alcalá de Henares, Spain

A. Rienzo Istituto Nazionale per lo Studio e la Cura dei Tumori "Fondazione Giovanni Pascale," IRCCS, Naples, Italy

F. Rigo dell'Angelo Hospital, Venice, Italy

D. Rodríguez Muñoz University Hospital Ramón y Cajal, Madrid, Spain

V. Sánchez Doce de Octubre University Hospital, Madrid, Spain

C. Santoro Federico II University Hospital, Naples, Italy

M. Scherrer-Crosbie Massachusetts General Hospital, Boston, MA, United States

R. Sicari Institute of Clinical Physiology, Pisa, Italy

M. Sollini Nuclear Medicine Unit, IRCCS MultiMedica, Sesto San Giovanni, Italy

R. Sorrentino Federico II University Hospital, Naples, Italy

N. Tiwari Montefiore-Einstein Center for Heart and Vascular Care, Bronx, NY, United States

J.L. Zamorano Gómez University Hospital Ramón y Cajal, Madrid, Spain; University of Alcalá, Alcalá de Henares, Spain

Foreword

It was in early 2000 that a 60-year old woman was admitted to my service at the University Hospital in Bern because of severe heart failure. The patient was diagnosed with breast cancer 2 years earlier and treated with surgery and adjuvant chemotherapy. Unfortunately, several metastases were discovered at the end of 1999 and since the tumor was HER2-positive she was one of the first to be treated with a new, promising drug called *trastuzumab*. We quickly found out that the reason for her heart failure was a severely reduced left ventricular ejection fraction but her left ventricle was not dilated. We also knew that her cardiac function was normal prior to the start of *trastuzumab* and that she was previously treated with doxorubicin and cyclophosphamide. We had no evidence for any common reasons for acute heart failure and the dynamic of the events spoke against anthracycline cardiotoxicity. So we started to search for a more unusual cause for cardiac dysfunction and it took us a while to suspect *trastuzumab* as the key to explain what was going on. The literature about *trastuzumab* cardiotoxicity was scarce at that time and, not knowing if we would harm the patient more than helping, we opted for stopping *trastuzumab*. The patient improved quickly and her cardiac function recovered to normal within 6 weeks. It was a difficult decision to stop *trastuzumab* since the patient seemed to profit from the drug and therapeutic alternatives were limited—and our concerns became a harsh reality when the patient died a few months later because of progressive cancer.

These events prompted us to look deeper into the case of cancer drug-induced cardiotoxicity. The cardiac biopsies from the unfortunate patient gave us an opportunity to further investigate possible mechanisms and we found myocardial messenger RNA encoding for HER2 and HER4, establishing a potential link between the cancer drug and cardiac side effects. We also found that trastuzumab alone did not induce myocardial cell death in human cardiac tissue, explaining the reversibility of cardiac dysfunction in our patient. Many years later we have a substantially better understanding of trastuzumab-induced cardiac dysfunction and cancer treatment and cardiotoxicity in general. We have learned that some cancer drugs cause irreversible and progressive cardiotoxicity while others lead only to temporary, stunning-like dysfunction without long-term consequences for the patient.

But daily clinical decision-making in cancer patients experiencing cardiotoxicity remains complex. Most cancer regimens contain several drugs and it is frequently difficult to identify those that cause side effects. And what should we do if these side effects become manifest? Should we immediately stop the potentially lifesaving cancer drugs and risk that the patient dies of cancer like our unfortunate woman? Or should we risk that the patient eventually experiences progressive cardiac disease introducing another life limiting health problem? We need to become smarter about the decision-making for our patients experiencing cardiotoxicity. We need experts who understand the complex pathophysiology of cardiotoxicity and clinicians and scientists who develop risk–benefit analysis tools to guide decision-making in clinical practice.

And this is where *Anticancer Treatments and Cardiotoxicity* comes to help. Patrizio Lancellotti and a dedicated group of experts have written a comprehensive book covering all aspects of cardio-oncology, including the important side effects of radiation therapy. This is one of few books that will help the clinician to come to the right conclusion when faced with a patient experiencing cardiotoxicity. But the authors do not stop here. They observe the tremendous progress in oncology with new drugs and treatments available at an exceedingly high pace. Several of these treatments bear the potential to cause cardiovascular harm. The book therefore also looks into the future and discusses research priorities to tackle these issues. I can only hope that every oncologist, every cardiologist, and every aspiring scientist in the area of cardio-oncology will read this book.

Thomas M. Suter

Preface

The goals of anticancer therapies are to prevent recurrence, prolong life, and provide cure. Partly due to improvements in treatment, the population of cancer survivors is large and growing. However, cancer treatment-related cardiotoxicity is the leading cause of treatment-associated mortality in cancer survivors. It is one of the most common posttreatment issues among 5–10-year survivors of adult cancer. Moreover, patients treated with cardiotoxic cancer therapies often develop multiple risk factors, further worsening cardiovascular reserve and increasing the likelihood of subsequent cardiotoxicity. The extent of cardiotoxicity is variable, depending on the type of drug used, combination with other drugs, prior mediastinal radiotherapy, and the presence of cardiovascular risk factors or history of heart disease. Early detection of the patients prone for developing cardiotoxicity is the key issue to decrease morbidity and mortality. It also facilitates more tailored therapeutic interventions. Therefore, the collaboration and interaction of cardiology and oncology may contribute to reducing the cardiovascular adverse effects and improving the results in the treatment of patients with cancer. Effective therapies to treat cancer and cancer therapy-induced cardiotoxicity must either take advantage of tissue-specific differences or affect the downstream mediators of toxicity, and there are active studies under way to develop new targeted therapies. Other effective therapies for cardioprotection include typical pharmacologic therapies used in cardiovascular disease that promote increased cardiac reserve and reverse remodeling under the stress of cancer therapy.

This book on *Anticancer Treatments and Cardiotoxicity* discusses the different aspects of cardiac effects of both radiotherapy and chemotherapy as well as diagnostic and imaging studies to evaluate/predict the development of cardiac dysfunction. New guidelines on imaging for the screening and monitoring of these patients are discussed. The book is highly illustrated. Most chapters contain a number of illustrations and tables.

Patrizio Lancellotti
Maurizio Galderisi
Jose L. Zamorano Gómez

Preamble

In the last decade, the therapeutic management of patients with cancer, traditionally including multiple combination of drugs, radiation therapy, and surgery, has been strongly enriched by the introduction of molecularly targeted therapies. This has led to an important reduction of morbidity and mortality of several kinds of cancer, increasing remission rate and often converting cancer into a chronic disease [1]. Nowadays, millions of cancer patients around the world are surviving long enough to develop adverse cardiovascular complications, which may become the cause of premature mortality and alter substantially the quality of life of these patients [2]. Therefore, cancer and heart are inextricably associated, including in relation to shared risk factors and diseases coexistence.

Both conventional chemotherapeutic agents, such as anthracyclines, and newer targeted agents, such as trastuzumab, can cause varying degrees of cardiac dysfunction [3]. Type I cardiac toxicity, typical of anthracyclines, may be acute or chronic, appearing even several years after therapy completion. It is dose-dependent and largely irreversible since it induces cellular necrosis. Type II cardiac toxicity, typical of newer targeted agents such as trastuzumab, is not dose-dependent and is generally reversible with cessation of the drug since it does not lead to cellular necrosis. It is noteworthy that types I and II cardiac toxicity can be associated sequentially in the same cancer patient (e.g., breast cancer) cumulating the effect of one of the drugs to the other. Accordingly, several cardiovascular adverse effects can become clinically overt years or even decades after receiving the cancer therapy: congestive heart failure, myocardial ischemia, systemic and/or pulmonary arterial hypertension, thromboembolic complications, arrhythmias, and conduction disturbances can all be clinical manifestations of these adverse effects [1,2,4]. This is particularly true for adult survivors of childhood cancers.

Also, the effect of radiation therapy shall not be underevaluated, in particular in some kinds of cancers, which are managed by irradiation of the neck and/or thorax (mainly, lymphoma and breast cancer). Radiation-induced heart disease comprises a spectrum of cardiac pathology including myocardial fibrosis and cardiomyopathy, coronary and carotid artery disease, valvular disease, pericardial disease, and arrhythmias. Tissue fibrosis is a common mediator in radiation-induced heart disease. Multiple pathways converge with both acute and chronic cellular, molecular, and genetic changes to result in fibrosis [5]. The total cumulative dosage of radiation is a function of the number of treatments and the dose of irradiation. Although they may acutely develop, the manifestations of radiotherapy most often become clinically evident several years after irradiation.

In addition to the adverse cardiac effects produced by cancer and radiation therapies, some kinds of cancers can themselves produce detrimental effects on the cardiovascular system inducing alterations of pericardium (mainly pericardial effusion till cardiac tamponade) myocardium (myocarditis), and cardiac valves (primary or secondary localization on valve structures), with a varying degrees of hemodynamic impairment, but also producing cardiac metastasis [4].

In this panorama, the substantial importance of diagnosing the onset of clinically overt toxicity on the heart is equal to the importance of detecting subclinical cardiotoxicity in order to develop cardioprotective strategies and avoid, whenever possible, cancer therapy withdrawal. Monitoring of cardiotoxicity exclusively based on symptoms onset assessment may in fact miss the opportunity to identify early cardiac injury that is still in a reversible stage. Potential strategies to mitigate the risks of cardiac complications for cancer patients include physical examination, electrocardiogram, and use of biomarkers and/or cardiac imaging [4]. Echocardiography and biomarkers such as cardiac troponins and, to a lesser extent, brain natriuretic peptide, are current means to detect presymptomatic cardiac damage and evaluate cardioprotective treatments. The next standard echocardiography, advanced ultrasound techniques can provide an additional diagnostic power. Speckle tracking echocardiography-derived global longitudinal strain has been demonstrated in fact to be altered as the effect of cancer therapy when left ventricular ejection fraction is still normal [4]. When compared to standard 2D echo, real-time 3D echocardiography provides much more reproducible estimation of ejection fraction and can therefore be used successfully to achieve early detection of cardiotoxicity in cancer patients [4]. The more sophisticated cardiovascular magnetic resonance can be taken into account in selected cases to highlight the presence of subtle cardiac abnormalities and myocardial fibrosis (late gadolinium enhancement) or when echocardiographic images are not adequate. While the more prominent role of biomarkers or cardiac imaging remains controversial, combined use of both approaches can also be suggested since the two strategies have already shown a complimentary diagnostic power, which is superior to that of the two separate approaches [4].

The treatment of cardiac toxicity is largely influenced by the comorbities in which the damage is diagnosed. The general principles utilized in the treatment of cardiac dysfunction in all cardiac patients (i.e., adequate diet, exercise and weight control, use of cardiac drugs such as beta-blockers and renin–angiotensin system inhibitors, selective use of aldosterone antagonists) can be considered equally important in cancer survivors experiencing cardiac toxicity. Nevertheless, conclusive data supporting the efficacy of these interventions are limited.

The reflection of strategies able to unmask subclinical cardiotoxicity on the cardiac management of patients undergoing cancer therapy has to be still definitely proven in the clinical setting. Data in selected centers highlight however that early detection of cardiotoxicity can lead to an early aggressive pharmacologic approach based on the use of ACE inhibitors and/or beta-blockers, which has been shown to be successful in anthracycline-related cardiotoxicity [6]. Data on the efficacy of cardiac drugs among childhood cancer patients are much more limited.

True prevention of overt cardiotoxicity begins before cancer therapy administration: a baseline assessment of cardiovascular health and effective treatment of cardiovascular conditions and effective treatment of cardiovascular risk factors are needed to prevent most late cardiac toxicities. Aspirin, effective control of dyslipidemia and of blood pressure in hypertensive patients, as well as cigarette smoking cessation are interventions that should be aggressively promoted when needed.

Combined together, all the above-mentioned findings, suggestions, and/or recommendations emphasize that an increased collaboration between cardiologists and oncologists is needed to determine the best treatment and the best preventive strategies that could improve the cardiac health of individual patients [7]. This means increased knowledge of the mechanisms responsible for cardiotoxicity of traditional and novel cancer therapeutics from the cardiologic side and the search for a continuous interaction with cardiologists from the oncologic side, in order to achieve the best methodology for cardiovascular prediction and risk stratification. A growing clinical demand is now producing the planning of dedicated cardio-oncology programs, which include diagnostic, interventional, and advanced heart failure services.

The present textbook has been created and developed on these grounds, to give access to both cardiologists and oncologists on the state of the art and perspectives of the interdisciplinary cardio-oncology clinical care. It includes general considerations on epidemiology and description of mechanisms underlying cardiotoxicity and radiotherapy, of detection of clinical and subclinical toxicity due to cancer therapeutics by both cardiovascular imaging and biomarkers in both adults and in childhood, presentation of traditional and innovative nonpharmacological and pharmacological management of anticancer drug-related cardiotoxicity as well as of a multidisciplinary approach to cardiac disease in cancer patients. Future research priorities, including pharmacogenomic screening, cardiac monitoring during clinical trials, and novel preventive therapies will be also presented as the new frontiers of a cardio-oncology approach to cancer patients and survivors.

Maurizio Galderisi and Patrizio Lancellotti

REFERENCES

[1] Todaro MC, Oreto L, Qamar R, Paterick TE, Carerj S, Khandheria BK. Cardioncology: state of the heart. Int J Cardiol 2013;168:680–7.

[2] Lenihan DK, Olive S, Chow EJ, Cardinale D. Cardiac toxicity in cancer survivors. Cancer 2013;119(Suppl. 11):2131–42.

[3] Bowles EJ, Wellman R, Feigelson HS, Onitilo AA, Freedman AN, Delate T, et al. Risk of heart failure in breast cancer patients after anthracycline and trastuzumab treatment: a retrospective cohort study. J Nat l Cancer Inst 2012;104:1293–305.

[4] Plana JC, Galderisi M, Barac A, Ewer MS, Ky B, Scherrer-Crosbie M, et al. Expert consensus for multimodality imaging evaluation of adult patients during and after cancer therapy: a report from the American Society of Echocardiography and the European Association of Cardiovascular Imaging. Eur Heart J Cardiovasc Imaging 2014;15:1063–93.

[5] Lancellotti P, Nkomo VT, Badano LP, Bergler-Klein J, Bogaert J, Davin L, et al. Expert consensus for multi-modality imaging evaluation of cardiovascular complications of radiotherapy in adults: a report from the European Association of Cardiovascular Imaging and the American Society of Echocardiography. Eur Heart J Cardiovasc Imaging 2013;14:721–40.

[6] Cardinale D, Colombo A, Lamantia G, Colombo N, Civelli M, De Giacomi G, et al. Anthracycline-induced cardiomyopathy: clinical relevance and response to pharmacologic therapy. J Am Coll Cardiol 2010;55:213–20.

[7] Barac AC, Murtagh G, Carver JR, Chen MH, Freeman AM, Hermann J, et al. Cardiovascular health of patients with cancer and cancer survivors. A roadmap to the next level. J Am Coll Cardiol 2015;65:2739–46.

How Big Is the Problem? The Oncologist's View

Fortunately, over time, the chance of cure after the diagnosis of cancer is improving. This is related to earlier diagnosis by screening or by earlier consultations and improved diagnostic procedures and more effective treatment options. Today, the oncologists are more and more concerned by the long-term side effects. Cardiac side effects are among the most frequent severe long-term side effects. Historically, it is well known that chemotherapy, radiotherapy and in particular the combination of both treatments exposes the patient to increased risk of cardiac morbidity and mortality. It has been shown more recently that some targeted therapies are also associated with increased risk of cardiac events [1,2]. Treatment decisions in the metastatic setting take mainly the short-term poor oncological prognosis into account. However, the situation is more complicated in the adjuvant setting. We frequently see now small tumors with an 80–90% probability of cure without using cardiotoxic chemotherapy or radiotherapy. The adjuvant therapies can further increase the chance of cure by 3–10% but we have to take into consideration treatment-related short- and long-term morbidity and mortality.

One of the problems is that some of these events are observed very late after the initial therapy. Consequently, it takes a very long time before these late side effects of alternative treatment options are known. Treatment modalities have changed over time in part because the awareness of cardiac side effects has increased. Chemotherapy regimens tend to include a lower cumulative dose of anthracyclines and radiotherapy fields try to avoid the cardiac region. We speculate that these modifications will have a major impact on a decrease of long-term cardiac side effects but we will really know only many years later. Unfortunately, we are facing also major problems with funding in long-term patient follow-up. Industry-sponsored clinical trials cut in general any support after 10 years of follow-up. The organization of clinical trials in the field of radiotherapy is even more challenging as there is no financial support coming from the industry either for the initiation or for the long-term follow-up. Administrative work in clinical trials is continuously increasing, even in academic trials, making clinical research more and more expensive.

We have only limited follow-up for targeted therapies used more recently also in the adjuvant setting, such as trastuzumab in breast cancer. For the earliest studies we have a 10-year follow-up. Nevertheless, longer follow-up is needed. We have also to take into account that patients included in these studies are highly selected and in particular younger than the average patient population. Results concerning cardiac outcome in less selected patient populations including in particular a higher number of older patients are also urgently needed. This need is further illustrated by an Italian multicenter prospective evaluation of trastuzumab-induced cardiotoxicity [3]. Four hundred and ninety-nine consecutive HER2-positive patients suffering from early-stage breast cancer were treated with adjuvant trastuzumab and chemotherapy at 10 Italian institutions. Clinical heart failure occurred in 6% of the patients older than 60, compared to 2% of the younger patients. A reduction in left ventricular ejection fraction (LVEF) of >10 points was detected in 33% of the older compared to 23% of the younger patients. They have also observed that anticancer therapy was interrupted in 10% of the older patients compared to 4% of the younger patients. Another even larger population-based study using the SEER-Medicare and the Texas Cancer Registry-Medicare databases in women at least 66 years old suffering from early-stage breast cancer treated with chemotherapy reported a very high rate of congestive heart failure (CHF) [4]. Among a total of 9535 patients who were evaluated, including 23.1% receiving trastuzumab, the incidence of CHF was 29.4% if they received trastuzumab and 18.9% in those who did not received trastuzumab.

We should better identify the high-risk patients because long-term side effects become an increasing concern in oncology. Multidisciplinary treatment planning is a standard in oncology. However, currently, the experts participating in multidisciplinary discussions are mainly experts in the field of diagnosis and treatment in oncology. It is easy to have access to imaging procedures such as heart ultrasound or MUGA. It is much more challenging to have access to a consultation of a geriatrician or cardiologist with special interest in oncology at the time of treatment planning.

Most patients don't present cardiac abnormalities at the time of diagnosis but they appear during long-term follow-up. Even oncologists well aware of the cardiotoxicity of our treatments need the help of cardiologists to best interpret the available literature and to predict the cardiac risk for an individual patient. Age is not the only risk factor [5]. Data from retrospective studies also suggest an association between cardiovascular risk factors such as history of hypertension, diabetes, or known coronary artery disease and cardiotoxicity of anticancer therapy [6–7]. Sometimes, based on this advice and according to the oncological risk, we will consider either cancellation of adjuvant therapy or, at least for systemic therapy, consideration of alternative therapy regimens which are less cardiotoxic, even if the relative risk reduction of cancer relapse may be a little lower. Time has come to create real cardio-oncology units where cardiologists and oncologists work closely together. All aspects should be considered: identification of patients at risk of developing cardiotoxicity, close monitoring of patients during treatment (such as patients receiving trastuzumab as adjuvant therapy for HER2-positive breast cancer) and long-term follow-up, including in particular optimal therapy in patients who develop toxicity.

Currently, this close collaboration mainly exists already for monitoring of cardiotoxicity during treatment. Clear guidelines for monitoring and therapy interruption exist in particular for adjuvant therapy with trastuzumab. Fortunately, these guidelines are largely followed in the clinic because cardiotoxicity is reversible in most cases if identified early. In many patients treatment can even be successfully reintroduced after interruption without observing a new event of cardiotoxicity [8]. Nevertheless, we still identify a need for earlier identification. Current guidelines are mainly based on decrease of LVEF or CHF. Serum biomarkers and more sensitive imaging techniques should be further evaluated [9]. LVEF recovery and cardiac event reduction may be more frequently achieved when cardiac dysfunction is detected early and a modern heart failure treatment is promptly initiated [10]. In addition, it is useful to point out that these guidelines are not really evidence-proofed but the reproduction of cardiac monitoring during the evaluation of a new potentially cardiotoxic drug in the registration trials. Cost-effectiveness has not been evaluated. More individualized monitoring according to risk factors should also be considered.

Among the major open questions is the role of angiotensin-converting enzyme (ACE) inhibitors in the prevention of trastuzumab-related cardiotoxicity [11]. Beta-blockers are other candidates for preventive treatments [12]. Today we consider anthracycline-free regimens and sequential use of chemotherapy and trastuzumab in patients with higher risk of cardiotoxicity but many consider this not the best treatment, in particular for high-risk patients [13]. If a preventive therapy by an angiotensin-converting enzyme inhibitor would be effective, this could be an alternative if physicians prefer the use of anthracycline-based chemotherapy followed by combined therapy with taxanes and trastuzumab in all high-risk patients. Close collaboration between oncologists and cardiologists is needed if we wish to further develop this kind of treatment strategy.

Patients with a history of cardiovascular disease are excluded from clinical trials evaluating cardiotoxic drugs. As life expectancy is increasing, many of these patients develop cancer. Sometimes, in the real world, the only remaining treatment options are based on cardiotoxic drugs. Unfortunately, no data are available to better differentiate between relative and absolute contraindications. We need the help of cardiologists in order to decide on an individual basis the anticancer therapy and cardiovascular monitoring. There is an urgent need for a prospective register of outcome in these difficult clinical situations.

Guy Jerusalem, Pierre Frères and Philippe Coucke

REFERENCES

[1] Swain SM, Whaley FS, Ewer MS. Congestive heart failure in patients treated with doxorubicin: a retrospective analysis of three trials. Cancer 2003;97:2869–79.

[2] Bird BR, Swain SM. Cardiac toxicity in breast cancer survivors: review of potential cardiac problems. Clin Cancer Res 2008;14:14–24.

[3] Tarantini L, Gori S, Faggiano P, Pulignano G, Simoncini E, Tuccia F, et al. On behalf of ICARO (Italian CARdio-Oncologic) network: adjuvant trastuzumab cardiotoxicity in patients over 60 years of age with early breast cancer: a multicenter cohort analysis. Ann Oncol 2012;23:3058–63.

[4] Chavez-MacGregor M, Zhang N, Buchholz TA, Zhang Y, Niu J, Elting L, et al. Trastuzumab-related cardiotoxicity among older patients with breast cancer. J Clin Oncol 2013;31:4222–8.

[5] Accordino MK, Neugut AI, Hershman DL. Cardiac effects of anticancer therapy in the elderly. J Clin Oncol 2014;32:2654–61.

[6] Grenier MA, Lipshultz SE. Epidemiology of anthracycline cardiotoxicity in children and adults. Semin Oncol 1998;4(Suppl. 10):72–85.

[7] Yeh ET. Cardiotoxicity induced by chemotherapy and antibody therapy. Annu Rev Med 2006;57:485–98.

[8] Ewer MS, Vooletich MT, Durand J-B, Woods ML, Davis JR, Valero V, et al. Reversibility of trastuzumab-related cardiotoxicity: new insights based on clinical course and response treatment. J Clin Oncol 2005;23:7820–6.

[9] Tocchetti CG, Ragone G, Coppola C, Rea D, Piscopo G, Scala S, et al. Detection, monitoring, and management of trastuzumab-induced left ventricular dysfunction: an actual challenge. Eur J Heart Fail 2012;14:130–7.

[10] Cardinale D, Colombo A, Lamantia G, Colombo N, Civelli M, De Giacomi G, et al. Anthracycline-induced cardiomyopathy: clinical relevance and response to pharmacologic therapy. J Am Coll Cardiol 2010;55:213–20.

[11] Hahn VS, Lenihan DJ, Ky B. Cancer therapy-induced cardiotoxicity: basic mechanisms and potential cardioprotective therapies. J Am Heart Assoc 2014;3:e000665.

[12] Kalay N, Basar E, Ozdogru I, Er O, Cetinkaya Y, Dogan A, et al. Protective effects of carvedilol against anthracycline-induced cardiomyopathy. J Am Coll Cardiol 2006;48:2258–62.

[13] Costa RB, Kurra G, Greenberg L, Geyer CE. Efficacy and cardiac safety of adjuvant trastuzumab based chemotherapy regimens for HER2-positive early breast cancer. Ann Oncol 2010;21:2153–60.

How Big Is the Problem? The Cardiologists' View

Increasing concerns have been expressed regarding the cardiac complications of cancer therapy over the last decade [1]. Cardiologists have traditionally been involved in the management of late stages of complications from cancer therapy. In addition to heart failure (HF)—which mainly relates to the fibrosis and apoptosis leading to myocardial dysfunction and arrhythmias—a number of chemotherapeutic agents cause disturbances of microvascular function. In addition, premature coronary artery disease, and valvular and pericardial disease are important sequelae of radiotherapy.

Of these conditions, the one that is the biggest problem for cardiologists is HF. While the incidence of HF remains relatively stable, the improving survival with this condition is fueling an epidemic of prevalent cases—which 15 years ago was already >23 million people worldwide [2]. In the United States, >550,000 new cases are diagnosed each year, contributing to a prevalent group of >5 million people, and a cost of >$30 billion [3]. The most common etiologies of HF are ischemic heart disease, hypertension, and diabetes—all of which attract major preventive efforts. Although not a major cause of the HF epidemic, HF due to cancer therapy has gained attention because it is potentially preventable, and seems more malignant than many other causes of HF [4]. From a research standpoint, especially younger patients with this problem present a relatively "clean" causal pathway to HF, which is more commonly multifactorial in most HF patients.

However, the recognition that there are limited opportunities for meaningful alteration of the course of late-stage disease has driven more interest in the recognition of early disease. A major catalyst for this engagement has been the development of sophisticated new imaging tools, including myocardial strain, that are sensitive markers for early myocardial dysfunction and have been shown to have prognostic value [5]. There is good evidence for the prevention of HF with cardioprotective therapy in asymptomatic left ventricular (LV) dysfunction of other etiologies [6–9], as well as specifically in patients at risk because of chemotherapy [10].

The definition of what constitutes "cardiotoxicity" is clearly of pivotal importance. The term is usually understood to reflect HF or LV dysfunction as a consequence of chemotherapy, and most definitions involve symptom status, as well as the degree of decrease and the final level of systolic function. The US National Cancer Institute's Common Terminology Criteria for Adverse Events (CTCAE) limits the condition to HF or LV ejection fraction (EF) <50% [11]. A more detailed definition involves a LVEF reduction of >10% points with a final LVEF <50% or an LVEF reduction greater than 15% points with a final LVEF >50% [12]. The use of EF is certainly problematic, as changes in this parameter are considered to reflect disease that is quite advanced [13]. An alternative and more widely inclusive approach has been proposed by Cardinale et al. [14] and includes HF, asymptomatic LV dysfunction, arrhythmia requiring treatment, and sudden cardiac death. Unfortunately, all of these neglect the approximately half of HF associated with normal EF [15]. The recent American Society of Echocardiography/European Association of Cardiovascular Imaging guidelines for the diagnosis of cardiotoxicity strongly support the use of LV strain for this purpose [16].

Defining the frequency of this problem has been challenging. Limited archival data exist because HF was not a codable diagnosis in the initial versions of the CTCAE, and clinical trials formerly documented only grade 3 toxicity (symptomatic LV systolic dysfunction with an LVEF <20%) [13]. Moreover, the frequency of HF among patients in cancer trials can be expected to be lower than among the general chemotherapy population, as those at risk of HF based on previous cardiac problems were excluded. Indeed, cancer trial participants who developed HF symptoms might drop out of chemotherapy trials and not undergo follow-up. Conversely, HF due to cardiotoxicity is underrepresented in most HF studies, as cancer survivors are excluded from these trials. Even in epidemiologic studies, HF due to cardiotoxicity may be underestimated because of the long interval between chemotherapy and clinical findings. Thus, the best clues originate from linkages between SEER (Surveillance, Epidemiology, an End Results) with Medicare administrative data in the United States [14,15], albeit in an older population, as well as the adult survivors of childhood cancer—many of whom were exposed to anthracyclines and radiotherapy [16,17].

However, cancer and HF are highly prevalent conditions, and their association doesn't necessarily infer causality.

The required time-course for development of HF poses challenges for the recognition of cardiotoxicity, not just because of the latency from the initial injury but also because of the interaction with other possible causes as the patients' age and the presence of cardiovascular risk factors, or due to the difficulty to discriminate HF symptoms from cancer treatment-related fatigue and shortness of breath [18–22].

In practice, cardiologists and oncologists should collaborate more to ensure appropriate prevention, early detection, and prevention of progression HF. A new clinical discipline has given birth, namely cardio-oncology, over

TABLE 1 **Definition of Cardiotoxicity**

References	Definition of Cardiotoxicity	Drug	Results and Cardiotoxicity
Tan-Chiu et al. [23]	0.10 decline LVEF to <0.55	Trastuzumab	3-year cardiac events: 4.1% (doxorubicin, cyclophosphamide, docetaxel and trastuzumab) versus 0.8% (doxorubicin, cyclophosphamide, docetaxel)
Perez et al. [24]	≥0.15 decline in LVEF to below LLN (toxicity grade 2)	Doxorubicin and cyclophosphamide	Grade 2 toxicity, 6.6%
Suter et al. [25]	>0.15 decline of LVEF to <0.50	Trastuzumab	Threshold attained in 6.5% with trastuzumab, 0.7% without trastuzumab
O'Brien et al. [26]	>0.20 decline in LVEF to >0.50 or >0.10 decline to <0.50 or clinical CHF	Doxorubicin	18.8% decline in LVEF (of whom 21% had HF) 0.8% HF without LVEF decline
Smith et al. [27]	>0.10 decline in LVEF from baseline to <0.50	Trastuzumab after adjuvant or neoadjuvant chemotherapy	Unadjusted HR = 0.64 (95% CI, 0.54–0.76; $p < 0.0001$)
Romond et al. [28]	>0.16 decline of LVEF or <LLN	Doxorubicin and cyclophosphamide followed by trastuzumab	31.4% discontinued trastuzumab because of toxicity
Ryberg et al. [29]	0.15 decline of LVEF or LVEF <0.45	Epirubicin	Developed cardiotoxicity: 11.4%

LVEF, left ventricular ejection fraction; LLN, lower limit of normal.

the last few years. Cardio-oncology brings together expert cardiologists and oncologists to provide optimal cardiovascular care for the cancer patient (Table 1 and references within).

Tom Marwick and Patrizio Lancellotti

REFERENCES

[1] Carver JR, Shapiro CL, Ng A, et al. American Society of Clinical Oncology clinical evidence review on the ongoing care of adult cancer survivors: cardiac and pulmonary late effects. J Clin Oncol 2007;25:3991–4008.

[2] McMurray JJ, Petrie MC, Murdoch DR, et al. Clinical epidemiology of heart failure: public and private health burden. Eur Heart J 1998;19(Suppl. P): 9–16.

[3] Hunt SA, Abraham WT, Chin MH, et al. Focused update incorporated into the ACC/AHA 2005 guidelines for the diagnosis and management of heart failure in adults. J Am Coll Cardiol 2009;2009(53):e1–e90.

[4] Felker GM, Thompson RE, Hare JM, et al. Underlying causes and long-term survival in patients with initially unexplained cardiomyopathy. New Engl J Med 2000;342:1077–84.

[5] Kalam K, Otahal P, Marwick TH. Prognostic implications of global LV dysfunction: a systematic review and meta-analysis of global longitudinal strain and ejection fraction. Heart 2015;100(21):1673–80.

[6] SOLVD Investigators. Effect of enalapril on mortality and the development of heart failure in asymptomatic patients with reduced left ventricular ejection fractions. The SOLVD investigators. N Engl J Med 1992;327:685–91.

[7] Yusuf S, Sleight P, Pogue J, et al. Effects of an angiotensin-converting-enzyme inhibitor, ramipril, on cardiovascular events in high-risk patients. The heart outcomes prevention evaluation study investigators. N Engl J Med 2000;342:145–53.

[8] Pfeffer MA, Braunwald E, Moye LA, et al. Effect of captopril on mortality and morbidity in patients with left ventricular dysfunction after myocardial infarction. Results of the survival and ventricular enlargement trial. The SAVE Investigators. N Engl J Med 1992;327:669–77.

[9] Vantrimpont P, Rouleau JL, Wun CC, et al. Additive beneficial effects of beta-blockers to angiotensin-converting enzyme inhibitors in the Survival and Ventricular Enlargement (SAVE) Study. SAVE investigators. J Am Coll Cardiol 1997;29:229–36.

[10] Kalam K, Marwick TH. Role of cardioprotective therapy for prevention of cardiotoxicity with chemotherapy: a systematic review and meta-analysis. Eur J Cancer 2013;49:2900–9.

[11] US Department of Health and Human Services, National Institutes of Health, National Cancer Institute. Common Terminology Criteria for Adverse Events (CTCAE), version 4.0. Available at: http://evs.nci.nih.gov/ftp1/CTCAE/CTCAE_4.03_2010-06-14_QuickReference_5x7.pdf. [accessed 28.05.09].

[12] Bird BR, Swain SM. Cardiac toxicity in breast cancer survivors: review of potential cardiac problems. Clin Cancer Res 2009;14:14–24.

[13] Ewer MS, Lenihan DJ. Left ventricular ejection fraction and cardiotoxicity: is our ear really to the ground? J Clin Oncol 2008;26:1201–3.

[14] Cardinale D, Sandri MT, Colombo A, et al. Prognostic value of troponin I in cardiac risk stratification of cancer patients undergoing high-dose chemotherapy. Circulation 2004;109:2749–54.

[15] Owan TE, Hodge DO, Herges RM, et al. Trends in prevalence and outcome of heart failure with preserved ejection fraction. N Engl J Med 2006;355:251–9.

[16] Plana JC, Galderisi M, Barac A, et al. Expert consensus for multimodality imaging evaluation of adult patients during and after cancer therapy: a report from the American Society of Echocardiography and the European Association of Cardiovascular Imaging. Eur Heart J Cardiovasc Imaging 2014;15:1063–93.

[17] Lenihan DJ, Oliva S, Chow EJ, Cardinale D. Cardiac toxicity in cancer survivors. Cancer 2013;119(Suppl. 11):2131–42.

[18] Chen J, Long JB, Hurria A, et al. Incidence of heart failure or cardiomyopathy after adjuvant trastuzumab therapy for breast cancer. J Am Coll Cardiol 2012;60:2504–12.

[19] Pinder MC, Duan Z, Goodwin JS, et al. Congestive heart failure in older women treated with adjuvant anthracycline chemotherapy for breast cancer. J Clin Oncol 2007;25:3808–15.

[20] Oeffinger KC, Mertens AC, Sklar CA, et al. Chronic health conditions in adult survivors of childhood cancer. N Engl J Med 2006;355:1572–82.

[21] Reulen RC, Winter DL, Frobisher C, et al. Long-term cause-specific mortality among survivors of childhood cancer. JAMA 2002;304:172–9.

[22] Schultz-Hector S, Trott KR. Radiation-induced cardiovascular diseases: is the epidemiologic evidence compatible with the radiobiologic data? Int J Radiat Oncol Biol Phys 2007;67:10–18.

[23] Tan-Chiu E, Yothers G, Romond E, Geyer Jr CE, Ewer M, Keefe D, et al. Assessment of cardiac dysfunction in a randomized trial comparing doxorubicin and cyclophosphamide followed by paclitaxel, with or without trastuzumab as adjuvant therapy in node-positive, human epidermal growth factor receptor 2-overexpressing breast cancer: NSABP B-31. J Clin Oncol 2005;23:7811–19.

[24] Perez EA, Suman VJ, Davidson NE, Kaufman PA, Martino S, Dakhil SR, et al. Effect of doxorubicin plus cyclophosphamide on left ventricular ejection fraction in patients with breast cancer in the North Central Cancer Treatment Group N9831 Intergroup Adjuvant Trial. J Clin Oncol 2004;22:3700–4.

[25] Suter TM, Cook-Bruns N, Barton C. Cardiotoxicity associated with trastuzumab (Herceptin) therapy in the treatment of metastatic breast cancer. Breast 2004;13:173–83.

[26] O'Brien ME, Wigler N, Inbar M, Rosso R, Grischke E, Santoro A, et al. CAELYX Breast Cancer Study Group. Reduced cardiotoxicity and comparable efficacy in a phase III trial of pegylated liposomal doxorubicin HCl (CAELYX/Doxil) versus conventional doxorubicin for first-line treatment of metastatic breast cancer. Ann Oncol 2004;15:440–9.

[27] Smith I, Procter M, Gelber RD, Guillaume S, Feyereislova A, Dowsett M, et al. HERA study team. 2-year follow-up of trastuzumab after adjuvant chemotherapy in HER2-positive breast cancer: a randomised controlled trial. Lancet 2007;369:29–36.

[28] Romond EH, Perez EA, Bryant J, Suman VJ, Geyer Jr CE, Davidson NE, et al. Trastuzumab plus adjuvant chemotherapy for operable HER2-positive breast cancer. N Engl J Med 2005;353:1673–84.

[29] Ryberg M, Nielsen D, Cortese G, Nielsen G, Skovsgaard T, Andersen PK. New insight into epirubicin cardiac toxicity: competing risks analysis of 1097 breast cancer patients. J Natl Cancer Inst 2008;100:1058–67.

Section I

General Considerations

Chapter 1

Epidemiology and Trend of Prognosis in Cancer Patients

G. Jerusalem, P. Freres and M. Moonen

Chapter Outline

Cancer is the leading cause of death in economically developed countries and the second leading cause of death in the developing world. The global burden of cancer continues to increase as a result of population aging and lifestyle choices, including smoking, physical inactivity, and poor diet [1,2].

Based on GLOBOCAN statistics, 12.7 million cancer cases and 7.6 million cancer deaths occurred globally in 2008. Although overall cancer incidence in developed countries is nearly twice as high as in economically developing countries in both sexes, mortality rates are generally similar. Cancer survival tends to be poorer in the developing world, partly due to late-stage diagnosis and limited access to standard treatments [1–3].

Breast and lung cancers are the most frequently diagnosed cancers worldwide, among females and males, respectively. In developed countries, lung cancer is preceded by prostate cancer as the most frequent cancer among males. For 2014, in the United States, breast cancer alone was forecast to account for 29% of cancer incidence in women and prostate cancer for 27% of cancer incidence in men [1–4].

Cancer epidemiology closely mirrors risk factor spread in various countries. Hepatocellular carcinoma is rare in the West but is the main cancer in China and neighboring countries, most likely due to the endemic presence of hepatitis B and aflatoxin in that population. Similarly, with tobacco smoking becoming more common in various developing countries, lung cancer incidence has increased in a parallel fashion [1–4].

Anticancer Treatments and Cardiotoxicity. DOI: http://dx.doi.org/10.1016/B978-0-12-802509-3.00001-7

Between 2006 and 2010, in the United States, the overall cancer incidence rates tend to decrease by 0.6% per year among males but remain stable in females. The decrease in men is driven by rapid declines in colorectal, prostate, and lung cancers, reflecting improvements in cancer prevention (colorectal and lung cancer). On the other hand, among women, breast cancer incidence has remained relatively stable since 2003. Lung cancer incidence began decreasing in the mid-1980s in males, but only in the late 1990s in females, reflecting the historical difference in tobacco use [1–5].

In contrast to the declining trends for most cancer types, incidence rates are increasing for melanoma of the skin, esophageal adenocarcinoma, cancers of the thyroid, liver, kidney, anus, pancreas, and human papillomavirus-positive oropharyngeal cancers [6].

In industrialized countries, the cancer mortality rate increased for most of the 20th century as a consequence of the major rise in lung cancer deaths among males. Then, there has been a 20% decline since the 1990s as a result of prevention, including tobacco control interventions, and early detection. As an example, in the first part of the 20th century, the leading cause of cancer deaths in women was uterine cancer. Then, the mortality of uterine cancer decreased more than 80% due to improved diagnostic techniques. The same decline was observed for stomach cancer due to improved food hygiene and control of infections by *Helicobacter pylori* [1–4].

Since about 2010, annual cancer death rates have decreased regardless of gender, ethnicity, or cancer site. This decrease is related to the earlier detection and treatment of the four major cancers (lung, breast, prostate, and colorectal cancers). In women, breast and colorectal cancers had favorable trends, but predicted lung cancer mortality still rises, reaching and possibly overtaking breast cancer rates in 2015 [1–4,7,8].

Only a few decades ago, the prognosis for people facing cancer was not nearly as favorable as it is today. The 5-year overall survival rates have improved since the mid-1970s. Survival was improved especially for leukemia and nonHodgkin lymphomas, whereas the benefits are more modest for cancers of the lung and pancreas. The survival benefit observed in developed countries is lower among black people, probably related to a lower socioeconomic status. Now, more than two of three people diagnosed with cancer survives at least 5 years. The improvement in cancer cure rates is especially high in the pediatric population. The number of cancer survivors in the United States has exceeded 12 million and is increasing [1–4].

Because more people are surviving cancer, more attention is focused on the quality of life and long-term outcomes of these cancer survivors. Cardiovascular disease is the leading noncancer cause of late mortality among survivors of childhood and adolescent cancer. Among many adult cancer patients in remission, the risk of cardiovascular death is higher than the actual risk of cancer recurrence. Survivors of cancer have a 7-fold higher mortality than the general population, with a 15-fold increased risk of developing heart failure and a 10-fold increased risk of myocardial ischemia. These patients also have a higher risk of atherosclerosis, hypertension, pericardial disease, valvular heart disease, and dyslipidemia. The higher cardiovascular death rate in cancer survivors is secondary to a combination of cancer treatment risk factors (ionizing irradiation, cytotoxic agents, surgery), native risk factors and health behavior. The risks were particularly high among survivors who had received anthracyclines containing chemotherapy or high-dose radiation therapy to the heart as part of their cancer treatment. There is an urgent need to educate cancer survivors and their physicians about the risk of cardiovascular disease. These patients need appropriate surveillance so that late side effects of cancer therapy can be diagnosed early and treated accurately. Practical arrangements for this long-term clinical monitoring should still be a consensus [9,10].

REFERENCES

[1] World Health Organization. The global burden of disease: 2004 update. Geneva: Word Health Organization; 2008.

[2] Jemal A, Bray F, Center M, Ferlay J, Ward E, Forman D. Global cancer statistics. CA Cancer J Clin 2011;61(2):69–90.

[3] Ferlay J, Shin HER, Bray F, Forman D, Mathers CD, Parkin D. GLOBOCAN 2008, cancer incidence and mortality worldwide: IARC CancerBase No. 10. Lyon: International Agency for Research on Cancer; 2010. Available at: <http://globocan.iarc.fr>.

[4] Siegel R, Ma J, Zou Z, Jemal A. Cancer statistics, 2014. CA Cancer J Clin 2014;64:9–29.

[5] Weiss W. Cigarette smoking and lung cancer trends. A light at the end of the tunnel? Chest 1997;111:1414–16.

[6] Simard EP, Ward EM, Siegel R, Jemal A. Cancers with increasing incidence trends in the United States: 1999 through 2008. CA Cancer J Clin 2012;62:118–28.

[7] Howlader N, Noone AM, Krapcho M, et al. SEER cancer statistics review, 1975–2010. Bethesda, MD: National Cancer Institute; 2013.

[8] Malvezzi M, Bertuccio P, Rosso T, Rota M, Levi F, La Vecchia C, et al. European cancer mortality predictions for the year 2015: does lung cancer have the highest death rate in EU women? Ann Oncol 2015;26(4):779–86.

[9] Diller L, Chow E, Gurney J, Hudson M, Kadin-Lottick N, Kawashima T, et al. Chronic disease in the Childhood Cancer Survivor Study cohort: a review of published findings. J Clin Oncol 2009;27:2339–55.

[10] Carver J, Shapiro C, Ng A, Jacobs L, Schwartz C, Virgo K, et al. American Society of Clinical Oncology clinical evidence review on the ongoing care of adult cancer survivors: cardiac and pulmonary late effects. J Clin Oncol 2007;25(25):3991–4008.

Chapter 2

Categories of Anticancer Treatments

P. Freres, G. Jerusalem and M. Moonen

Chapter Outline

Chemotherapy is one of the cornerstones of cancer treatment. Cytotoxic agents have been used for a very long time as palliative treatment for metastatic disease. Since the 1990s, chemotherapy has also been administered with curative intent in addition to surgery and radiotherapy. Neoadjuvant chemotherapy is given preoperatively to decrease tumor size and facilitate surgery, in addition to the systemic effect. Adjuvant chemotherapy is performed postoperatively to eliminate microscopic metastases and increase the chance of long-term disease-free survival and cure. Sometimes, such as for the treatment of some lymphomas, chemotherapy is the only treatment modality without any local therapy but still with cure as the goal of treatment.

The major mechanism of action of chemotherapy is interruption of cell division and/or promotion of apoptosis in tumor cells. This mechanism of action is not specific to tumor cells but the rationale is that tumor cells divide more rapidly than normal cells. Many chemotherapy-associated adverse events are consequences of this lack of selectivity. Cytotoxic agents will disrupt cell division in several ways and they can be roughly classified by their activities relative to the cell generation cycle.

Phase-specific drugs are only effective during a particular phase of the cell cycle. For example, methotrexate specifically acts on the S-phase to disturb DNA synthesis, while alkaloid agents (vinca alkaloids) are M-phase-specific, inhibiting spindle formation and alignment of chromosomes. A linear dose-dependent activity is not observed with these cytotoxic agents:

Anticancer Treatments and Cardiotoxicity. DOI: http://dx.doi.org/10.1016/B978-0-12-802509-3.00002-9

above a fixed plasma level, further increase in dose does not result in more cell killing; in addition, a minimum plasma level is needed before any antitumor activity is seen.

Phase-independent drugs can be cycle-independent, allowing the killing of cells that are not dividing. Cycle-specific, phase-independent drugs are effective at any point in the cycle (e.g., alkylating agents) but the cell has to be in the active phase of the cell cycle. Phase nonspecific drugs generally have, at least in vitro, a linear dose–response curve: the greater the amount of drug given, the greater is the fraction of cells killed.

Alkylating agents are cytotoxic, which produces alkylation through the formation of covalent links between DNA strands. Alkylation results in abnormal nucleotide sequences, miscoding of messenger RNA, blockade of DNA replication, and breakage of DNA strands. Tumor cells are thus unable to divide and enter into apoptosis. Alkylating agents include cyclophosphamide, ifosfamide, lomustine, dacarbazine, temozolomide, and procarbazine. Platinum derivatives, including cisplatin, carboplatin, and oxaliplatin, are organic heavy metal complexes, which covalently bond to proteins, RNA and, especially, DNA, to form intra- and inter-DNA strand adducts.

Antimetabolites are structural analogs of natural substances such as vitamins, nucleosides, or amino acids, which are essential for cell growth and division. They compete with the natural substrate for the active site on an essential enzyme or receptor, interfering with the DNA synthesis. Some are incorporated directly into DNA or RNA. Most are phase-specific, acting during the S-phase of the cell cycle. In general, these agents have been most effective when cell proliferation is rapid. Their efficacy is furthermore greater over a prolonged period of time, so they are usually given continuously or at least over several days. Among antimetabolites, we distinguish the antifolates (methotrexate and pemetrexed) and the pyrimidine analogue (cytarabine, hydroxyurea, 5-fluorouracil, capecitabine, and gemcitabine).

Topoisomerase inhibitors are agents designed to interfere with the action of topoisomerase enzymes I and II. Topoisomerases are enzymes that control the changes in DNA tridimensional structure by catalyzing the breaking and rejoining of the phosphodiester backbone of DNA strands during the normal cell cycle. Inhibition of topoisomerases interferes with transcription and replication by causing DNA damage, inhibition of DNA replication, failure to repair strand breaks, and then, cell death. Camptothecin derivatives (irinotecan, topotecan) exert their cytotoxic effect by inhibiting topoisomerase I. Epipodophyllotoxin derivatives (etoposide, teniposide) inhibit topoisomerase II.

Antitumor antibiotics are drugs derived from microorganisms. They usually are cycle-nonspecific agents and are especially useful in slowly growing tumors. They act by several mechanisms: induction of DNA strand breaks, intercalation between DNA base pairs, and inhibition of topoisomerase 2.

This family of cytotoxic agents includes anthracyclines (daunorubicin, doxorubicin, liposomal doxorubicin, epirubicin, idarubicin), bleomycin, mitomycin, and mitoxantrone.

Mitotic spindle toxic agents include vinca alkaloids and taxanes. The vinca alkaloids have been identified from substances isolated from the Madagascar periwinkle. These drugs bind to microtubular proteins, thus inhibiting microtubule assembly (M-phase of the cell cycle) and resulting in dissolution of the mitotic spindle structure. They include vinblastine, vincristine, vindesine, and vinorelbine. Taxanes (paclitaxel, docetaxel, and cabazitaxel) not only bind to microtubules but also promote microtubule assembly and resistance to depolymerization, resulting in the production of nonfunctional microtubules. Paclitaxel was originally derived from the Pacific yew tree.

Recent advances in technology have provided an unprecedented opportunity to implement precision and personalized medicine in cancer. Targeted therapies, in contrast to chemotherapy, inhibit tumor growth by acting on specific molecular targets involved in tumor progression. Targeted therapies use specific genetic or protein abnormalities present only or mostly in the tumor cells. In general, targeted therapies are only cytostatic, i.e., they block cell division without causing cell death. Many drugs are already registered and in addition numerous clinical and preclinical studies evaluating targeted agents are currently ongoing in the field of oncology.

The oldest targeted agents used in cancer are the endocrine therapies. Endocrine agents can slow down or stop the growth of cancer by either stopping the synthesis of hormones or by preventing the action of hormones by blocking their receptors. These endocrine therapies are mainly prescribed in hormone-sensitive cancers, such as breast cancer (including tamoxifen, aromatase inhibitors, and luteinizing hormone-releasing hormone analogs) or prostate cancer (including antiandrogens and luteinizing hormone-releasing hormone analogs). Mitotane, which directly suppresses the adrenal cortex and alters cortisone metabolism, is used in the treatment of adrenocortical carcinoma.

Currently, the main categories of recent targeted therapies are tyrosine kinase inhibitors (TKIs) and monoclonal antibodies (mAb).

Small molecules inhibit tyrosine kinases, which are enzymes responsible for the activation of proteins involved in signal transduction cascades. In general, TKIs can block multiple tyrosine kinases involved in cell growth, such as epidermal growth factor receptors (EGFR), vascular endothelial growth factor receptors (VEGFR), platelet-derived growth factor receptors (PDGF), or fibroblast growth factor receptors (FGF).

By targeting cancer cells, mAb can: (1) activate the immune system; (2) block growth signals; (3) block the angiogenesis; (4) deliver radiation to cancer cells (e.g., ^{90}yttrium ibritumomab tiuxetan in nonHodgkin's lymphomas); or (5) deliver chemotherapy to cancer cells (antidrug conjugate, such as trastuzumab emtansine in HER2-positive breast cancers).

The use of a targeted therapy requires the identification of a target specifically dysregulated inside the tumor tissues. An example of such a differentially expressed target is the human epidermal growth factor receptor 2 protein (HER2) in breast and stomach cancers. HER2 is expressed at high levels on the surface of these cancer cells, promoting cell growth and division. Several targeted agents are directed against HER2, including mAb (trastuzumab and pertuzumab), TKI (lapatinib), and antidrug conjugate (trastuzumab emtansine). EGFR is frequently overexpressed in colon, non small-cell lung, head and neck and pancreatic cancers. EGFR can be targeted by TKIs (erlotinib and gefitinib) or a monoclonal antibody (cetuximab). VEGF pathway, especially amplified in kidney, ovarian or nonsmall-cell lung cancers, may also be inhibited by TKIs (sunitinib, sorafenib, axitinib, pazopanib) or a monoclonal antibody (bevacizumab).

Another approach to identify potential targets is to determine whether cancer cells produce mutant proteins that drive cancer progression. For example, the cell growth-signaling protein BRAF is present in an altered form (known as BRAFV600E) in half of melanomas. Vemurafenib and dabrafenib are enzyme inhibitors that target BRAFV600E protein. These molecules are approved in inoperable or metastatic melanoma with a mutated BRAF protein. Sometimes, abnormalities in chromosomes are present in cancer cells but not in normal cells. These chromosome abnormalities result in the creation of a fusion gene whose product, called a fusion protein, may drive cancer growth. Such fusion proteins are potential targets for targeted cancer therapies. For example, imatinib mesylate targets the BCR-ABL fusion protein present in Philadelphia chromosome-positive chronic myelogenous leukemia and crizotinib targets the EML4-ALK fusion protein in non small-cell lung cancers.

Immunotherapies use the immune system to destroy cancer cells. In fact, some cancers are able to avoid detection and destruction by the immune system. Immunotherapies therefore restore or enhance the immune system's ability to fight cancer. One immunotherapy approach is to block the activity of certain proteins that limit the strength of immune responses. These proteins normally keep immune responses in check to prevent overly strong responses that might damage normal cells. In cancer cells, these "checkpoint" proteins may be abnormal and may help tumors to evade the immune response. The first immune checkpoint modulator to gain Food and Drug Administration approval is called ipilimumab. Ipilimumab is a monoclonal antibody that blocks the activity of CTLA4 and allow cytotoxic T lymphocytes to destroy cancer cells. The programmed death 1 protein (PD-1) is another key immune checkpoint receptor expressed by activated T cells. PD-1 binds to its ligands PD-L1 (B7-H1) and PD-L2 (B7-DC), which are expressed on tumor cells, thereby preventing the immune system from rejecting the tumor. mAb targeting both PD-1 (pembrozilumab, nivolumab) and PD-L1 are being developed to interrupt this pathway. These immunotherapies have demonstrated significant clinical activity against several tumor types, particularly in metastatic melanoma.

The use of cancer treatment vaccines is another approach to immunotherapy. Sipuleucel-T is used in some men with metastatic prostate cancer. Peripheral blood mononuclear cells, obtained from patients, are exposed to a recombinant protein that consists of prostatic acid phosphatase (PAP) fused to granulocyte macrophage colony-stimulating factor (GM-CSF). These activated cells are then infused back into the patient to cause an immune response against cancer cells carrying the PAP antigen.

About half of all cancer patients receive some type of radiation therapy sometime during the course of their treatment. Radiation therapy or radiotherapy uses high-energy radiation to shrink tumors and kill cancer cells. X-rays, gamma rays, and charged particles are types of radiation used for cancer treatment. The radiation may be delivered by a machine outside the body (external-beam radiation therapy), or it may come from radioactive material placed in the body near cancer cells (internal radiation therapy, also called brachytherapy). Systemic radiation therapy uses radioactive substances, such as radioactive iodine, that travel in the blood to kill cancer cells. Radiation therapy kills cancer cells by damaging their DNA. Radiation therapy can either damage DNA directly or create free radicals within the cells that can in turn damage the DNA. As with chemotherapy, radiation therapy is given with curative or palliative intent and may be used alone or in combination with surgery, chemotherapy, or both.

FURTHER READING

[1] DeVita V, Lawrence T, Rosenberg S. DeVita, Hellman, and Rosenberg's cancer: principles & practices of oncology. 10th ed. Philadelphia, PA: Lippincott Williams & Wilkins; 2014. Print.

[2] Casciato D, Territo M. Manual of clinical oncology. 7th ed. Philadelphia, PA: Lippincott Williams & Wilkins; 2012. Print.

[3] National Cancer Institute. Targeted cancer therapies, <http://www.cancer.gov/cancertopics/treatment/types/targeted-therapies/targeted-therapies-fact-sheet>; 2014.

[4] National Cancer Institute. Immunotherapy: using the immune system to treat cancer, <http://www.cancer.gov/researchandfunding/areas/treatment/immunotherapy-using-immune-system>; 2014.

[5] National Cancer Institute. Radiation therapy for cancer, <http://www.cancer.gov/cancertopics/treatment/types/radiation-therapy/radiation-fact-sheet>; 2010.

Chapter 3

Classification by Mechanisms of Cardiotoxicity

D. Kerkhove, I. Paciolla and G. Arpino

Chapter Outline

INTRODUCTION

Strict pathophysiological classification of the cardiotoxicity mechanisms is difficult because of several reasons:

1. A single agent can damage the myocardium through different mechanisms or pathways.
2. In some cases, thresholds must be reached before measurable damage occurs.
3. Additive and synergistic toxic effects exist, which can cause confusion about the true origin of the aggressor [1].
4. Some effects need catalyzation by surrounding factors, called risk factors, like arterial hypertension [2], smoking [3], and irradiation [4,5], or are influenced by genetic predisposition [6].
5. Confounding factors might cause delayed toxic effects which might increase the unanticipated long-term toxic load.

Nevertheless, classification itself and application in clinical practice is fundamental since it undoubtfully guides diagnostic and therapeutic strategy, and consequently cardio-oncological prevention. For example, since anthracyclines kill myocardial cells and myocardium is a postmitotic tissue with poor regenerative capacity, early recognition of this necrosis and apoptosis is

Anticancer Treatments and Cardiotoxicity. DOI: http://dx.doi.org/10.1016/B978-0-12-802509-3.00003-0

crucial in the further limitation of myocardial damage. Therefore, a very appropriate one-liner in cardio-oncology that "*time is muscle*" [7].

Anthracycline cardiotoxicity has been known of since the 1970s [8] but introduction of trastuzumab, an antibody directed against human endothelial growth factor receptor B2 (ErbB2), in the late 1990s seemed to increase the incidence of cardiotoxicity [9].

It took more than 10 years to understand that trastuzumab's cardiotoxicity is triggered mainly by earlier or concomitant administration of anthracyclines, introducing the concept of synergistic cardiotoxicity [1]. This discovery changed again oncotherapeutic strategies in an attempt to enhance cardio-oncological prevention, which was illustrated in the HERA trial [10].

The classification is based on either specific pathophysiological features or clinical findings. Grossly, we identify three types of cardiotoxic mechanisms. A fourth group collects the remainder of toxic mechanisms. An overview is given in Table 3.1. Types 1 and 2 cardiotoxicity will be discussed in

TABLE 3.1 Types of Cardiotoxic mechanisms

	Type I	Type II	TKI
Prototype	**Anthracycline**	**Trastuzumab**	**Sunitinib**
Predominant pathological feature	Cell destruction	Interference with growth/repair Disinhibition of apoptosis "stunning"	Inhibition of VEGF signaling pathway
Histology	Vacuolization Sarcomere disarray and rupture Necrosis	Normal ultrastructure	Microvascular rarefaction, Endothelial dysfunction, Thrombotic microangiopathy
Cumulative dose dependency	++++	–	–
Reversibility	Poor and only in early phase	High (few data)	High (few data)
Effect of rechallenge	Enhances cardiotoxicity (cumulative effect)	Probably none (few data)	Probably none
Prognostic impact	Yes: CHF and death	No?	Yes: high risk of thrombotic events

detail, as well as tyrosine kinase inhibition-related and antivascular endothelial growth factor signaling-related toxicity.

TYPE I CARDIOTOXICITY

Type 1 cardiotoxicity concerns drugs causing myocardial apoptosis and necrosis in a cumulative dose-related fashion. Since anthracyclines are the archetypal example of this type of cardiotoxicity, it is more popularly called anthracycline cardiotoxicity. It is the oldest known mechanism and consequently the best studied. Besides being the most frequent, related to the widespread use of anthracyclines for several malignancies, it is also the most feared because of its poor reversibility, especially when not caught in an early phase, and potentially leading to end-stage congestive heart failure [11].

1. Pathophysiological mechanisms
   a. Main mechanisms

      Fe ion in the anthracycline complex produces free O^{-} radicals, inducing oxidative stress in the myocardial cell membranes. This results in increased permeability of the inner myocardial cell membranes [12,13] and makes it more vulnerable for further damage and consequently apoptosis.

      Depletion of GATA-4, a survival transcription factor, enhances apoptosis [14].

   b. Accessory mechanisms

      Accumulation of 8-OH- guanosine adducts in mitochondrial DNA causes mitochondrial dysfunction [15].

      Doxorubinicol, an active metabolite of doxorubicin, induces structural and functional changes in the cardiomyocytes, enhancing iron-mediated cardiotoxic effects [16].

      It is important to stress that the cardiotoxic mechanisms of anthracyclines are, at least in part, distinct of their oncotherapeutic or cytostatic effect: the inhibition of DNA and RNA synthesis and protein synthesis that triggers DNA cleavage by topoisomerase II. If this were not the case, the cardiotoxic effect would always equal the cytotoxic effect and abolish the net and global prognostic gain of such treatment for the patient!
2. Cumulative dose relationship

   The exponential relation between the cumulative anthracycline dose and the incidence of congestive heart failure, illustrated in Fig. 3.1, was first identified in the late 1970s [17] by Von Hoff and colleagues. Swain confirmed this fact 25 years later, and additionally derived that a cumulative dose of 550 mg/m^2 doxorubicin was the threshold for a risk of congestive heart failure exceeding 5% [18].

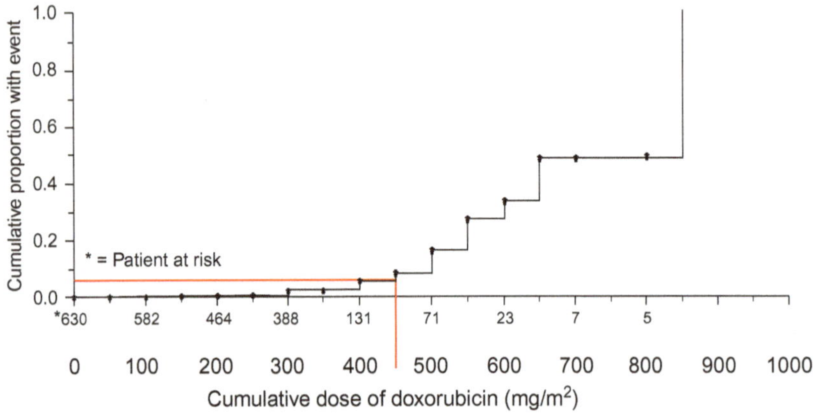

FIGURE 3.1 Exponential relationship between the cumulative dose of administered doxorubicin and the cardiac event rate, expressed as the risk for developing congestive heart failure (CHF); above the threshold of 400–450 mg/m^2, that risk exceeds 5% (cf. red line). *From Swain S, et al. Congestive heart failure in patients treated with doxorubicin: a retrospective analysis of three trials. Cancer 2003;97(11):2869–79.*

The exponential cumulative dose relationship led to additional clinical key insights:

a. Extrapolation to the intersection made clear that a good balance between oncotherapeutic and cardiotoxic effect implies the oncocell damage or cytostatic effect must appear at much lower doses than myocardial cell damage.
b. Correlation with cardiac biopsies confirmed that structural myocardial changes preceed functional changes [19].
c. A mathematical relationship could be derived, leading to approximation or prediction of cardiotoxicity [20].

3. Characteristic structural abnormalities induced by type I agents

The anthracycline-induced ultrastructural myocardial changes are typical and were first described by Billingham [21], shortly after the appearance of the first cardiotoxicity reports in anthracycline-treated patients. These are illustrated in Fig. 3.2. The observed variety in severity of those changes permitted the authors to develop a grading scale between 0 and 3, based on their progressiveness. Since those changes do not occur uniformly in all myocytes, Mackay refined the grading scale to allow an appreciation of this heterogeneous spreading in a more accurate and quantifiable way, by adding grades 0.5 and 1.5 [22,23]. This grading system, illustrated in Table 3.2, was shown to correlate well with cumulative doxorubicin dose, an anthracycline analogue, as illustrated in Fig. 3.3. Consequently, it became the first tool and gold standard in the clinical evaluation of anthracycline-induced cardiotoxicity.

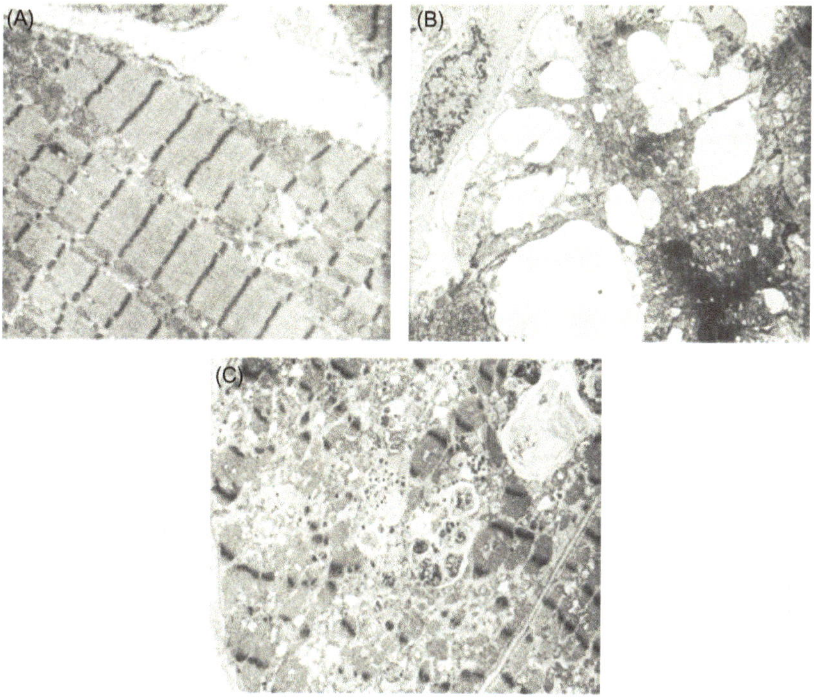

FIGURE 3.2 Electronmicrographs from patients who have received anthracyclines. (A) Normal myocardium without evidence of anthracycline damage. (B) Abundant vacuolization and disarray of myocardial fibrils. (C) High-grade myocardial necrosis with unrecognizable myocardium. *From Ewer MS, Suter TM. Diagnostic aspects of cardiovascular toxicity of antitumor drugs. In: Minotti G (ed.).* Cardiotoxicity of non-cardiovascular drugs. *John Wiley & Sons Ltd; 2010.*

TABLE 3.2 Electronmicroscopic Grading of Cardiac Biopsy Specimens: Number of Muscle Fibers Showing Changes[a,b]

Grade	Vacuoles	Myofibrillar Dropout	Necrosis
0.5	<4	0	0
1.0	4–10	<3	0
1.5	>10	3–5	<2
2.0	varies[c]	6–8	2–5
3[d]	varies[c]	>8	>5

[a] *Reflects average number of abnormal muscle fibers per grid based on an examination of a minimum of six grids obtained from six blocks.*
[b] *The highest biopsy grade based on any category is assigned. If two or more categories indicate the same grade, the grade is increased by half a point.*
[c] *Any number of vacuoles.*
[d] *With present dosing and schedules, a biopsy grade of 3 is seldom achieved.*
Source: Adapted from Billingham M, Bristow M. Endomyocardial biopsy findings in Adriamycin-treated patients. Proc. Am. Soc. Clin. Oncol. 1976;17:281 (abstract); and from Billingham M, Bristow M. Evaluation of Anthracyclin cardiotoxicity: predictive ability and functional correlation of endomyocardial biopsy. Cancer Treat. Symp. 1984;3:71–76.

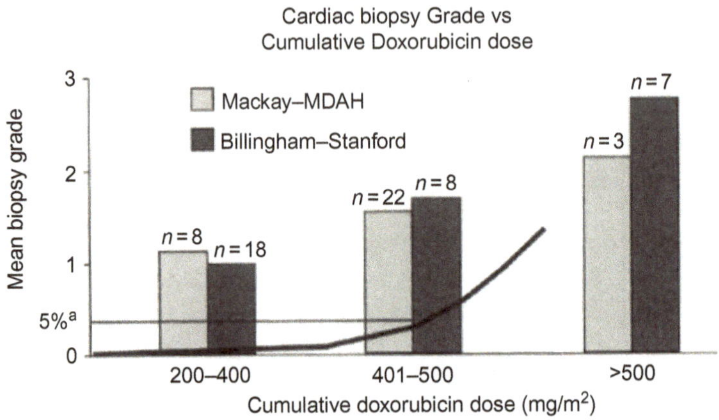

FIGURE 3.3 Correlation between cumulative doxorubicin dose and myocardial biopsy grades collected from two different series. *From Ewer M, et al. A comparison of cardiac biopsy grades and ejection fraction estimations in patients receiving adriamycin. J Clin Oncol 1984;2 (2):112–17.*

Even though those structural changes appear at much lower cumulative doses than global left ventricle systolic function change does, cardiac biopsy has lost its diagnostic importance in daily clinical practice due to its invasiveness and the development of noninvasive cardiac imaging, especially the possibility to monitor accurately global systolic function. Unfortunately, this "switch of the pendulum" causes the actual failure in the conventional detection strategies for cardiotoxicity: focusing almost all diagnostic attention to the monitoring of left ventricular ejection fraction (LVEF) alone, as evident from the most "accurate" CREC (Clinical Research Ethics Committee) criteria for defining cardiotoxicity [24], excludes at least partially cardio-oncological prevention abilities [7]. This urged the birth of a new discipline, which can either be called cardio-oncology or onco-cardiology [25].

4. Clinical spectrum of cardiotoxicity due to type I agents

Traditionally, anthracycline or type I cardiotoxicity was considered to appear either early or late, with "early" being characterized by transient ECG changes and discrete troponin rises but no changes in systolic left ventricular (LV) function. This form was ought to be "benign" and consequently neglected in literature and daily clinical practice. The late form, in contrast, was studied more profound and could be characterized by a variable reduction in systolic LV function, ranging from asymptomatic to a dilated cardiomyopathy with overt congestive heart failure and death.

Since we tend to forget the results of the myocardial biopsy for cardiotoxicity studies, and since we can only quantify biomarkers of myocardial injury in routine for 10 years, we mistakenly thought that there was no relation between the early and late forms of type I cardiotoxicity. Better understanding of the functional cardioanatomy and cardiac mechanics, and the integration of this knowledge with the evidence of troponin release during and early after anthracycline administration, should promptly lead to the conclusion that there is probably only one pathological entity with different stages and severities, influenced by chemotherapy regimen and sequence, a multitude of risk factors like genetic predisposition for cardiotoxicity, age, arterial hypertension (AHT), cardiac irradiation, underlying heart disease, and especially coronary artery disease (CAD), and a multitude of cardioprotective measures like heart failure therapy, statins, and radical scavengers like dexrazoxane.

a. Risk factors for enhanced type I cardiotoxicity

   As stated in section above, the risk for developing type I cardiotoxicity is enhanced by several clinical factors, which can be considered as risk factors. Those known in the literature are listed in Table 3.3 with their corresponding hazard ratio (HR) if calculated.

   Prior anthracycline therapy was the first to be discovered, and is a logical consequence of the cumulative dose relationship. Further important risk factors (HR above 2.0) are age and especially CAD, because it is detectable and modifiable before instauration of type I agents! The impact of combining anthracycline with trastuzumab will be discussed in type II CT.

b. The role of biomarkers in the detection of type I cardiotoxicity

   A troponin rise is considered as the gold standard biomarker for myocardial injury from any cause. Its strengths are related to an almost absolute cardiac specificity, high sensitivity, wide diagnostic window, and a robust biochemical assay [26]. In conclusion, the

TABLE 3.3 Risk Factors for Anthracycline Cardiotoxicity

Risk Factors	HR	References
Prior anthracycline use	NA	[17]
cardiac irradiation	NA	[4]
Other heart disease	1.53	[2]
AHT	1.58	[2]
CAD	2.21	[2]
Age > 65 years	2.25	[18]
Smoking	NA	[3]
Combination with HER	NA	[1]

troponin rise during and after anthracycline-based chemotherapy is the biochemical confirmation of drug-related myocardial cell necrosis and apoptosis.

Meanwhile, multiple papers have illustrated the relationship between a troponin rise during or shortly after anthracycline-based chemotherapy and later LVEF drop [27–29]. Additionally, Cardinale et al. found that troponin I was successful in differentiating reversible from irreversible myocardial injury and negative troponin I during and after chemotherapy had a negative predictive value of 99% for excluding cardiotoxicity, expressed as a 10% drop in LVEF [29]. Residual issues for the routine use of troponin rise in cardio-oncological prevention are discussed in Chapter 24, Other Biomarkers.

Evidence for the use of natriuretic peptides in identifying cardiotoxicity is much less impressive and abundant. It reflects the potential hemodynamic impact of myocardial injury due to chemotherapy rather than the myocardial injury itself.

5. Mitigation of type I CT

The fact that the cytotoxic and cardiotoxic mechanisms clearly differ, offers the opportunity to reduce cardiotoxic aggression of the drugs without necessarily reducing its oncologic efficacy. Several cardioprotective methods have been tested with variable success (for further details see Kalam and Marwick [30]). They can be divided into four groups on the basis of their specific effect/goal.

a. Biochemical changes in anthracycline structure

Several epimers of doxorubicin, the parent compound, have been developed in an attempt to reduce cardiotoxicity without compromising oncological efficacy.

Epirubicine is the semisynthetic 4-epimer of doxorubicin. It appears to be half as cardiotoxic as doxorubicin (5% risk of CHF at 900 mg/m^2 compared to 450 mg/m^2 for doxorubicin) but because of its lesser myelosuppressive capacity, necessitating the administration of higher doses compared to doxorubicin, the net prognostic might be limited. This was confirmed in a meta-analysis which showed only a strong trend to but no significant reduction in cardiac events [31]. Nevertheless, it adds to the cumulative dose relationship of the native compound doxorubicin.

Mitoxantrone is an anthracendione, structurally related to anthracyclines. It causes similar ultrastructural changes to anthracyclines and also exhibits a cumulative dose relationship [32]. Consequently, crossing over from anthracycline therapy to mitoxantrone does not offer any cardioprotection [33].

b. Modification of the administration schedule

Since it is recognized that peak plasma levels are more related to doxorubicin cardiotoxicity than to oncological efficacy, extended infusion duration is cardioprotective [34]. Prolonged infusion schemes have not been widely used for agents other than doxorubicin.

c. Liposomal encapsulation

Encapsulation of doxorubicin into a liposomal delivery system increases the size of this complex, resulting in lower penetration into tissues with normal vascular beds like myocardium, and increased diffusion and penetration in immature vascular beds like tumor mass [35,36].

Secondly, this process prolongs the half-life of the molecule.

Both mechanisms allow to approximately double the number of chemotherapy cycles compared with the nonencapsulated compound [35], but unfortunately this also changes the oncologic spectrum.

d. Cardioprotective agents

Dexrazoxane is a free radical scavenger that, after hydrolysis to form ADR-925 inside the cardiomyocyte, removes the iron from the anthracycline complexes to prevent its cardiotoxic effect. It has not been used in daily practice yet because of concerns about reduced oncological efficacy [37–39].

Any molecule directly reducing myocardial injury, slowing consecutive myocardial remodeling, or promoting myocardial repair might prove to be relatively cardioprotective. This has been the case for ACE-inhibition and/or β-blockade [40–43].

Additionally, Seican's paper suggested that statins might be cardioprotective in the context of anthracycline treatment for breast cancer [44] through its pleiotropic effects, thereby reducing vascular inflammation [45] and oxidative stress [46].

TYPE II CARDIOTOXICITY

This cardiotoxic mechanism was only discovered in the very beginning of this century with the publication of a pivotal trial combining anthracyclines with trastuzumab for treatment of metastatic breast cancer [9]. Meanwhile, another group of targeted oncotherapies with tyrosine kinases seems to have similar cardiotoxic potential through resembling mechanisms [47]. There is still debate about whether they should be considered as alternative type II agents, or rather as a separate class with distinct cardiotoxic mechanisms. Therefore, those small molecules like lapatinib, sunitinib and sorafenib will be discussed in the section Molecules, later in this chapter, and we will focus here on trastuzumab cardiotoxicity.

1. Mechanism of trastuzumab cardiotoxicity

   Trastuzumab is a monoclonal antibody, acting as an antagonist of the human epidermal growth factor receptor tyrosine kinase HER2 (Erb B2). This causes interference with neoangiogenesis and adaptation of cells to physiological or pathological stress. It is not only overexpressed in HER2-positive breast cancer, but is also present in normal cardiomyocytes. It was proven to promote survival and growth of cardiomyocytes [48] and selective inhibition in animal models initiated structural and functional changes leading to dilated cardiomyopathy [49].
2. Absence of structural changes

   Ewer [48] proved, in a very limited cohort though, that the typical ultrastructural cardiomyocyte changes, as seen during or early after anthracycline treatment, do not appear after trastuzumab administration, as illustrated in Fig. 3.4. Despite this apparently reassuring fact, that cohort did develop reduced LV systolic function, expressed as a significant drop in LVEF [50]!
3. Clinical presentation of type II cardiotoxicity: domination by the synergistic cardiotoxic properties of anthracyclines and trastuzumab

   The absence of ultrastructural myocardial changes in trastuzumab-treated patients suggests that type II cardiotoxicity is much less aggressive than type I cardiotoxicity. Several clinical data support this statement.

   The first is that one arm of the BCIRG-006 study, administering trastuzumab only, showed a 5.1-fold lower incidence of NYHA class III–IV heart failure (0.40% vs 2%, $P < 0.001$) and a 2.1-fold lower incidence of

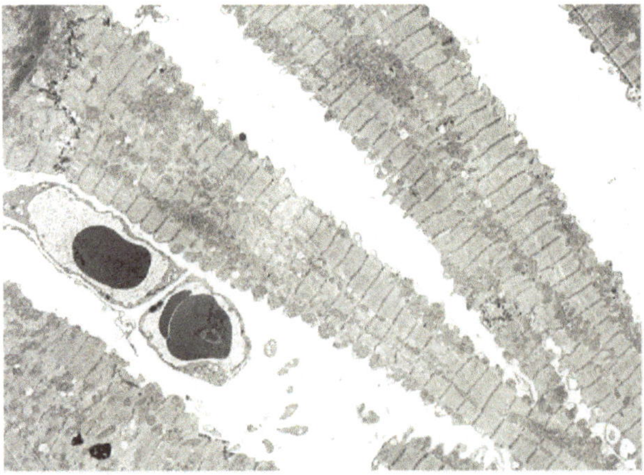

FIGURE 3.4 Typical biopsy (×4000) from a patient with left ventricular dysfunction on trastuzumab alone. Representative biopsy specimen from a patient with trastuzumab-related cardiotoxicity demonstrating no ultrastructural changes. *From Ewer MS, et al. Reversibility of trastuzumab-related cardiotoxicity: new insights based on clinical course and response to medical treatment. J Clin Oncol 2005;23(31):7820–26.*

an absolute drop in LVEF (9.4% vs 18.6%, $P < 0.001$) compared to the anthracycline-treated arm (mean dose 240 mg/m^2) for an equal distribution of the risk factors, left-sided breast irradiation, diabetes, and AHT among both groups [51]. Second, only one cardiac death has been reported in the more than 10,000 patients who received trastuzumab in the various adjuvant trials in the north central cancer treatment group N9831 [52] and none in the formerly mentioned BCIRG-006 study including 2174 trastuzumab-treated patients with mean follow up of 65 months[51]! Third, and in contrast with what is seen in type I cardiotoxicity, reversibility of type II cardiotoxicity is higher and more frequent [50,53–55]. Fourth, there are no arguments supporting a cumulative dose relationship between trastuzumab treatment and the risk of cardiac events. Fifth, and even though with little evidence, trastuzumab rechallenge after withdrawal and stabilization of LV systolic function, either with heart failure therapy or spontaneously, did not further reduce LVEF nor caused CHF symptoms [50]. Finally, Cardinale brought the most convincing proof of the more benign type II cardiotoxicity: in her paper on clinical and prognostic implications of troponin I elevation in "trastuzumab-induced" cardiotoxicity, all patients showing troponin I rises after or during trastuzumab therapy had been treated formerly with anthracyclines. None of the patients having had trastuzumab without prior anthracyclines developed any troponin rise during the study [56]!

All these arguments generate the clinical hypothesis that anthracyclines and trastuzumab have synergistic cardiotoxic properties. Additional evidence for this statement is delivered by the results of a metastatic trial in which anthracyclines and trastuzumab are given simultaneously, resulting in a considerable increase in cardiac events including heart failure and an asymptomatic decline in systolic LV function [9]. Ewer helped to better establish this synergism hypothesis by correlating the incidence of heart failure with the time elapsed between anthracycline and trastuzumab initiation in several trials, as illustrated in Fig. 3.5. The incidence of cardiac morbidity was higher in those trials in which there was no or only a short interval between both drugs [57]. This is in conjunction with what is expected from the pathophysiological viewpoint: first, anthracyclines cause not only cardiomyocyte necrosis and apoptosis, but make it vulnerable to further damage [58]. This induces upregulation of HER2 [59] in an attempt to repair ultrastructure and recover normal function. If trastuzumab is administered simultaneously or too short after anthracyclines, cardiomyocyte repair is inhibited, leading to enhanced apoptosis and thus augmented cardiotoxicity. The augmenting cardiotoxic effect of risk factors like smoking, AHT, chest irradiation, and underlying myocardial ischemia could simply be explained by the fact that this additional myocardial aggression cannot be compensated by the already trastuzumab-induced inhibition of myocardial repair.

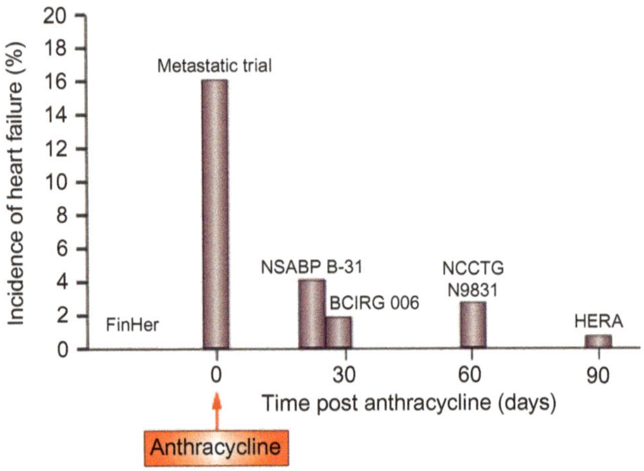

FIGURE 3.5 Incidence of heart failure following doxorubicin and trastuzumab therapy. Incidence of NYHA class III or class IV heart failure as a factor of the interval of time between the completion of doxorubicin and administration of trastuzumab, as reported in the major adjuvant trials. In a pivotal metastatic trial, the drugs were given concomitantly, and in the FinHer trial, trastuzumab administration preceded anthracycline. A higher incidence of heart failure was observed in the trials that administered trastuzumab with or shortly after anthracycline. *From Ewer MS, Ewer SM. Cardiotoxicity profile of trastuzumab. Drug Safety 2008;31(6):459–67.*

4. Mitigation of type II cardiotoxicity

   Ewer nicely illustrated that postponing the administration of trastuzumab after former anthracycline treatment can prevent or reduce the above-discussed synergistic cardiotoxicity [57]. Furthermore, temporal withdrawal and reinitiation after stabilization of LV systolic function, either with heart failure therapy or spontaneously, have been partially successful in the prevention of cardiotoxicity [50]. Monitoring of troponin release has proven to be the first and most sensitive test in detecting early signs of cardiotoxicity with a proven impact on cardiac prognosis [60], especially after anthracycline therapy. Comparable data for trastuzumab (after prior anthracycline) therapy are scarce, not to say absent.

CARDIOTOXICITY INDUCED BY TKI, VEGF INHIBITORS

In addition to the well-known anthracycline and anti-her2 cardiotoxicity, there is toxicity induced by a newer class of anticancer drugs, namely tyrosine kinase inhibitors (TKI) and antibodies inhibiting vascular endothelial growth factor (VEGF).

Constitutive VEGF signaling is important in normal adult cardiovascular physiology, and its abrogation by antiangiogenic therapies can result in vasoconstriction and microvascular rarefaction. Cardiovascular toxicity associated with specific antiangiogenic therapies has been reported at higher than anticipated rates and may be more prevalent when applied in unselected patient populations.

Molecules

Bevacizumab

Bevacizumab is a humanized monoclonal anti-VEGF antibody composed of a human IgG1 scaffold upon which the six complementarity-determining regions of the murine monoclonal antibody are engrafted. Bevacizumab binds to all biologically active isoforms of VEGF, and it is used in many types of tumors (breast, ovarian, colorectal, and lung cancer).

The effects of bevacizumab on the cardiovascular system are various, but in particular induce hypertension and thromboembolic events. In the three phase II clinical trials [61–63] that investigated the toxicity and efficacy of single agent bevacizumab, 11.2% of patients developed grade ≥ 3 hypertension (common toxicity criteria), and in combination with conventional or targeted therapies, the incidence of grade 3–4 hypertension was in the range of 0–28%. The median interval from initiation of bevacizumab to development of hypertension was 4.5–6 months. A pooled analysis of five randomized trials demonstrated a higher risk for angina pectoris, myocardial or cerebral ischemia/infarct, or arterial thrombosis in patients treated with bevacizumab and chemotherapy than in those treated with chemotherapy alone and a meta-analysis of 15 randomized trials also demonstrated that this antibody was associated with a significantly higher risk for venous thromboembolism.

Sorafenib

Sorafenib is a small-molecule tyrosine kinase inhibitor designed to inhibit C-type Raf-kinase (CRAF), LT-3, KIT, and BRAF. Besides targeting VEGFR-2, VEGFR-3, and platelet-derived growth factor receptor (PDGFR)-β, resulting in a robust proapoptotic effect on endothelial cells.

This small molecule is used in renal cell carcinoma, and in a prospective study of sorafenib a persistent increase in blood pressure was observed in most patients within 3 weeks of treatment, and vascular stiffness increased significantly for up to 10 months of observation. In patients treated with sunitinib there is a high incidence of ischemia/infarction too.

Sunitinib

Sunitinib is an oral antiangiogenic small-molecule tyrosine-kinase inhibitor. It inhibits VEGFR-1-2-3, PDGFR-α and -β, rearranged during transfection and FLT-3.

By targeting VEGFR-3 and PDGFR-β, sunitinib leads to impaired angiogenic sprouting and impairs vessel stabilization through pericyte recruitment and maturation. The use of sunitinib in GIST and renal cell cancer induced an increase in blood pressure with secondarily increased risk of left ventricular dysfunction (LVD) and heart failure [64].

Pathogenetic Mechanisms

The effects of anti-VEGF on normal tissues are described in Fig. 3.6.

The pathogenetic mechanism underlying the side effects is the inhibition of VEGF signaling, which can cause hypertension by inhibition of the vasomotor effects of VEGF and promotion of microvascular rarefaction. The vasomotor effects of VEGF are mediated through VEGFR-2. VEGFR-2 activation leads to upregulation of endothelial nitric oxide synthase through the Src and Akt signaling pathways.

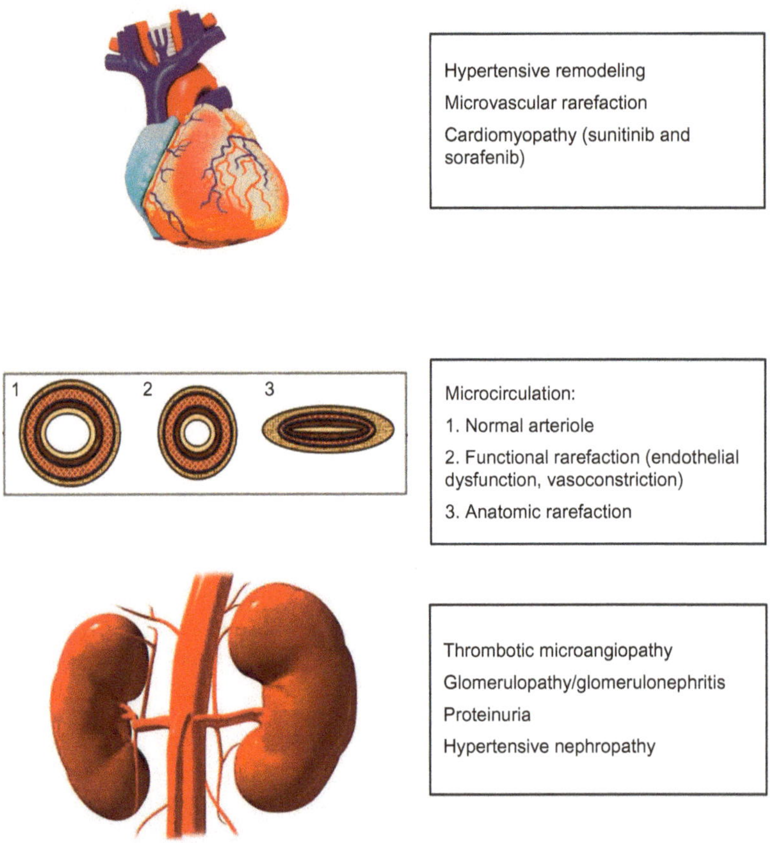

FIGURE 3.6 VEGF inhibition by the approved anti-VEGF therapies has differential effects on the VEGF–VEGFR axis in tumor cells and normal tissues. In noncancer tissues, endothelial dysfunction and microvascular rarefaction set the stage for the development of hypertension, cardiomyopathy, and thrombotic microangiopathy and proteinuria in the kidney.

Microvascular rarefaction is the extinction of small blood vessels that comprise the microcirculation and it is a consistent feature encountered in primary and secondary hypertension. It has been described in individuals with genetic propensity for high blood pressure, predating the onset of hypertension. Elimination of constitutive baseline VEGF signaling may therefore lead to endothelial dysfunction and vasoconstriction to the extent of nonperfusion. This functional rarefaction sets the stage for anatomic rarefaction, i.e., the frank extinction of microvessels. VEGF is upregulated in hypertension and mediates compensatory responses, which may be abrogated by anti-VEGF therapy.

The anti-VEGF drugs can cause cardiotoxicity because hypertension is associated with left ventricular hypertrophy, a strong and independent predictor of cardiovascular morbidity and mortality. The net decline in microvascular density leads to hypertension-associated cardiovascular events. Indeed, in animal models, promotion of capillary growth with VEGF reduced apoptosis and preserved contractile function in hypertrophied, pressure-loaded hearts. Finally, experiments in animal models have shown that VEGF signaling in normal cardiac physiology mediates important compensatory responses to stress and injury too.

VEGF abrogation is related to both hemorrhage and thrombosis. Selective knockout of VEGF in endothelial cells increases apoptosis and compromises the junctions between endothelial cells. The increased abnormalities in apoptosis have a prothrombotic effect. Targeting the VEGF-signaling pathway can also adversely affect the production of platelet inhibitors, such as prostaglandin I–II and nitric oxide.

Kinases are enzymes that catalyze the transfer of phosphate from ATP to a protein substrate. Through these phosphorylation reactions, kinases act as critical mediators of cellular signal transduction involved in cell cycle progression, metabolism, transcription, and apoptosis. A major problem is that kinases act through interconnected networks rather than via distinct linear pathways. Therefore, the range of potential adverse cellular effects that could arise through inhibition of kinase targets is enormous. In cancer cells, many kinases, particularly receptor tyrosine-kinases (RTKs), are constitutively active, often through mutation or translocation, and act as drivers of cancer cell proliferation and survival. For this reason, kinases have emerged as key therapeutic targets in the area of oncology in the last 10 years. An important question is whether the common mechanisms of action of these drugs can cause cardiac dysfunction.

Mitochondria play a crucial role in the cell, providing the majority of the cell's energy, through electron transport and oxidative phosphorylation. Cardiac muscle is highly reliant upon aerobic metabolism and therefore is susceptible to drugs that perturb mitochondrial homeostasis or metabolism. Drug-induced mitochondrial toxicity can be evoked via inhibition of numerous processes, and there are several kinases localized in and regulating mitochondrial function, including c-Jun N-terminal kinase (JNK), pyruvate dehydrogenase kinase (PDK), branched-chain α-ketoacid dehydrogenase kinase, and protein kinase A (PKA) [65]. JNK appears to be a frequent off-target of small molecule kinase inhibitors [66]. With respect to specific kinase inhibitors, direct mitochondrial effects of sorafenib have been reported as a potential mechanism of cardiotoxicity. Histopathological examination of endomyocardial biopsies from sunitinib-treated patients who developed heart failure revealed cardiomyocyte hypertrophy and mitochondrial abnormalities including swelling, membrane whorls, and effaced cristae. Since mitochondria are a central component of the intrinsic apoptotic process, mitochondrial functional and structural changes will be a common outcome of adverse interactions between drug molecules and cells. Mitochondrial morphological changes, such as aggregation and remodeling of the cristae, are common in apoptotic cells . Therefore, caution should be taken not to overinterpret any observed "mitochondrial effects" occurring as a consequence of drug treatment as representing direct drug-induced mitochondrial toxicity. With regard to sunitinib cardiotoxicity, it has been hypothesized that it could be mediated through inhibition of AMP-activated protein kinase (AMPK), an important regulator of cellular energy metabolism required to maintain normal cardiac contractility. ATP reserves in cardiac tissue are small, and given the critical role of AMPK as regulator of cellular ATP homeostasis, myocytes could be particularly sensitive to AMPK inhibition.

Imatinib, sunitinib, sorafenib, dasatinib, and nilotinib all inhibit PDGFR. Although the full picture is not yet elucidated, data indicate that for some malignancies, the anticancer effects of these drugs are dependent upon PDGFR inhibition. It remains a possibility that inhibition of PDGFR in the heart may be a contributory factor in the cardiotoxicity associated with the use of some of these small-molecule inhibitors.

Recently, evidence has emerged that some RTKs directly modulate ion channel activity. In whole-cell patch clamp experiments, the EGFR inhibitor AG556, the Src family inhibitor PP2, and the broad-spectrum RTK inhibitor genistein all inhibited tyrosine phosphorylation of human ether-a-go-go related gene and reduced channel activity.

Inhibition of adenosine receptors represents another potential, but largely underexplored, mechanism of kinase inhibitor-induced cardiotoxicity. In response to insults such as cardiac ischemia, the extracellular adenosine concentration rises, leading to enhanced activation of the adenosine receptors A_1 and A_3 in cardiomyocytes. The resulting downstream activation of phospholipases C and D has a cardioprotective effect. In the rabbit heart, adenosine has been shown to activate the PI3K/Akt signaling pathway.

CARDIOTOXICITY INDUCED BY OTHER CHEMOTHERAPY DRUGS

Several chemotherapy agents have been associated with cardiac dysfunctions though the molecular mechanisms underlying these side effects are not completely elucidated.

LVD has been associated with alkylating agents. Rates of LVD in patients receiving cyclophosphamide range from 7% to 28% and the risk of cardiotoxicity is dose-related. Higher rates of heart failure have been described with the use of ifosfamide too.

Some drugs might enhance myocardial toxicity by causing cardiac ischemia. Coronary artery thrombosis, arteritis, and vasospasm secondary to drug exposure have been proposed as the most likely underlying mechanisms. In patients treated with 5-fluorouracil, the incidence of cardiac events ranges from 1% to 68%. Cardiac toxicity typically occurs with early onset, within 2–5 days of starting therapy. Electrocardiogram changes have been reported in up to 68% of patients. However, the exact rate of cardiac myocyte damage is not completely known, as most of the studies have not included serum cardiac markers or echocardiographic data.

Cases of myocardial ischemia and infarction associated with paclitaxel administration have been reported, a retrospective study reviewed cardiac events in four clinical trials and reported manifestations of cardiac ischemia in 5% of patients.

REFERENCES

[1] Ewer MS. Cardiotoxicity of anticancer treatments: what the cardiologist needs to know. Nat Re Cardiol 2010;7:564–75.

[2] Hershman DL, et al. Doxorubicin, cardiac risk factors, and cardiac toxicity in elderly patients with diffuse B-cell non-Hodgkin's lymphoma. J Clin Oncol 2008;26:3159–65.

[3] Ho E, et al. Subclinical anthracycline- and trastuzumab induced cardiotoxicity in the long-term follow-up of asymptomatic breast cancer survivors: a speckle tracking echocardiographic study. Heart 2010;96:701–7.

[4] Steinherz LJ, et al. Cardiac toxicity 4 to 20 years aftervcompleting anthracycline therapy. JAMA 1991;266:1672–7.

[5] Tsai H, et al. Left ventricular function assessed by two-dimensional speckle tracking echocardiography in long-term survivors of Hodgkin's lymphoma treated by mediastinal radiotherapy with or without anthracycline therapy. Am J Cardiol 2011;107:472–7.

[6] Altena R, et al. Cardiovascular toxicity caused by cancer treatment: strategies for early detection. Lancet Oncol 2009;10:391–9.

[7] Kerkhove D, et al. How to monitor cardiac toxicity: time is muscle!. Heart 2014;100 1208–17.

[8] Lefrak EA, et al. A clinicopathologic analysis of adriamycin cardiotoxicity. Cancer 1973;32:302–14.

[9] Slamon DJ, et al. Use of chemotherapy plus a monoclonal antibody against HER2 for metastatic breast cancer that overexpresses HER2. N Engl J Med 2001;344:783–92.

[10] De Azambuja E, et al. Trastuzumab-associated cardiac events at 8 years of median follow-up in the Herceptin Adjuvant trial (BIG 1-01). J Clin Oncol 2014;32(20):2159–65.

[11] Lefrak EA, et al. A clinicopathological analysis of adriamycin cardiotoxicity. Cancer 1973;32:302–14.

[12] Link G, et al. Role of Iron in the potentiation of anthracycline cardiotoxicity: identification of heart cell mitochondria as a major site of iron-anthracycline interaction. J Lab Clin Med 1996;127:272–8.

[13] Gille L, Nohl H. Analysis of the molecular mechanism of Adriamycin-induced cardiotoxicity. Free Radical Biol Med 1997;23:775–82.

[14] Aries P, et al. Essential role of GATA-4 in cell survival and drug-induced cardiotoxicity. Proc Natl Acad Sci USA 2004;101((18):6975–80.

[15] Sacco G, et al. Chronic cardiotoxicity of anticancer anthracyclines in the rat: role of secondary metabolites and reduced toxicity by a novel anthracycline with impaired metabolite formation and reactivity. Br J Pharmacol 2003;139:641–51.

[16] Minotti G, et al. Doxorubicin irreversibly inactivates iron regulatory proteins 1 and 2 in cardiomyocytes: evidence for distinct metabolic pathways and implications for iron-mediated cardiotoxicity of antitumor therapy. Cancer Res 2001;61:8422–8.

[17] Von Hoff DD, Layard MW, Basa P, Davis Jr HL, Von Hoff AL, Rozencweig M, et al. Risk factors for doxorubicin-induced congestive heart failure. Ann Intern Med 1979;91 (5):710–17.

[18] Swain S, et al. Congestive heart failure in patients treated with doxorubicin: a retrospective analysis of three trials. Cancer 2003;97:2869–79.

[19] Ewer MS, et al. A comparison of biopsy grades and ejection fraction estimations in patients receiving Adriamycin. J Clin Oncol 1984;2:112–17.

[20] Ewer MS. A mathematical model for doxorubicin cardiotoxicity: added evidence for the concept of sequential stress. In: Paper presented at: Proceedings of the 40th Annual Meeting of the American Society of Clinical Oncology; 2004.

[21] Billingham M, et al. Endomyocardial biopsy findings in Adriamycin-treated patients. Proc Am Soc Clin Oncol 1976;17:281 (abstract).

[22] Mackay B, et al. Cardiac biopsy. Texas Soc Electron Microsc 1981;11(2):7–15.

[23] Mackay B, et al. Assessment of anthracycline cardiomyopathy by endomyocardial biopsy. Ultrastructural Pathol 1994;18:203–11.

[24] Seidman A, et al. Cardiac dysfunction in the Trastuzumab Clinical Trials Experience. J Clin Oncol 2002;20(5):1215–21.

[25] Albini A, et al. Cardiotoxicity of anti-cancer drugs: the need for cardio-oncology and cardio-oncological prevention. J Natl Cancer Inst 2010;102:14–25.

[26] O'Brien PJ. Cardiac troponin is the most effective translational safety biomarker for myocardial injury in cardiotoxicity. Toxicology 2008;245:206–18.

[27] Lipshultz S, et al. Changes in cardiac biomarkers during doxorubicin treatment of peadiatric patients with high-risk acute lymphoblastic leukemia: associations with longterm echocardiographic outcomes. J Clin Oncol 2012;30(10):1042–9.

[28] Kilickap S, et al. Troponin T can be a useful marker for early detection of anthracycline cardiotoxicity. Ann Oncol 2005;16(5):798–804.

[29] Cardinale D, et al. Prognostic value of troponin I in cardiac risk stratification of cancer patients undergoing high-dose chemotherapy. Circulation 2004;109:2749–54.

[30] Kalam K, Marwick TH. Role of cardioprotective therapy for prevention of cardiotoxicity with chemotherapy: a systematic review and meta-analysis. Eur J Cancer 2013;49 (13):2900–9.

[31] Van Dalen EC, et al. Different anthracycline derivatives for reducing cardiotoxicity in cancer patients. Cochrane Database of Systematic Reviews 2006;(4). Art.no.CD005006. doi:10.1002/14651858CD005006.pub4.

[32] Minotti G. Cardiotoxicity of non-cardiovascular drugs- Chapter 6:Diagnostic aspects of cardiovascular toxicity of antitumor drugs. Hoboken, NJ: John Wiley & Sons Ltd; 2010ISBN 978-0-470-77274-4.

[33] Ewer M, et al. Cardiac Safety of liposomal anthracyclines. Semin Oncol 2004;31 (Suppl. 13):161–81.

[34] Calabresi L, et al. High-density lipoproteins protect isolated rat hearts from ischaemia—reperfusion injury by reducing cardiac tumor necrosis factor alpha content and enhancing prostaglandin release. Circ Res 2003;92:330–7.

[35] Valero V, et al. Phase II trial of liposome-encapsulated doxorubicin, cyclophosphamide, and fluoro-uracil as first-line therapy in patients with metastatic breast cancer. J Clin Oncol 1999;17:1425–34.

[36] Swain S, et al. Cardioprotection with dexrazoxane for doxorubicine-containing chemotherapy for advanced breast cancer. J Clin Oncol 1997;15(4):1318–32.

[37] Speyer JL, et al. Protective effect of the bispiperazinedione ICRF-187 against doxorubicine-induced cardiac toxicity in women with advanced breast cancer. N Engl J Med 1988;319:117–21.

[38] Cardinale D, et al. Prevention of high dose chemotherapy-induced cardiotoxicity in high risk patients by ACE-inhibition. Circulation 2006;114:2474–81.

[39] Cardinale D, et al. Prevention and treatment of cardiomyopathy and heart failure in patients receiving cancer chemotherapy. Curr Treat Cardiovasc Med 2008;10:186–95.

[40] Blaes AH, et al. Angiotensin converting inhibitors may be protective against cardiac complications following anthracycline chemotherapy. Breast Cancer Res Treat 2010;122: 585–90.

[41] Kalay N, et al. Protective effects of carvedilol against anthracycline-induced cardiomyopathy. J Am Coll Cardiol 2006;48:2258–62.

[42] Seicean S, et al. Effect of statin therapy on the risk for incident heart failure in patients with breast cancer receiving anthracycline chemotherapy. J Am Coll Cardiol 2012;60: 2384–90.

[43] Ridker P.M. et al. for the Air Force/Texas Coronary Atherosclerosis Prevention Study Investigators. Measurement of C-reactive protein for the targeting of statin therapy in the primary prevention of acute coronary events. N Engl J Med 2011;344:1959-1965.

[44] Jones SP, et al. Simvastatin attenuates oxidant-induced mitochondrial dysfunction in cardiac myocytes. Circulation Res 2003;93:697–9.

[45] Cheng H, et al. Why do kinase inhibitors cause cardiotoxicity and what can be done about it? Prog Cardiovasc Dis 2010;53:114–20.

[46] Zhao YY, et al. Neuregulins promote survival and growth of cardiac myocytes. Persistence of ErbB2 and ErbB4 expression in neonatal and adult ventricular myocytes. J Biol Chem 1998;273:10261–9.

[47] Crone SA, et al. ErbB2 is essential in the prevention of dilated cardiomyopathy. Nat Med 2002;8:459–65.

[48] Ewer MS, et al. Reversibility of trastuzumab-related cardiotoxicity: new insights based on clinical course and response to medical treatment. J Clin Oncol 2005;23:7820–6.

[49] Slamon D, et al. Adjuvant trastuzumab in HER2-positive breast cancer. N Engl J Med 2011;365(14):1273–83.

[50] Perez EA, et al. Cardiac safety analysis of doxorubicin and cyclophosphamide followed by paclitaxel aith or without trastuzumab in the North Central Cancer Research Group N9831 adjuvant breast cancer trial. J Clin Oncol 2008;26:1231–8.

[51] Yoon GJ, et al. Left ventricular dysfunction in patients receiving cardiotoxic cancer therapies: are clinicians responding optimally? J Am Coll Cardiol 2010;56:1644–50.

[52] Thavendiranathan P, et al. Reproducibility of echocardiographic techniques for sequential assessment of left ventricular ejection fraction and volumes: application to patients undergoing cancer chemotherapy. J Am Coll Cardiol 2013;61:77–84.

[53] Negishi K, et al. Use of speckle strain to assess left ventricular responses to cardiotoxic chemotherapy and cardioprotection. Eur Heart J Cardiovasc Imaging 2013, sept 20; epub.

[54] Cardinale D, et al. Trastuzumab-induced cardiotoxicity: clinical and prognostic implications of troponin I evaluation. J Clin Oncol 2010;28:3910–16.

[55] Ewer SM, et al. Cardiotoxicity profile of trastuzumab. Drug Safety 2008;31:459–67.

[56] Mann DL. Mechanisms and models in heart failure : a combinational approach. Circ 1999;100:999–1008.

[57] De Korte MA, et al. Indium-trastuzumab visualizes myocardial human epidermal growth factor receptor 2 expression shortly after anthracycline treatment but not during heart failure: a clue to uncover the mechanisms of trastuzumab-related cardiotoxicity. Eur J Cancer 2007;43:2046–51.

[58] Mele D, Tocchetti CG, Pagliaro P, Madonna R, Novo G, Pepe A, et al. Pathophysiology of anthracycline cardiotoxicity. J Cardiovasc Med (Hagerstown) 2016;17(Suppl 1):S3–11.

[59] de Korte MA, de Vries EG, Lub-de Hooge MN, Jager PL, Gietema JA, van der Graaf WT, et al. 111Indium-trastuzumab visualises myocardial human epidermal growth factor receptor 2 expression shortly after anthracycline treatment but not during heart failure: a clue to uncover the mechanisms of trastuzumab-related cardiotoxicity. Eur J Cancer 2007;43(14):2046–51.

[60] Henri C, Heinonen T, Tardif JC. The role of biomarkers in decreasing risk of cardiac toxicity after cancer therapy. Biomark Cancer 2016;8(Suppl 2):39–45.

[61] Siegel AB, Cohen EI, Ocean A, et al. Phase II trial evaluating the clinical and biologic effects of bevacizumab in unresectable hepatocellular carcinoma. J Clin Oncol 2008;26: 2992–8.

[62] Burger RA, Sill MW, Monk BJ, Greer BE, Sorosky JI. Phase II trial of bevacizumab in persistent or recurrent epithelial ovarian cancer or primary peritoneal cancer: AGynecologic Oncology Group study. J Clin Oncol 2007;25:5165–71.

[63] Cannistra SA, Matulonis UA, Penson RT, et al. Phase II study of bevacizumab in patients with platinum-resistant ovarian cancer or peritoneal serous cancer. J Clin Oncol 2007;25: 5180–6.

[64] Rock EP, Goodman V, Jiang JX, et al. Food and Drug Administration drug approval summary: sunitinib malate for the treatment of gastrointestinal stromal tumor and advanced renal cell carcinoma. The Oncologist 2007;12:107–13.

[65] Thomson M. Evidence of undiscovered cell regulatory mechanisms: phosphoproteins and protein kinases in mitochondria. Cell Mol Life Sci 2002;59:213–19.

[66] Fabian MA, Biggs III WH, Treiber DK, Atteridge CE, Azimioara MD, Benedetti MG, et al. A small molecule-kinase interaction map for clinical kinase inhibitors. Nat Biotechnol 2005;23:329–36.

[67] Swain S, et al. Delayed administration of dexrazoxane provides cardioprotection for patients with advanced breast cancer treated with doxorubicine-containing chemotherapy. J Clin Oncol 1997;15(4):133–40.

[68] Lenihan DJ. Tyrosine kinase inhibitors: can promising new therapy associated with cardiac toxicity strengthen the concept of teamwork? J Clin Oncol 2008;26:5154–5.

[69] Mourad JJ, des Guetz G, Debbabi H, et al. Blood pressure rise following angiogenesis inhibition by bevacizumab. A crucial role for microcirculation. Ann Oncol 2008;19:927–34.

[70] Di Lorenzo G, Figg WD, Fossa SD, et al. Combination of bevacizumab and docetaxel in docetaxel-pretreated hormone-refractory prostate cancer: a phase 2 study. Eur Urol 2008;54:1089–94.

[71] Nalluri SR, Chu D, Keresztes R, et al. Risk of venous thromboembolism with the angiogenesis inhibitor bevacizumab in cancer patients: a metaanalysis. JAMA 2008;300:2277–85.

[72] Tammela T, Zarkada G, Wallgard E, et al. Blocking VEGFR-3 suppresses angiogenic sprouting and vascular network formation. Nature 2008;454:656–60.

[73] Bergers G, Song S, Meyer-Morse N, et al. Benefits of targeting both pericytes and endothelial cells in the tumor vasculature with kinase inhibitors. The J Clin Invest 2003;111:1287–95.

[74] Chu TF, Rupnick MA, Kerkela R, et al. Cardiotoxicity associated with tyrosine kinase inhibitor sunitinib. Lancet 2007;370:2011–19.

[75] Khakoo AY, Kassiotis CM, Tannir N, et al. Heart failure associated with sunitinib malate: a multitargeted receptor tyrosine kinase inhibitor. Cancer 2008;112:2500–8.

[76] Veronese ML, Mosenkis A, Flaherty KT, et al. Mechanisms of hypertension associated with BAY 43–9006. J Clin Oncol 2006;24:1363–9.

[77] Kane RC, Farrell AT, Saber H, et al. Sorafenib for the treatment of advanced renal cell carcinoma. Clin Cancer Res 2006;12:7271–8.

[78] Henry TD, Annex BH, McKendall GR, et al. The VIVA trial: vascular endothelial growth factor in Ischemia for Vascular Angiogenesis. Circulation 2003;107:1359–65.

[79] Nachman RL, Rafii S. Platelets, petechiae, and preservation of the vascular wall. N Engl J Med 2008;359:1261–70.

[80] Elice F, Rodeghiero F, Falanga A, et al. Thrombosis associated with angiogenesis inhibitors. Best Pract Res Clin Haematol 2009;22:115–28.

[81] Scappaticci FA, Skillings JR, Holden SN, et al. Arterial thromboembolic events in patients with metastatic carcinoma treated with chemotherapy and bevacizumab. J Natl Cancer Inst 2007;99:1232–9.

[82] Gschwind A, Fischer OM, Ullrich A. The discovery of receptor tyrosine kinases: targets for cancer therapy. Nat Rev Cancer 2004;4:361–70.

[83] Wallace KB. Mitochondrial off targets of drug therapy. Trends Pharmacol Sci 2008;29:361–6.

[84] Kerkela R, Grazette L, Yacobi R, Iliescu C, Patten R, Beahm C, et al. Cardiotoxicity of the cancer therapeutic agent imatinib mesylate. Nat Med 2006;12:908–16.

[85] Force T, Krause DS, Van Etten RA. Molecular mechanisms of cardiotoxicity of tyrosine kinase inhibition. Nat Rev Cancer 2007;7:332–44.

[86] Lage R, Dieguez C, Vidal-Puig A, Lopez M. AMPK: a metabolic gauge regulating whole-body energy homeostasis. Trends Mol Med 2008;14:539–49.

[87] Zhang P, Hu X, Xu X, Fassett J, Zhu G, Viollet B, et al. AMP activated protein kinasealpha2 deficiency exacerbates pressure-overload-induced left ventricular hypertrophy and dysfunction in mice. Hypertension 2008;52:918–24.

[88] Krause DS, Van Etten RA. Tyrosine kinases as targets for cancer therapy. N Engl J Med 2005;353:172–87.

[89] Van den Akker NM, Winkel LC, Nisancioglu MH, Maas S, Wisse LJ, Armulik A, et al. PDGF-B signaling is important for murine cardiac development: its role in developing atrioventricular valves, coronaries, and cardiac innervation. Dev Dyn 2008;237 494–503.

[90] Yang JC, Haworth L, Sherry RM, Hwu P, Schwartzentruber DJ, Topalian SL, et al. A randomized trial of bevacizumab, an anti-vascular endothelial growth factor antibody, for metastatic renal cancer. N Engl J Med 2003;349:427–34.

[91] Bhargava P. VEGF kinase inhibitors: how do they cause hypertension? Am J Physiol Regul Integr Comp Physiol 2009;297:R1–5.

[92] Sica DA. Angiogenesis inhibitors and hypertension: an emerging issue. J Clin Oncol 2006;24:1329–31.

[93] Verheul HM, Pinedo HM. Possible molecular mechanisms involved in the toxicity of angiogenesis inhibition. Nat Rev Cancer 2007;7:475–85.

Chapter 4

Cardiotoxicity of Oncologic Treatments: Is There a Uniform Definition?

M. Scherrer-Crosbie

Chapter Outline

Cardiotoxicity is defined as "toxicity that affects the heart" by the US National Cancer Institute [1]. Although simple to understand in theory, this definition is very broad and in the case of cancer treatments, may encompass many effects, such as cardiac dysfunction and heart failure, myocardial ischemia or infarction, valvular abnormalities, pericardial disease, hypertension, and arrhythmias [2]. A large body of research has been generated on chemotherapy and in particular anthracycline-induced cardiotoxicity. In that field of research, cardiotoxicity generally refers to cardiac dysfunction and failure. However, the new cancer therapies, in particular the vascular endothelial growth factor (VEGF) inhibitors such as bevacizumab, sunitinib, and sorafenib, also increase the occurrence of myocardial ischemia [3,4] and have indirect cardiotoxic effects through the development of hypertension. Radiotherapy has even broader cardiotoxic effects, including significant increases in cardiac ischemia [5,6], valvular abnormalities [7], and pericardial disease.

The largest body of research that has been done on the cardiotoxicity of cancer treatments has involved anthracycline-induced cardiac effects. Anthracycline-induced cardiotoxicity was first described in the 1970s and was initially thought of as a cumulative dose-related form of congestive heart failure that occurred during treatment [8]. Subsequently, both acute reversible cardiotoxicity during treatment and late progressive cardiotoxicity were

Anticancer Treatments and Cardiotoxicity. DOI: http://dx.doi.org/10.1016/B978-0-12-802509-3.00004-2

also identified. The direct cardiac specific effects of anthracyclines are quite pleiotropic, however, heart failure is the most recognized [2]. The effects of anthracyclines have been further categorized based on whether complications present during treatment (acute), within a year of treatment discontinuation (early), or subsequently (late) [9,10]. Acute and late complications are believed to arise from different pathological mechanisms.

By far the most confusing aspect of the definition of cardiotoxicity is whether only clinical, clinical and subclinical, or only subclinical events are considered. In the case of heart failure, these subclinical events can include histological changes, changes in left ventricular ejection fraction (LVEF), changes in more subtle parameters of cardiac injury and function such as myocardial deformation indices (strain) and serum biomarkers. The degree to which the subclinical events are included in the definition of cardiotoxicity represents the most flagrant difference in the definition of cardiotoxicity adopted by the cardiology and oncology societies. The American College of Cardiology/American Heart Association guidelines for the diagnosis and management of congestive heart failure recommend that patients exposed to cardiotoxic drugs (stage A) be carefully monitored and their risk factors treated. Any detectable sign of cardiac remodeling or structural abnormality (stage B), even if asymptomatic, warrants therapeutic intervention. In particular, any LVEF impairment requires treatment with angiotensin-converting enzyme inhibitors and beta-blockers [11]. In contrast, the Common Terminology for Adverse Events developed by the National Cancer Institute does not recognize left ventricular (LV) dysfunction unless it is symptomatic [12]. Biomarkers or imaging abnormalities without symptoms are recorded as a low-severity event on the heart failure classification; in theory low-severity effects do not require treatment.

Finally, even the magnitude of the LVEF decrease that defines cardiotoxicity is a matter of intense discussion. The definitions include a decrease in LVEF by >20% to a value <50%, a decrease in LVEF by >10 % (or ≥10%) to a value <55%, a decrease in LVEF by >10% (or ≥10%) to a final value of <50% [13]. The percentage is generally implied as units rather than true percentage. One of the most used definitions of cardiotoxicity has been formulated by the cardiac review and evaluation committee supervising trastuzumab clinical trials, which defined drug-associated cardiotoxicity as one or more of the following: (1) cardiomyopathy in terms of a reduction in LVEF, either global or more severe in the septum; (2) symptoms associated with heart failure; (3) signs associated with heart failure, such as S3 gallop, tachycardia, or both; and (4) reduction in LVEF from baseline that is in the range of ≥5% to <55% with accompanying signs or symptoms of heart failure, or a reduction in LVEF in the range of ≥10% to <55%, without accompanying signs or symptoms [14].

Recently, the American Society of Echocardiography and European Association for Cardiovascular Imaging published an expert consensus for multimodality imaging of the adult patient during and after cancer therapy and defined the following terms:

A. *Cancer therapeutics-related cardiac dysfunction (CTRCD):* CTRCD is defined as a decrease in the LVEF of >10 percentage points, to a value lower than the limit of normal for 2D echocardiography. This decrease should be confirmed by repeated cardiac imaging 2–3 weeks following the baseline diagnostic study showing the initial decrease in LVEF [15].
B. *Subclinical LV dysfunction:* In the absence of CTRCD, subclinical LV dysfunction is defined as a $>15\%$ decrease in global longitudinal myocardial deformation (strain) during treatment, as compared to baseline.

The absence of a clear definition of cardiotoxicity has a tremendous effect on the reported incidence and prevalence of cancer treatment-related cardiotoxicity. This confusion is further compounded by the fact that studies report cardiotoxicity in widely different populations, with different risk factor profiles and heterogeneous treatments. As the field of cardio-oncology is growing in size and relevance, standardization of the definition of cardiotoxicity is an essential issue.

REFERENCES

[1] National Cancer Institute NIOH. NCI Dictionary of Cancer Terms [Internet]. Available from <www.cancer.gov/dictionary>; [cited 2014 Aug 22].

[2] Yeh ETH, Bickford CL. Cardiovascular complications of cancer therapy: incidence, pathogenesis, diagnosis, and management. J Am Coll Cardiol 2009;53:2231–47.

[3] Choueiri TK, Schutz FAB, Je Y, Rosenberg JE, Bellmunt J. Risk of arterial thromboembolic events with sunitinib and sorafenib: a systematic review and meta-analysis of clinical trials. J Clin Oncol 2010;28:2280–5.

[4] Ranpura V, Hapani S, Chuang J, Wu S. Risk of cardiac ischemia and arterial thromboembolic events with the angiogenesis inhibitor bevacizumab in cancer patients: a meta-analysis of randomized controlled trials. Acta Oncol 2010;49:287–97.

[5] Heidenreich PA, Schnittger I, Strauss HW, Vagelos RH, Lee BK, Mariscal CS, et al. Screening for coronary artery disease after mediastinal irradiation for Hodgkin's disease. J Clin Oncol 2007;25:43–9.

[6] Nilsson G, Holmberg L, Garmo H, Duvernoy O, Sjögren I, Lagerqvist B, et al. Distribution of coronary artery stenosis after radiation for breast cancer. J Clin Oncol 2012;30:380–6.

[7] Heidenreich PA, Hancock SL, Lee BK, Mariscal CS, Schnittger I. Asymptomatic cardiac disease following mediastinal irradiation. J Am Coll Cardiol 2003;42:743–9.

[8] Rahman AM, Yusuf SW, Ewer MS. Anthracycline-induced cardiotoxicity and the cardiac-sparing effect of liposomal formulation. Int J Nanomed 2007;2:567–83.

[9] Floyd JD, Nguyen DT, Lobins RL, Bashir Q, Doll DC, Perry MC. Cardiotoxicity of cancer therapy. J Clin Oncol 2005;23:7685–96.

[10] Monsuez J-J, Charniot J-C, Vignat N, Artigou J-Y. Cardiac side-effects of cancer chemotherapy. Int J Cardiol 2010;144:3–15.

[11] Writing Committee Members, Yancy CW, Jessup M, Bozkurt B, Butler J, Casey DE, Drazner MH, et al. American College of Cardiology Foundation/American Heart Association Task Force on Practice Guidelines. 2013 ACCF/AHA guideline for the management of heart failure: a report of the American College of Cardiology Foundation/American Heart Association Task Force on practice guidelines. 2013. p. e240–327.

[12] National Cancer Institute NIOH. Common Terminology for Adverse Events version 4.0 [Internet]. Available from <http://evs.nci.nih.gov/ftp1/CTCAE>; 2011 [cited 2015 Feb 10].

[13] Ganz WI, Sridhar KS, Forness TJ. Detection of early anthracycline cardiotoxicity by monitoring the peak filling rate. Am J Clin Oncol 1993;16:109–12.

[14] Seidman A, Hudis C, Pierri MK, Shak S, Paton V, Ashby M, et al. Cardiac dysfunction in the trastuzumab clinical trials experience. J Clin Oncol 2002;20:1215–21.

[15] Plana JC, Galderisi M, Barac A, Ewer MS, Ky B, Scherrer-Crosbie M, et al. Expert consensus for multimodality imaging evaluation of adult patients during and after cancer therapy: a report from the American Society of Echocardiography and the European Association of Cardiovascular Imaging. J Am Soc Echocardiogr 2014;27:911–39.

Chapter 5

The Impact of Radiotherapy

B. Cosyns and R. Dulgheru

Chapter Outline

MECHANISMS OF TOXICITY

The cardiovascular system has been shown to be more sensitive to radiation than previously expected. The main effects of radio-induced toxicity are seen on the vascular system (coronary and carotid artery disease), the myocardium itself, the pericardium, the valves, and the conduction system.

Although the toxicity of irradiation shares a common pathway, some specific mechanisms can be seen in these various cardiovascular target-structures and will be reviewed systematically.

The primary basic mechanism behind radiation-induced damage appears to be endothelial dysfunction [1]. Then, endothelial cell swelling, increased permeability, interstitial fibrin deposition, and development of platelet thrombi ultimately lead to fibrosis. Significant increase in superoxides and peroxides represents another mechanism of radiation-induced endothelial dysfunction via production of these reactive oxygen species [2] and also via nuclear factor-kappa B [3]. Moreover, cytokines and growth factors, such as transforming growth factor β1 and Interleukin 1 beta (IL-1β), may stimulate radiation-induced endothelial proliferation, fibroblast proliferation, collagen deposition, and fibrosis leading to advanced lesions [4]. Secondary systemic inflammation with elevated levels of the proinflammatory cytokines IL-6, c-reactive protein (CRP), tumor necrosis factor-α, and interferon-γ and also increased levels of the antiinflammatory cytokine IL-10 have also been observed [5]. On the other hand, the monocyte chemoattractant protein-1 (MCP-1) chemoattractant concentration increases, mainly driven by radiation-induced monocyte death [6]. The endothelial cell neutrophil

Anticancer Treatments and Cardiotoxicity. DOI: http://dx.doi.org/10.1016/B978-0-12-802509-3.00005-4

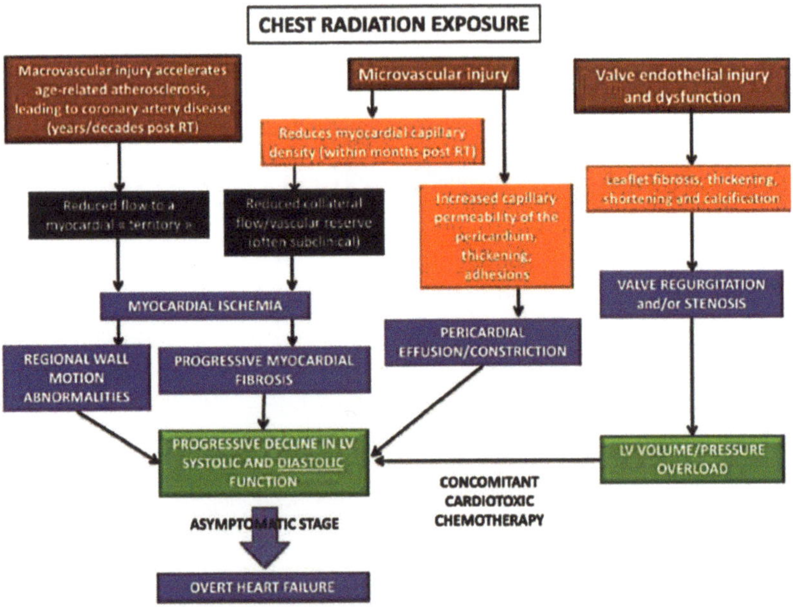

FIGURE 5.1 The mechanisms of radio-induced cardiovascular toxicity. *From Lancellotti P, et al. Expert consensus for multi-modality imaging evaluation of cardiovascular complications of radiotherapy in adults: a report from the European Association of Cardiovascular Imaging and the American Society of Echocardiography. Eur Heart J Cardiovasc Imag 2013 Aug;14(8):721–40.*

chemotactic activity is increased, with greater adherence of polynuclear leukocytes to irradiated endothelial cells [7]. The main mechanisms of radio-induced cardiovascular toxicity are summarized in Fig. 5.1.

The Vascular System

Coronary Artery Disease

In irradiated coronary vessels, intimal proliferation and fibrosis lead to luminal narrowing [9]. Although there is some overlap between typical coronary artery disease (CAD) and radiation-induced CAD, media are more often severely destroyed and the adventitia markedly thickened or fibrotic in radiation-induced CAD [10]. In irradiated coronary vessels, a loss of smooth muscle cells from the media and adventitial fibrosis may also be more frequently observed [9]. The combined effect of irradiation and traditional clinical risk factors may significantly accelerate radiation-induced atherosclerosis [11]. The proximal coronary vessels, which are in the range of radiation, are mainly involved [9,12]. The decrease in capillary density several months after the onset of radiotherapy may in return increase the risk of ischemia, symptomatic or not, that will lead to secondary fibrosis and systolic/diastolic myocardial dysfunction.

Carotid Vascular Disease

The mechanisms have been described above. Radio-induced carotid lesions are usually more extensive, long stenosis, with an atypical area distribution, and characterized by greater intima–media thickness [13]. Note that other vessels exposed to irradiation may also exhibit the typical features of radio-induced lesions. Extended calcification of the aorta may lead to porcelain aorta in the areas of exposure at more advanced stages.

The Myocardium

A direct effect of radiation may be seen at the level of the myocardium. There is an increase in collagen synthesis, and the proportion of type I collagen increases proportionally to type III. This may contribute to impaired diastolic function [14]. The most common pattern of fibrosis is pericellular and perivascular [12]. The loss of myocardium results in renin–angiotensin–aldosterone and adrenergic system-driven myocardial remodeling, which is usually progressive. Microvascular damage to the myocardium, which over time may lead to myocardial fibrosis and diastolic dysfunction, is also frequently observed [15]. Even if acute myocardial damage is only moderate, the process of myocardial remodeling can lead to progressive myocardial dysfunction over years, leading to symptoms and signs of heart failure sometimes only at the latest stages.

The Pericardium

The mechanisms of pericardial toxicity are reviewed in detail in Chapter 10, Pericardial Damage.

The Valves

The cusps or leaflets of the valves thicken due to fibrosis. The toxicity is related to endothelial injury and follows similar mechanisms as in other target-structures. The cusps may be partially calcified, radiation is a potent stimulate for procalcifying factors such as osteopontin, RUNX2, and alkaline phosphatase. It may occur very early after acute exposure and is also mediated by the inflammation process in the chronic phase [16,17]. The phenotypic dystrophic and calcified pattern of radiation-induced valvular disease may take several years to appear and the incidence increase with time (up to 20 years after exposure). The left-side heart valves are more often involved (related to mechanical and pressure factors). The presence of severe valvular lesions may increase hemodynamic instability and precipitate heart failure in these patients.

The Conduction System

Right bundle branch block is commonly associated with mediastinal irradiation because the right bundle lies close to the endocardium on the right side [18]. Injury to the bundle may occur either directly from radiation or indirectly from associated myocardial fibrosis and ischemia.

FACTORS MODULATING RADIOSENSITIVITY

The main factors modulating the effect of radiation on the heart are summarized in Table 5.1. From a historical point of view, over the two last decades, the practice of radiation oncology has dramatically changed. The evidence of heart side effects related to radiation has led to a more multidisciplinary management of cancer as a standard of care. The endpoint for complications analysis and modeling has considerably altered practice. Many changes in the technology, the radiotherapy itself but also the CT simulation, have become routine, along with the fusion of other modalities (magnetic resonance imaging, PET scan, etc.), and the new 3D technologies have improved the array of these evaluation tools. Therefore, dose distributions have become very complex. While, in doses >30 Gy, the risk of radiation-induced heart disease (RIHD) becomes apparent, even at lower radiation doses, there appears to be an excess risk of cardiovascular disease, as shown in the Japanese atomic bomb survivors [19]. Therefore a precise threshold dose is difficult to define. Nevertheless, recently there has been a trend to decrease the cumulative dose of exposure as much as possible. There is now clear evidence that the incidence of cardiovascular complications is proportional to the radiation dose [20]. Conversely, little is known about the effect of dose reduction during recent years. Since heart side effects occur late after exposure, the effects of new protocols will be evaluable only in a number of years from now. It is not well established whether reducing the doses of radiation will decrease side effects or only delay them.

The volume of the heart exposed is also of critical importance, and eccentric fields of irradiation to avoid as much as possible heart exposure are

TABLE 5.1 Main Factors Influencing Radiotherapy-Induced Tissue Toxicity

1. Total radiation dose (>30 Gy)
2. The dose per fraction (>2 Gy/day)
3. The volume of the heart irradiated
4. Concomitant administration of cardiotoxic systemic agents
5. Patient-related factors:
    a. Younger age (<50 years)
    b. Other CV risk factors (hypertension, smoking, etc.)
    c. Previous heart disease

proposed based on the dosimetric simulation. The absence of standard anatomy sometimes makes it challenging. Breath hold is systematic and new protocols using supine versus prone irradiation are under investigation, especially for left breast cancer complementary treatment. Radiation increases the risk of cardiotoxic effects of certain chemotherapeutic agents, such as anthracyclines [21]. This interaction appears to be dependent on the total cumulative dose of anthracyclines [22].

Clinical or patient-related factors are also of importance: younger age at irradiation for breast cancer has been shown to influence the risk, with a relative risk of 6.5 compared to the general population of RIHD [23]. Smoking also increases the relative risk. Other risk factors such as diabetes, hypertension, overweight, and hypercholesterolemia influence the overall risk [24]. The combination of several risk factors with radiotherapy increases the risk even further [20]. Therefore, an aggressive preventive approach to all the risk factors is highly recommended. Furthermore, the presence of prior heart disease increases the risk for developing cardiac events and should be taken into account when assessing the individual risk of the patient.

REFERENCES

[1] Paris F, Fuks Z, Kang A, et al. Endothelial apoptosis as the primary lesion initiating intestinal radiation damage in mice. Science 2001;293(5528):293–7.

[2] Hatoum OA, Otterson MF, Kopelman D, et al. Radiation induces endothelial dysfunction in murine intestinal arterioles via enhanced production of reactive oxygen species. Arterioscler Thromb Vasc Biol 2006;26(2):287–94.

[3] Weintraub NL, Jones WK, Manka D. Understanding radiation-induced vascular disease. J Am Coll Cardiol 2010;55(12):1237–9.

[4] Basavaraju SR, Easterly CE. Pathophysiological effects of radiation on atherosclerosis development and progression, and the incidence of cardiovascular complications. Med Phys 2002;29(10):2391–403.

[5] Hayashi T, Morishita Y, Kubo Y, et al. Long-term effects of radiation dose on inflammatory markers in atomic bomb survivors. Am J Med 2005;118(1):83–6.

[6] Little MP, Gola A, Tzoulaki I. A model of cardiovascular disease giving a plausible mechanism for the effect of fractionated low-dose ionizing radiation exposure. PLoS Comput Biol 2009;5(10). Article ID e1000539.

[7] Dunn MM, Drab EA, Rubin DB. Effects of irradiation on endothelial cell-polymorphonuclear leukocyte interactions. J Appl Physiol 1986;60(6):1932–7.

[8] Lancellotti P, Nkomo VT, Badano LP, Bergler-Klein J, Bogaert J, Davin L, et al. Expert consensus for multi-modality imaging evaluation of cardiovascular complications of radiotherapy in adults: a report from the European Association of Cardiovascular Imaging and the American Society of Echocardiography. Eur Heart J Cardiovasc Imag 2013 Aug;14(8):721–40.

[9] Brosius FC, Waller BF, Roberts WC. Radiation heart disease. Analysis of 16 young (aged 15 to 33 years) necropsy patients who received over 3,500 rads to the heart. Am J Med 1981;70(3):519–30.

[10] Virmani R, Farb A, Carter AJ, Jones RM. Pathology of radiation-induced coronary artery disease in human and pig. Cardiovasc Rad Med 1999;1(1):98–101.

[11] Amromin GD, Gildenhorn HL, Solomon RD, Nadkarni BB. The synergism of X-irradiation and cholesterol-fat feeding on the development of coronary artery lesions. J Atheroscler Res 1964;4:325–34.

[12] Veinot JP, Edwards WD. Pathology of radiation-induced heart disease: a surgical and autopsy study of 27 cases. Human Pathol 1996;27(8):766–73.

[13] Bilora F, Pietrogrande F, Petrobelli F, Polato G, Pomerri F, Muzzio PC. Is radiation a risk factor for atherosclerosis? An echo-color Doppler study on Hodgkin and non-Hodgkin patients. Tumori 2006;92(4):295–8.

[14] Chello M, Mastroroberto P, Romano R, Zofrea S, Bevacqua I, Marchese AR. Changes in the proportion of types I and III collagen in the left ventricular wall of patients with post-irradiative pericarditis. Cardiovasc Surg 1996;4(2):222–6.

[15] Adams MJ, Hardenbergh PH, Constine LS, Lipshultz SE. Radiation-associated cardiovascular disease. Crit Rev Oncol/Hematol 2003;45(1):55–75.

[16] Brand MD, Abadi CA, Aurigemma GP, Dauerman HL, Meyer TE. Radiation-associated valvular heart disease in Hodgkin's disease is associated with characteristic thickening and fibrosis of the aortic-mitral curtain. J Heart Valve Dis 2001;10(5):681–5.

[17] Katz NM, Hall AW, Cerqueira MD. Radiation induced valvulitis with late leaflet rupture. Heart 2001;86(6):E20.

[18] Totterman KJ, Pesonen E, Siltanen P. Radiation-related chronic heart disease. Chest 1983;83(6):875–8.

[19] Shimizu Y, Pierce DA, Preston DL, Mabuchi K. Studies of the mortality of atomic bomb survivors. Report 12, part II. Noncancer mortality: 1950–1990. Radiat Res 1999;152 (4):374–89.

[20] Darby SC, Ewertz M, Hall P. Ischemic heart disease after breast cancer radiotherapy. N Engl J Med 2013 Jun 27;368(26):2527.

[21] Meyer R, Gospodarowicz M, Connors J, Pearcey R, Wells W, Winter J, et al. ABVD alone versus radiation-based therapy in limited-stage Hodgkin's lymphoma. N Engl J Med 2012;366:399–408.

[22] Shapiro C, Hardenbergh P, Gelman R, Blanks D, Hauptman P, Recht A, et al. Cardiac effects of adjuvant doxorubicin and radiation therapy in breast cancer patients. J Clin Oncol 1998;16:3493–501.

[23] Hooning M, Botma A, Aleman B, Baaijens M, Bartelink H, Klijn J, et al. Long-term risk of cardiovascular disease in 10-year survivors of breast cancer. J Natl Cancer Inst 2007;99:365–75.

[24] King V, Constine L, Clark D, Schwartz R, Muhs A, Henzler M, et al. Symptomatic coronary artery disease after mantle irradiation for Hodgkin's disease. Int J Radiat Oncol Biol Phys 1996;36:881–9.

Section II

Detrimental Effects of Anticancer Drugs and Radiotherapy on the Heart

Chapter 6

Lessons From Preclinical Models

M. Scherrer-Crosbie

Chapter Outline

Preclinical models are invaluable in research as they allow dissection of the mechanisms that underlie physiology and the pathogenesis of diseases. The simplest models that have been commonly used to study anticancer treatment toxicity are isolated cardiomyocytes, especially rat neonatal cardiomyocytes or immortalized cardiomyocyte-derived cell lines, for their ease of use [1,2]. These allow the testing of the direct effects of drugs or radiation on cells.

In contrast, intact animal models, although more complex, permit to integrate the effect of the treatment on the whole biology system. Mice in particular are extensively used, as they are cheap, their genome is more than 98% similar to that of humans, and they can be genetically modified to overexpress or lack a gene of interest. Some obstacles in cardiovascular research, however, involve the small size of the mouse heart, its rapid rate (500–700 bpm), and the exquisite sensitivity of the mouse heart rate and cardiac function to sedation and anesthesia [3]. Two types of model exist in rodents, an acute model, in which 15–25 mg/kg of doxorubicin is injected and the effect measured in the next few days and a chronic model, in which repeated weekly injections of doxorubicin of 3–6 mg/kg are performed for a duration of approximately 4–6 weeks. Doxorubicin is most commonly injected intraperitoneally, and peritonitis is frequent, increasing the variability of the absorption of the drug. Intravenous injections are also described, although very difficult chronically. A few studies have used Alzet pumps [4] but skin necrosis is frequent. Although the acute model can bring some information on the triggers and mechanisms of cardiotoxicity, including an increase in reactive oxidant species (ROS) and subsequent apoptosis, its clinical relevance is controversial. In this model, as is noted in humans, the LV function remains either unchanged or very slightly decreased, a change that can be mostly detected using sensitive parameters of LV systolic function, such as strain rate [5]. In the chronic

Anticancer Treatments and Cardiotoxicity. DOI: http://dx.doi.org/10.1016/B978-0-12-802509-3.00006-6

model, the left ventricular ejection fraction (LVEF) decrease is noted starting 6–8 weeks after the completion of the doxorubicin injections and is accompanied by high mortality. Other animal models include normotensive and hypertensive rats (the latter, as in humans, appear to be more sensitive to the effects of doxorubicin than normotensive) [6]. In addition to rodents, large animals (pigs [6,7], nonhuman primates [8,9]) have been used to study anthracycline cardiotoxicity because of a greater similarity in cardiac anatomy and physiology with humans. These models have largely been discontinued for mechanistic studies, because of their cost, but remain important in drug development.

As mentioned above, consensus exists that the production of ROS plays a crucial role in the development of cardiotoxicity [10,11]. Experimental models (including cell-free in vitro chemical models) can study the chemical reactions involved in the production of ROS by anthracyclines, a process catalyzed by the presence of iron. Further studies, in isolated mitochondria, in cells, or in intact animals allow to detect this surge in ROS and to investigate the location of their production, in particular in the cell membrane and in mitochondria [11]. The increase in intracellular calcium produced by anthracyclines and its further toxic effect on mitochondria can be documented, underlining other processes that can be targeted in cardioprotection. In cells and animals, the effect of anthracyclines can be traced on proapoptotic processes and on the degradation of intracellular proteins [10,11]. Finally, anthracyclines have been shown to interact with multiple genes. Topoisomerase 2β is a target of doxorubicin, and the Top2–doxorubicin–DNA ternary cleavage complex can induce DNA double-strand breaks, leading to cell death [12]. Using mice deficient in topoisomerase 2β, Zhang et al. demonstrated that this deficiency protected against doxorubicin-induced cardiotoxicity [13].

Recently, studies have developed models of trastuzumab-associated cardiomyopathy in mice [14,15]. Using a genome-wide gene expression microarray analysis in mice treated with trastuzumab or placebo, ElZarrad et al. [15] demonstrated that trastuzumab treatment altered the expression of genes involved in adaptability to cardiac contractility, hemodynamic stress, DNA repair mechanisms, apoptosis, and mitochondrial function, and resulted in an increase in oxidative stress and apoptosis.

Experimental models have also been used to clarify the mechanisms involved in radiation-induced toxicity. Common doses used in preclinical models of localized heart irradiation are either a single dose between 5 and 25 Gy, or fractionated schedules (e.g., five daily fractions of 9 Gy). Although these models are imperfect reflections of clinical scenarios, they have revealed that microvascular disease and endothelial dysfunction play a crucial role in radiation-induced cardiotoxicity [16].

In summary, preclinical models of cancer treatments, although not always perfectly reproducible and relevant in humans, are a significant help in elucidating the mechanisms by which cancer treatments affect the cardiovascular system.

REFERENCES

[1] Barnabé N, Zastre JA, Venkataram S, Hasinoff BB. Deferiprone protects against doxorubicin-induced myocyte cytotoxicity. Free Radic Biol Med 2002;33:266–75.

[2] Sawyer DB, Fukazawa R, Arstall MA, Kelly RA. Daunorubicin-induced apoptosis in rat cardiac myocytes is inhibited by dexrazoxane. Circ Res 1999;84:257–65.

[3] Yang XP, Liu YH, Rhaleb NE, Kurihara N, Kim HE, Carretero OA. Echocardiographic assessment of cardiac function in conscious and anesthetized mice. Am J Physiol 1999;277:H1967–74.

[4] Slate DL, Fraser-Smith EB, Rosete JD, Freitas VR, Kim YN, Casey SM. Modulation of doxorubicin efficacy in P388 leukemia following co-administration of verapamil in mini-osmotic pumps. In Vivo 1993;7:519–23.

[5] Neilan TG. Tissue Doppler imaging predicts left ventricular dysfunction and mortality in a murine model of cardiac injury. Eur Heart J 2006;27:1868–75.

[6] Herman EH, el-Hage AN, Ferrans VJ, Ardalan B. Comparison of the severity of the chronic cardiotoxicity produced by doxorubicin in normotensive and hypertensive rats. Toxicol Appl Pharmacol 1985;78:202–14.

[7] Van Vleet JF, Greenwood LA, Ferrans VJ. Pathologic features of adriamycin toxicosis in young pigs: nonskeletal lesions. Am J Vet Res 1979;40:1537–52.

[8] Gralla EJ, Fleischman RW, Luthra YK, Stadnicki SW. The dosing schedule dependent toxicities of adriamycin in beagle dogs and rhesus monkeys. Toxicology 1979;13:263–73.

[9] Sieber SM, Correa P, Young DM, Dalgard DW, Adamson RH. Cardiotoxic and possible leukemogenic effects of adriamycin in nonhuman primates. Pharmacology 1980;20:9–14.

[10] Khouri MG, Douglas PS, Mackey JR, Martin M, Scott JM, Scherrer-Crosbie M, et al. Cancer therapy-induced cardiac toxicity in early breast cancer: addressing the unresolved issues. Circulation 2012;126:2749–63.

[11] Štěrba M, Popelová O, Vávrová A, Jirkovský E, Kovaříková P, Geršl V, et al. Oxidative stress, redox signaling, and metal chelation in anthracycline cardiotoxicity and pharmacological cardioprotection. Antioxid Redox Signal 2013;18:899–929.

[12] Lyu YL, Kerrigan JE, Lin C-P, Azarova AM, Tsai Y-C, Ban Y, et al. Topoisomerase IIbeta mediated DNA double-strand breaks: implications in doxorubicin cardiotoxicity and prevention by dexrazoxane. Cancer Res 2007;67:8839–46.

[13] Zhang S, Liu X, Bawa-Khalfe T, Lu L-S, Lyu YL, Liu LF, et al. Identification of the molecular basis of doxorubicin-induced cardiotoxicity. Nat Med 2012;18:1639–42.

[14] Milano G, Raucci A, Scopece A, Daniele R, Guerrini U, Sironi L, et al. Doxorubicin and trastuzumab regimen induces biventricular failure in mice. J Am Soc Echocardiogr 2014;27:568–79.

[15] ElZarrad MK, Mukhopadhyay P, Mohan N, Hao E, Dokmanovic M, Hirsch DS, et al. Trastuzumab alters the expression of genes essential for cardiac function and induces ultrastructural changes of cardiomyocytes in mice. PLoS One 2013;8:e79543.

[16] Boerma M, Hauer-Jensen M. Preclinical research into basic mechanisms of radiation-induced heart disease. Cardiol Res Pract 2011; Article ID 858262, 8 pages doi:10.4061/2011/858262.

Chapter 7

Genetic and Epigenetic Risk Factors

M. Scherrer-Crosbie

Chapter Outline

ANTHRACYCLINES

The strongest risk factor for the development of anthracycline-associated cardiomyopathy is the cumulative dose of anthracyclines [1–4], with an increase in the rate of symptomatic heart failure occurrence during a median of 2–3 years of follow-up exponentially related to the total dose (<5% of patients with a cumulative anthracycline exposure of <300 mg/m^2; approximately 15% at doses between 300 and 500 mg/m^2; >30% for doses >600 mg/m^2 [1,5–8]). In terms of LV dysfunction, the reported prevalence rates are markedly higher [9]. There is no known lower threshold of anthracyclines below which there is no cardiotoxic risk.

The rate of administration and formulation of the anthracycline treatment also influence the risk of cardiotoxicity; slower rates of infusion and possibly liposomal formulations are associated with lower rates of cardiotoxicity. The addition of other cancer therapies including chest radiotherapy [10] and additional chemotherapies such as trastuzumab increase the risk of cardiotoxicity.

In terms of patient characteristics, age at the time of therapy also influences the risk of cardiotoxicity. The highest risk exists in both the very young and old patients [1,2,4]. Women are typically at higher risk compared with men [2]. Traditional cardiovascular risk factors such as hypertension, smoking, diabetes, obesity, and renal dysfunction have also been implicated, as well as preexisting cardiovascular diseases, such as coronary artery disease and valvular disease [1,11,12]. The presence of a lower left ventricular ejection fraction (LVEF) prior to treatment [13,14], reflecting possible cardiac susceptibility to injury, is also a strong predictor of cardiotoxicity. Recently, low myocardial

Anticancer Treatments and Cardiotoxicity. DOI: http://dx.doi.org/10.1016/B978-0-12-802509-3.00007-8

strain before or after anthracyclines, and increased troponin plasma levels, have also been reported to be risk factors of subsequent cardiotoxicity [15–17].

The mechanisms involved in the innate sensitivity of subjects to anthracycline-induced cardiotoxicity are the topic of active research. Genetic mutations that may predispose to anthracycline-induced cardiotoxicity include mutations in nucleosides and ATP transporters in children [18] and in NADPH oxidase in adults [19]. The nucleosides include chemotherapeutic drugs, suggesting abnormalities in the transport of chemotherapies, and NADPH oxidase is a well-recognized enzyme involved in oxidative stress.

TRASTUZUMAB

Although trastuzumab-induced cardiotoxicity has generated extensive interest, it is difficult to tease out the impact of trastuzumab by itself as anthracyclines are commonly associated. Three small or medium-sized studies, however, implicate the polymorphism of the *HER2* gene (Ile655Val), i.e., a change of the isoleucine at codon 655 to valine, present in about 50% of patients with breast cancer, as an increased risk factor for trastuzumab-induced cardiotoxicity [20–22].

RADIOTHERAPY

As opposed to chemotherapy, radiotherapy is a local insult, therefore, exposure of the heart is necessary for cardiotoxicity. This exposure is found mainly in patients with lymphoma, however, patients with breast cancer and lower esophageal cancers can also be affected. Patients with left breast cancer are at risk of irradiation of both the left anterior descending and the right coronary artery and patients with right breast cancer or lower esophageal cancer can have right coronary irradiation [23,24]. The dose of radiotherapy is a strong risk factor of acute and chronic cardiac toxicity [25,26]. Both a high cumulative dose (>30 Gy) or fractionated dose (>2 Gy/day) are risk factors [25,26] but no lower dose exists below which there is no risk. Radiation exposure appears to have a synergistic cardiotoxic effect with anthracyclines [27]. Younger age (<35 years) at the time of irradiation, and cardiovascular risk factors may also increase the risk of radiation-induced cardiotoxicity [28,29]. Finally, a recent study in 442 women with breast cancer (87% who received radiotherapy) reported involvement of a polymorphism in the transforming growth factor β1 (TGFβ1) gene (namely TGFβ1 C29T) in the development of late cardiovascular disease ($P = 0.06$) [30]. TGFβ1 is involved in the development of fibrosis. As fibrosis plays an important role in radiation-induced cardiovascular disease, the investigators speculated that TGFβ1 C29T may be involved in the development of radiation-involved cardiotoxicity. It has to be noted, however, that a nonspecific cardiotoxic effect of the polymorphism in all women could not be excluded.

REFERENCES

[1] Hoff Von DD, Layard MW, Basa P, Davis HL, Hoff Von AL, Rozencweig M, et al. Risk factors for doxorubicin-induced congestive heart failure. Ann Intern Med 1979;91:710–17.

[2] Lipshultz SE, Colan SD, Gelber RD, Perez-Atayde AR, Sallan SE, Sanders SP. Late cardiac effects of doxorubicin therapy for acute lymphoblastic leukemia in childhood. N Engl J Med 1991;324:808–15.

[3] Steinherz LJ, Steinherz PG, Tan CT, Heller G, Murphy ML. Cardiac toxicity 4 to 20 years after completing anthracycline therapy. JAMA 1991;266:1672–7.

[4] Swain SM, Whaley FS, Ewer MS. Congestive heart failure in patients treated with doxorubicin: a retrospective analysis of three trials. Cancer 2003;97:2869–79.

[5] Giantris A, Abdurrahman L, Hinkle A, Asselin B, Lipshultz SE. Anthracycline-induced cardiotoxicity in children and young adults. Crit Rev Oncol Hematol 1998;27:53–68.

[6] Lipshultz SE, Lipsitz SR, Sallan SE, Dalton VM, Mone SM, Gelber RD, et al. Chronic progressive cardiac dysfunction years after doxorubicin therapy for childhood acute lymphoblastic leukemia. J Clin Oncol 2005;23:2629–36.

[7] Yahalom J, Portlock CS. Long-term cardiac and pulmonary complications of cancer therapy. Heart Fail Clin 2011;7:403–11.

[8] van Dalen EC, van der Pal HJH, Kok WEM, Caron HN, Kremer LCM. Clinical heart failure in a cohort of children treated with anthracyclines: a long-term follow-up study. Eur J Cancer 2006;42:3191–8.

[9] Hudson MM, Ness KK, Gurney JG, Mulrooney DA, Chemaitilly W, Krull KR, et al. Clinical ascertainment of health outcomes among adults treated for childhood cancer. JAMA 2013;309:2371–81.

[10] Tukenova M, Guibout C, Oberlin O, Doyon F, Mousannif A, Haddy N, et al. Role of cancer treatment in long-term overall and cardiovascular mortality after childhood cancer. J Clin Oncol 2010;28:1308–15.

[11] Tan-Chiu E, Yothers G, Romond E, Geyer CE, Ewer M, Keefe D, et al. Assessment of cardiac dysfunction in a randomized trial comparing doxorubicin and cyclophosphamide followed by paclitaxel, with or without trastuzumab as adjuvant therapy in node-positive, human epidermal growth factor receptor 2-overexpressing breast cancer: NSABP B-31. J Clin Oncol 2005;23:7811–19.

[12] Raj S, Franco VI, Lipshultz SE. Anthracycline-induced cardiotoxicity: a review of pathophysiology, diagnosis, and treatment. Curr Treat Options Cardiovasc Med 2014;16:315.

[13] Romond EH, Jeong J-H, Rastogi P, Swain SM, Geyer CE, Ewer MS, et al. Seven-year follow-up assessment of cardiac function in NSABP B-31, a randomized trial comparing doxorubicin and cyclophosphamide followed by paclitaxel (ACP) with ACP plus trastuzumab as adjuvant therapy for patients with node-positive, human epidermal growth factor receptor 2-positive breast cancer. J Clin Oncol 2012;30:3792–9.

[14] Wang L, Tan TC, Szymonifka J, Picard MH, Scherrer-Crosbie M. Value of left ventricular ejection fraction and its changes for the prediction of symptomatic heart failure in patients treated by anthracyclines. *Circulation* 2013; 128:A14921.

[15] Ky B, Putt M, Sawaya H, French B, Januzzi JL, Sebag IA, et al. Early increases in multiple biomarkers predict subsequent cardiotoxicity in breast cancer patients treated with doxorubicin, taxanes, and trastuzumab. J Am Coll Cardiol 2013;63:809–16.

[16] Sawaya H, Sebag IA, Plana JC, Januzzi JL, Ky B, Cohen V, et al. Early detection and prediction of cardiotoxicity in chemotherapy-treated patients. Am J Cardiol 2011;107:1375–80.

[17] Sawaya H, Sebag IA, Plana JC, Januzzi JL, Ky B, Tan TC, et al. Assessment of echocardiography and biomarkers for the extended prediction of cardiotoxicity in patients treated with anthracyclines, taxanes and trastuzumab. Circ Cardiovasc Imaging 2012;5:596–603.

[18] Visscher H, Ross CJD, Rassekh SR, Barhdadi A, Dube MP, Al-Saloos H, et al. Canadian pharmacogenomics network for drug safety consortium. pharmacogenomic prediction of anthracycline-induced cardiotoxicity in children. J Clin Oncol 2012;30:1422–8.

[19] Wojnowski L, Kulle B, Schirmer M, Schlüter G, Schmidt A, Rosenberger A, et al. NAD(P)H oxidase and multidrug resistance protein genetic polymorphisms are associated with doxorubicin-induced cardiotoxicity. Circulation 2005;112:3754–62.

[20] Roca L, Diéras V, Roché H, Lappartient E, Kerbrat P, Cany L, et al. Correlation of HER2, FCGR2A, and FCGR3A gene polymorphisms with trastuzumab related cardiac toxicity and efficacy in a subgroup of patients from UNICANCER-PACS 04 trial. Breast Cancer Res Treat 2013;139:789–800.

[21] Lemieux J, Diorio C, Côté M-A, Provencher L, Barabé F, Jacob S, et al. Alcohol and HER2 polymorphisms as risk factor for cardiotoxicity in breast cancer treated with trastuzumab. Anticancer Res 2013;33:2569–76.

[22] Beauclair S, Formento P, Fischel JL, Lescaut W, Largillier R, Chamorey E, et al. Role of the HER2 [Ile655Val] genetic polymorphism in tumorogenesis and in the risk of trastuzumab-related cardiotoxicity. Ann Oncol 2007;18:1335–41.

[23] Gayed IW, Liu HH, Yusuf SW, Komaki R, Wei X, Wang X, et al. The prevalence of myocardial ischemia after concurrent chemoradiation therapy as detected by gated myocardial perfusion imaging in patients with esophageal cancer. J Nucl Med 2006;47:1756–62.

[24] Nilsson G, Holmberg L, Garmo H, Duvernoy O, Sjögren I, Lagerqvist B, et al. Distribution of coronary artery stenosis after radiation for breast cancer. J Clin Oncol 2012;30:380–6.

[25] Darby SC, Ewertz M, McGale P, Bennet AM, Blom-Goldman U, Brønnum D, et al. Risk of ischemic heart disease in women after radiotherapy for breast cancer. N Engl J Med 2013;368:987–98.

[26] Hancock SL, Tucker MA, Hoppe RT. Factors affecting late mortality from heart disease after treatment of Hodgkin's disease. JAMA 1993;270:1949–55.

[27] Meyer RM, Gospodarowicz MK, Connors JM, Pearcey RG, Wells WA, Winter JN, et al. ABVD alone versus radiation-based therapy in limited-stage Hodgkin's lymphoma. N Engl J Med 2012;366:399–408.

[28] Heidenreich PA, Kapoor JR. Radiation induced heart disease: systemic disorders in heart disease. Heart 2009;95:252–8.

[29] Hooning MJ, Botma A, Aleman BMP, Baaijens MHA, Bartelink H, Klijn JGM, et al. Long-term risk of cardiovascular disease in 10-year survivors of breast cancer. J Natl Cancer Inst 2007;99:365–75.

[30] Hilbers FSM, Boekel NB, van den Broek AJ, van Hien R, Cornelissen S, Aleman BMP, et al. Genetic variants in TGFβ-1 and PAI-1 as possible risk factors for cardiovascular disease after radiotherapy for breast cancer. Radiother Oncol 2012;102:115–21.

Chapter 8

Changes of Myocardial Structure and Function

N. Maurea, C. Coppola and A. Rienzo

Chapter Outline

INTRODUCTION

In later years the survival rate of oncology patients has increased thanks to early diagnosis, development of new drugs, and aggressive therapies. These factors expose patients to severe complications, such as cardiovascular diseases, which seem to be the most relevant [1,2].

Cancer and cardiovascular diseases share a lot of risk factors (tabagism, obesity, diabetes, etc.) [3,4].

Patients exposed to treatment complications are still rising; in the United States, cancer survivors were estimated to be 14 million on January 2014 and they are likely to become 18 million by 2022 [5]. Sixty-seven percent of adults with cancer go beyond 5 years and 75% of children even more than 10 years [6].

Even if the oncological drugs and the target therapy have revolutionized the approach to the oncological patient, with good results in terms of healing and survival, the most common unfavorable effects are ventricular

Anticancer Treatments and Cardiotoxicity. DOI: http://dx.doi.org/10.1016/B978-0-12-802509-3.00008-X

dysfunction and heart failure (HF), which specialists must deal with daily. Targeted therapy can cause cardiac failure, systolic ventricular dysfunction, hypertension, thrombosis, and arrhythmia in a higher percentage than anthracyclines, another class of cancer drug. In addition, mediastinal radiotherapy could lead to alterations of myocardial function, with consequent development of acute myocarditis and restrictive cardiomyopathy. Cardiotoxicity represents one of the main limits of antineoplastic treatments, and has a strong effect on survival and patient quality of life.

To reduce the risk of cardiac diseases, cardiologists should be aware of the potential cardiotoxic effects of antitumor drugs. Finally, it is essential to follow cancer survivors over the years, as the damage induced by chemotherapy and radiotherapy can arise even many years after the end of treatments.

ANTHRACYCLINES

Anthracyclines can be defined as the oldest anticancer drugs. Doxorubicin and epirubicin are the most commonly used anthracyclines. They are able to induce acute, early, or late cardiotoxicity. According to the Ewer classification, anthracycline cardiotoxicity is defined as type I cardiotoxicity; it has been defined as permanent and characterized by histological alterations such as myofibrillar disorganization, myocyte apoptosis, and necrosis [7] (Fig. 8.1).

According to the same classification, type II cardiotoxicity, considered as reversible cardiotoxicity, has been mainly related to monoclonal antibodies [8]. The cardiotoxicity of antibodies has been associated with trastuzumab, a humanized anti-ErbB2 monoclonal antibody currently in clinical use for the therapy of breast carcinomas, which induces cardiac dysfunction when used in monotherapy, or in combination with anthracyclines [9,10]. Furthermore, recent retrospective studies have shown an increased incidence of HF and/or cardiomyopathy in patients treated with trastuzumab, which can persist many years after the conclusion of the therapy, thus suggesting that the side toxic effects are not always reversible as was initially proposed [7]. On the other hand, early detection and prompt therapy of anthracycline-associated cardiotoxicity can lead to substantial recovery of cardiac function. Furthermore, several in vitro and in vivo studies in human cardiac cell cultures and in mice, respectively, clearly indicate that trastuzumab induces apoptosis of cardiomyocytes, thus leading to irreversible cell death [11,12]. On the other hand, some data suggest that cardiotoxicity in patients treated with anthracyclines is not necessarily irreversible but it may become reversible if diagnosed early [13]. Furthermore, the reversibility of left ventricular (LV) dysfunction (both symptomatic and asymptomatic), in patients undergoing treatment with anthracyclines, depends critically on the timing of the initiation of cardioprotection therapy with β-blockers and angiotensin-converting

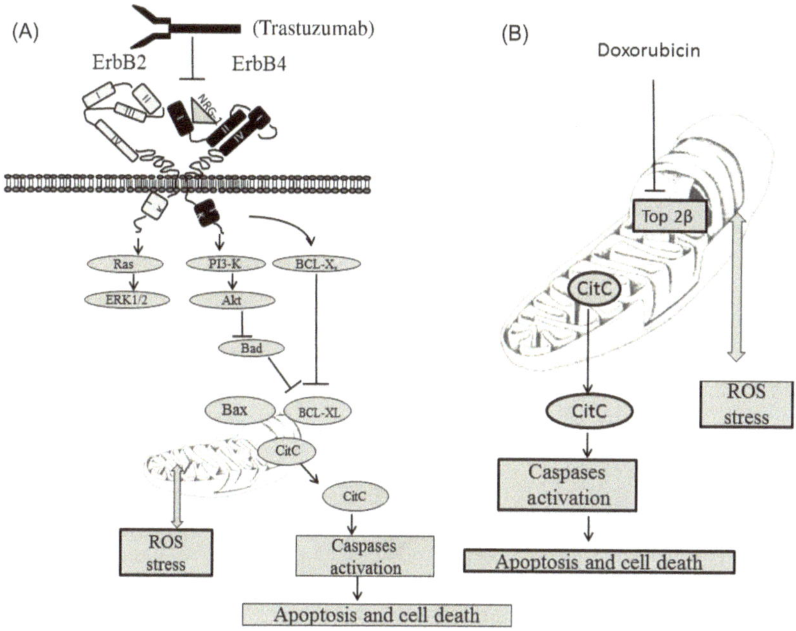

FIGURE 8.1 (A) Doxorubicin treatment triggers adverse effects similarly to trastuzumab treatment. (B) Oxidative stress and cytochrome C releases cause adverse effects in cardiomyocytes following doxorubicin treatment. *Modified from Riccio G, et al. Trastuzumab and target-therapy side effects: is still valid to differentiate anthracycline type I from type II cardiomyopathies? Hum Vaccin Immunother 2016;12(5):1124–31.*

enzyme inhibitors [14]. On the basis of these observations, we have proposed to find a new different classification for cardiotoxic side effects of drugs used in cancer therapy [15]. Accordingly, type I and type II classification, based on reversible or nonreversible cardiotoxicity, has become inappropriate as the reversibility concept is ambiguous. It has been demonstrated that ErbB2 inhibitors can be toxic for cardiomyocytes when used in monotherapy in a fashion similar to doxorubicin [16]. In particular, trastuzumab induces and promotes activation of the apoptotic pathway, thus triggering cell death [11,12,17]. These effects may lead to cardiomyopathy or HF in treated patients as described above, especially in elder patients [18–20].

We can distinguish multiple anthracycline-induced cardiomyopathy hypotheses; one refers to the generation of excess reactive oxygen species (ROS) by electron exchange between the anthracycline quinone moiety and oxygen molecules and other cellular electron donors [21,22] (Fig. 8.2).

In addition, anthracyclines form complexes with iron that undergo redox cycling and generate oxygen radicals [23].

The most recent hypothesis involves topoisomerase2ß (Top2ß), which normally unwinds deoxyribonucleic acid (DNA) strands, in all quiescent

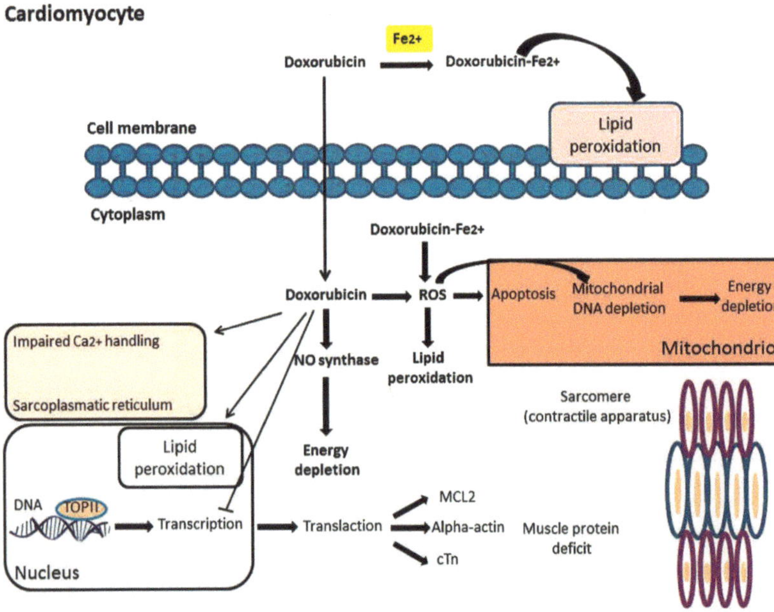

FIGURE 8.2 Effects of doxorubicin chemotherapy on cardiomyocytes.

cells, including cardiomyocytes [2,24–28] (Fig. 8.2). Top2 inhibition by anthracycline causes double-stranded breaks in DNA, which can lead to cardiomyocyte death [24]. The activation of p53 and the apoptotic pathway are implicated in doxorubicin-induced cardiotoxicity, involving Top2ß, as well as in anthracycline-induced ROS production, due to a reduction in antioxidant enzyme gene transcription [24,29].

Recent studies have shown that doxorubicin, throughout the production of ROS, can produce the hyperactivation of calcium-calmoduline (CaMKII). Hyperactivated CaMKII can determine diastolic overload of secondary cytosolic calcium with hyperaction of the late sodium current in cardiomyocytes. The overload of calcium, sodium-dependent, is able to determine, in cardiomyocytes, marked alterations, either mechanical or energetic.

Recently, in in vitro and in vivo studies, we have demonstrated that ranolazine, the most powerful inhibitor of late sodium current, protects from doxorubicin-induced oxidative stress and cardiac dysfunction, when administered before treatment [30]. In addition, we have demonstrated that ranolazine also protects when administered after the end of treatment [31].

CLINICAL ASPECTS

Acute cardiotoxicity due to anthracyclines is a rare event. It occurs in 1% of patients during, or a few hours after, anthracycline infusion, or within the first week of therapy [32]. Tachycardia, hypotension, electrocardiographic abnormalities, and arrhythmia are usually reversible in a few days. Rarely, anthracyclines may induce acute HF or acute pericarditis-myocarditis syndrome.

Early anthracycline-induced cardiotoxicity, characterized by asymptomatic LV dysfunction or acute HF, can occur during the first year after administration of the drug. The peak time is 3 months after the last infusion.

Late anthracycline-induced cardiotoxicity can occur from 1 year after the last administration and may not be apparent for years, or even decades, after the use of the drug. Also in this case, asymptomatic LV dysfunction and HF are the most common toxic events. The reported incidence of doxorubicin-induced HF varies from 4%, at a cumulative dose of 500–550 mg/m^2, to >36% in patients receiving 600 mg/m^2 of doxorubicin, but nowadays medical oncologists choose lower cumulative dose schedules. As a matter of fact, the overall current incidence rate of anthracycline-induced clinical HF is 1.6%, when doxorubicin is administered at a dose of 240–360 mg/m^2 in adjuvant chemotherapy. Adjuvant treatment means chemotherapy offered after a surgical procedure in order to improve the outcome of patients at high risk of relapse. However, even when a very low dose, such as 180 mg/m^2, of doxorubicin is administered, subclinical cardiac abnormalities are present in some patients, concomitantly with the microscopic evidence of myocardial tissue damage. Truthfully, in a retrospective study, among childhood cancer survivors, the cumulative incidence of cardiac disorders due to anthracyclines at 10, 20, and 30 years after diagnosis, was much higher in the case of a dosage >250 mg/m^2 [33].

To this end, several strategies have been employed to reduce the incidence of anthracycline-associated cardiovascular complications. These include: schedule modification of anthracycline administration (lower doses), screening for patient-related and treatment-related cardiac risk factors, careful monitoring for cardiac abnormalities, and adoption of an alternative strategy such as liposomal formulation. Anyway, the best predictor of cardiotoxicity is the total cumulative dose of anthracycline [34]. Before starting anthracyclines, it is necessary for a careful evaluation of medical history, baseline ejection fraction (EF), and correction of risk factors, while, during therapy, the monitoring should be closer with increasing dose [35].

TARGET THERAPY

The term target therapy refers to drugs that selectively target specific molecular pathways involved in tumorigenesis or tumor progression. Unfortunately, these pathways are not only involved in oncogenesis, but also in myocardial homeostasis. This cardiotoxicity is potentially life-threatening and necessitates limiting or discontinuing an otherwise-effective cancer treatment. Clinical management for target therapy-induced cardiotoxicity is needed [10]. It must be addressed to two new broad molecular target anticancer families: ErbB2 inhibitors and antiangiogenic inhibitors.

ERBB2 INHIBITORS

Trastuzumab is a monoclonal antibody that selectively binds to the human epidermal growth factor receptor 2 (HER2) protein, preventing epidermal growth factor (EGF) from binding and thus inhibiting the effects of HER2 overexpression. When trastuzumab binds to HER2 protein of cancerous cells, the HER2 protein no longer causes cells in the breast to reproduce uncontrollably. This improves the prognosis for women with this type of cancer.

Trastuzumab is overexpressed in 25% of women with breast cancer and it is used in one-quarter of cancer patients. Until 2005, it has been shown that the single or combined use of trastuzumab with chemotherapy reduced the risk of relapse by 50% and the risk of death by 33% in cancer patients [36]. Cardiotoxicity is related to the block of ErbB2 in cardiomyocytes and occurs with HF or asymptomatic LV dysfunction. It has been demonstrated that, also for this type of toxicity, the metabolism and overload of calcium seem to be involved, as is shown in Fig. 8.3 [37].

Recently, we have demonstrated that ranolazine is able to protect from trastuzumab toxicity, either if administered before the treatment or at the end of it [38,39].

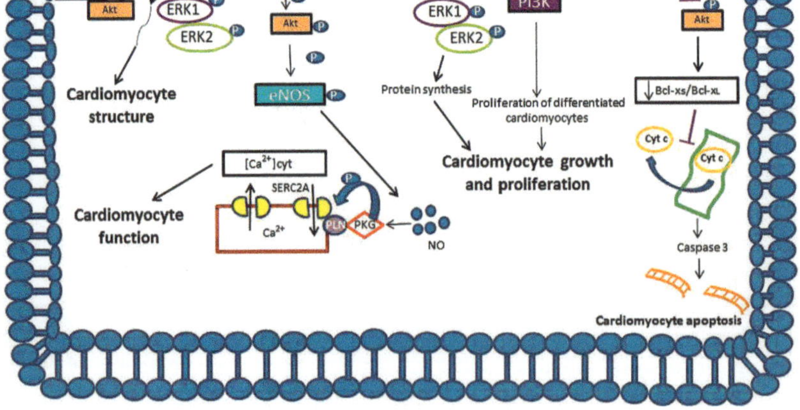

FIGURE 8.3 Metabolism and overload of calcium involved in cardiotoxicity, related to the block of ErbB2 in cardiomyocytes.

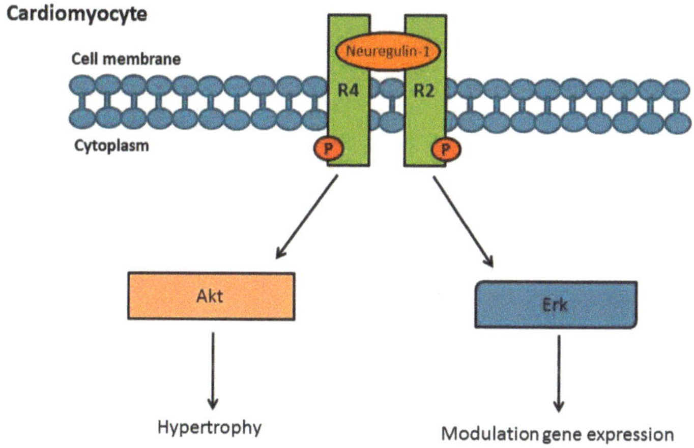

FIGURE 8.4 Molecular mechanism of ErbB2 and ErbB4 heterodimerization in cardiomyocytes. Neuregulin-1 activates ErbB by promoting its dimerization.

Clinical studies performed on lapatinib, a dual tyrosine kinase inhibitor of epidermal growth factor receptor (EGFR) and HER2, showed that the cardiac safety of anti-Erb-B2 is agent-specific, because lapatinib is less cardiotoxic than trastuzumab. It has also been demonstrated that therapy with pertuzumab leads to a reduction of EF in a percentage similar to those observed with trastuzumab therapy, according to the data obtained from experiments performed on mice [9,40,41]. The mechanisms by which trastuzumab causes cardiotoxicity are not completely clear, although it is known that they are different from those induced by anthracyclines. In Fig. 8.4 [42], we have summarized the mechanism of the heterodimerization of Erb-B2 and Erb-B4 in cardiomyocytes.

This mechanism is activated under stress conditions, thus providing an important method of survival. If this pathway is blocked, the stress induced by anthracyclines rapidly proceeds. There is a phase in which the myocytes are damaged due to the oxidative stress induced by anthracyclines. In this condition, the myocytes undergo apoptosis and necrosis processes. Therefore, the upregulation of the Erb-B2 receptor promotes cellular repair, and prevents apoptosis and necrosis. The blocking of the receptor, induced by trastuzumab, prevents the triggering pathway of protection and allows the cell damage to go on. Alteration of troponin dosage can be explained by the mechanism of cardiotoxicity induced by anthracyclines and trastuzumab [43,44].

Other studies have demonstrated that increased levels of troponin were present in some cancer patients receiving trastuzumab after treatment with anthracyclines [36].

Specifically, in these studies alterations in levels of troponin represented a measure of the damage induced by anthracyclines, mediated by trastuzumab, which blocks the cellular repair mechanisms. In particular, the same authors noticed that in patients treated only with trastuzumab, they never observed an alteration of troponin levels [36]. It is important to underline that classical echocardiographic parameters, used to evaluate cardiac function (such as EF), are not able to identify early the cardiac damage, leading to its underestimation. The EF is not a sensitive parameter to detect early cardiotoxicity, because myocardium contraction can be lost before EF reduction. The study of Fallah-Rad et al. describes well the utility of cardiac biomarkers, tissue Doppler imaging, strain imaging, and cardiovascular magnetic resonance (CMR) imaging in prediction of early LV dysfunction in patients with HER2-positive breast cancer treated with adjuvant trastuzumab therapy [45]. In this paper, the authors did not detect any plasma biomarker alternations, such as natriuretic peptide (BNP), troponin T (TnT), and C-reactive protein. Experiments performed on a mouse model of cardiotoxicity, allowed us to support the role of the strain, obtained by speckle tracking method, in the early detection of cardiotoxicity [45]. When the evaluation of cardiac damage, in cancer patients treated with target therapy, is performed, the timing of trastuzumab treatment with respect to doxorubicin administration is fundamental. In fact, during treatments in trial adjuvants, a higher rate of HF was found in cancer patients treated with trastuzumab in combination with anthracyclines (no longer used) or immediately after anthracycline administration. However, the incidence of HF observed in these trials was <4%, while a higher incidence of asymptomatic LV systolic dysfunction was also found in almost 18% of cases. We have to note that in HERA trials, in which trastuzumab was administered after 90 days from the anthracycline treatment, the incidence of HF was <2%.

These data all together suggest that if the EF of cancer patients is slightly reduced after treatment with anthracyclines, the oncologists have to wait for a few weeks or months, before starting with trastuzumab therapy.

It should be emphasized that the cardiotoxicity induced by trastuzumab is higher in real-world women with breast cancer, as reported in databases of cardiotoxicity: from 26% to 30% in patients with more cardiovascular risk factors [16]. In other studies, it was demonstrated that HF occurred in 2% of patients who did not take either angiotensin-converting enzyme inhibitors/angiotensin receptor blockers (ACEi/ARBs) or β-blockers, 8% of patients receiving ACEi/ARBs alone, 8% receiving β-blockers alone, and 19% receiving both medications [46,47]. These findings can be explained by assuming that these drugs, taken by cancer patients, are an indirect indicator of cardiovascular diseases, since it identifies patients who presented with a risk of cardiovascular disease before treatment with trastuzumab [18,46,47].

Pertuzumab. Pertuzumab is a humanized monoclonal antibody that binds and inhibits a different HER2 epitope than trastuzumab, thereby preventing the interaction of HER2 with other HER family members. In 2012, Baselga et al., in a study on patients with HER2-positive metastatic breast cancer (MBC), demonstrated that the addition of pertuzumab did not appear to

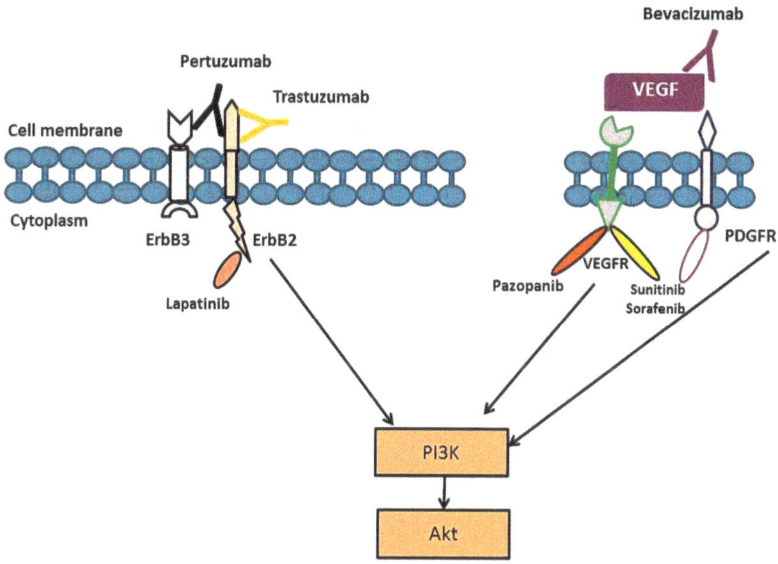

FIGURE 8.5 Mechanism of action of current target therapy, in HER2-positive cancer cells, and of antiangiogenic drugs.

affect the cardiac toxicity of the backbone regimen of trastuzumab plus docetaxel [48]. In addition, in 2015, Danese et al., run a simulation model over the previous 15 years, by using first-line trastuzumab in HER2-positive women with MBC, to estimate the life-years saved from using trastuzumab plus chemotherapy [49]. The same simulation was made over the future 15 years, to estimate the life-years that might be saved by adding pertuzumab, instead. The result of this study is very promising, suggesting a notable progress in the treatment of HER2-positive women [49,50].

Lapatinib. The tyrosine kinase inhibitor, lapatinib, targets both EGFR or ErbB1 and HER2 (Fig. 8.5). It is used in the treatment of HER2-positive MBC.

In the 2008, Perez et al. presented a large study of 3689 patients on lapatinib cardiac toxicity [51]. The review showed a 1.6% incidence of cardiac events and only 0.2% of the patients who experienced a cardiac event developed symptomatic congestive heart failure (CHF) [51].

For its reversible nature, lapatinib-induced cardiotoxicity is classified as type II cardiotoxicity; the cellular mechanism activated by this tyrosine kinase inhibitor may lead to the inability of myofibril contractile elements to coordinate their activity. Accordingly, the reduced incidence of cardiac events associated with lapatinib compared with trastuzumab may be due to an increase of ATP production with the consequent preservation of cardiomyocytes against apoptosis [52]. Moreover, in a recent study by Lorenzen et al., lapatinib showed insufficient activity in HER2-amplified pretreated advanced gastroesophageal GC [53].

MONOCLONAL ANTIBODIES

Alemtuzumab. Alemtuzumab is an anti-CD52 monoclonal antibody used in the treatment of various hematologic malignancies. Cardiac events and LV dysfunction are more common in patients who have received prior cardiotoxic anticancer agents [53] and acute coronary syndrome [54].

PROTEASOME INHIBITORS

Bortezomib. Bortezomib is a proteasome inhibitor. In a phase III study conducted on 669 multiple myeloma patients, only 2% of patients in each group developed CHF [55].

ANGIOGENESIS INHIBITORS

Antiangiogenic therapies are used in the treatment strategies of a variety of tumor types. Unfortunately, these therapies can cause significant systemic cardiovascular side effects. Angiogenesis plays a fundamental role in tumor progression [56]. Since VEGF is a crucial player in the maintenance of cardiovascular homeostasis, antiangiogenic drugs have been found to be associated with LV systolic dysfunction and HF (Fig. 8.5) [57].

Inactivation of endogenous VEGF led to a net reduction in capillary density, impaired cardiac hypertrophy, and loss of contractile function, after pressure overload in mice subjected to transverse aortic constriction [58].

The inhibition of the VEGF pathway blocks microvascular plasticity, contributing to maladaptive hypertrophy of cardiomyocytes [59]. To this end, Zentilin et al. showed that expression of VEGF, after myocardial infarction, improves contractility, prevents pathological remodeling, and preserves viable cardiac tissue [60]. Tumor angiogenesis is also regulated by another tyrosine kinase receptor (RTK), platelet-derived growth factor receptor (PDGFR), which plays a crucial role in the heart [61]. In the 2010, Chintalgattu et al. published a very interesting study showing how knockout of PDGFR-β in cardiomyocytes leads to cardiac dysfunction, HF, and stress-induced cardiac angiogenesis failure [62]. Indeed, the tyrosine kinase inhibitor, sunitinib, is the most powerful inhibitor of the PDGF pathway, and has the highest incidence of LV dysfunction and HF. Such a high incidence may also be explained by inhibition of off-target kinases.

These effects result in energy compromise and cardiomyocyte dysfunction [61]. To this end, Rainer et al. have shown direct contractile effects of sunitinib on different experimental myocardial preparations [63]. Sunitinib elicits a dose-dependent negative inotropic effect in myocardium, accompanied by a decline in intracellular Ca^{2+}. Moreover, myofilament Ca^{2+} sensitivity is not altered, while ROS generation increases.

The VEGF and PDGF pathways are inhibited not only by sunitinib, but also by sorafenib. This multitargeted kinase inhibitor also blocks RAF-1 and BRAF kinase activity, disrupting ERK signaling, important for myocyte survival during stress conditions [61]. Indeed, in a mouse model, cardiac deletion of RAF-1 brings dilation and reduces contractility, increasing myocyte apoptosis and fibrosis [64].

CLINICAL ASPECTS

Bevacizumab

Bevacizumab (Avastin) is a humanized neutralizing monoclonal antibody that blocks the binding of human VEGF to its receptors. It is used in a variety of tumor treatments, such as metastatic carcinoma of colon, rectum, lung, breast and kidney. It has been reported that bevacizumab induces HF only in 1, 6% of the cases. Global contractile dysfunction is due to decrease in myocardial capillary density, cardiac fibrosis. The pathogenesis of CHF is likely related to hypertension [65].

Sunitinib and Sorafenib

Sunitinib and sorafenib are small-molecule inhibitors of multiple intracellular and receptor protein kinases, involved in the signaling pathways that control tumor growth and angiogenesis. Sunitinib is used in the treatment of metastatic carcinoma of the kidney and in gastrointestinal stromal tumors (GISTs), while sorafenib is used in metastatic renal cell carcinoma and in the hepatocarcinoma. Evidence of sunitinib-associated HF, LV systolic dysfunction, and/or hypertension in imatinib-resistant GIST patients has been evidenced in a study conducted by Chu et al. [66]. Sunitinib-induced cardiotoxicity is mediated by cardiomyocyte mitochondrial damage and cytochrome-C-induced apoptosis [57]. One of the most risky consequences is CHF (8.0–12.5%). Particularly, a decrease in LV ejection fraction (LVEF) of 1.5–2.0% after each cycle of treatment has been observed [66–69]. Moreover, prior cardiac disease and preexisting hypertension must be considered as risk factors associated with LV dysfunction [66]. Another cardiovascular toxicity associated with the administration of sunitinib is hypertension, with an incidence of ~17–43%. In addition, in patients with metastatic renal cell cancer (mRCC), hypertension is considered a biomarker of efficacy. To this end, patients with mRCC and sunitinib-induced hypertension had better outcomes compared with those without treatment-induced hypertension [70]. Finally, sunitinib therapy could also compromise myocyte energy homeostasis and inhibit the compensatory upregulation of AMPK [71,72]. On the other hand, sorafenib has been shown to increase the susceptibility of cardiomyocytes to pathologic stress, but its treatment causes a lower incidence of HF [73].

OTHER TYROSINE KINASE INHIBITORS

Imatinib

Imatinib is a competitive tyrosine kinase inhibitor of the BCR–ABL enzyme approved by the Food and Drug Administration (FDA) for the treatment of chronic myeloid leukemia (CML), GISTs, and hypereosinophilic syndrome. The 2.0% of patients treated with imatinib may suffer from CHF [72,74]. In a study on heart biopsy samples from CHF patients, Kerkela et al. reported the presence of abnormal mitochondria, characteristics of toxin-induced myopathies as opposed to ischemic myopathy [74].

Dasatinib

Cardiac events associated with dasatinid treatment include CHF with LV dysfunction. Half of the patients who developed CHF or LV dysfunction had histories of cardiovascular disease.

Nilotinib

Nilotinib is an orally bioavailable inhibitor of the tyrosine kinase activity of ABL1 and BCR-ABL1 fusion protein. It has improved target specificity and potency compared with imatinib. Nilotinib is a BCR–ABL kinase inhibitor approved for Philadelphia chromosome-positive CML. In the heart, this drug inhibits the ion channel responsible for the delayed-rectifier K + . Nilotinib has been shown to cause QT prolongation in humans [75].

Pazopanib and Levantinib

Pazopanib is an orally active multitargeted kinase inhibitor that targets several kinases, including vascular endothelial growth factor receptors (VEGFR). It is used for the treatment of advanced renal cell carcinoma as well as soft tissue sarcoma. Levantinib is a multitargeted TKI that targets VEGFR, KIT, RET, PDGFRα, and fibroblast growth factor. It is used for treatment of refractory differentiated thyroid cancer. Reported complications are hypertension and cardiac dysfunction (decreased EF, cardiac failure, or pulmonary edema) in approximately 7% of cases.

RADIATION-INDUCED CARDIOMYOPATHY

Radiation-induced cardiomyopathy can be directly related to the exposition to radiation or can turn up consequent to coronary disease and/or postactinic valvulopathy.

Even if the relation between the dose and the type of cardiac damage is unknown, it seems that doses of about 35 Gy determine myocardial impairment [76]. Nevertheless, the real incidence of cardiomyopathy caused by radiotherapy (RT) is still unknown.

One of the side effects of irradiation is the onset of a restrictive cardiomyopathy, caused by fibrosis of the myocardium. Moreover, mediastinal RT appears to have a greater impact on diastolic rather than systolic cardiac function [77,78]. This is in contrast with the effects of anthracyclines, which predominantly cause systolic dysfunction.

The prevalence of dysfunction varies depending upon RT technique and dose, concomitant use of anthracyclines, length of follow-up, and method of screening.

In a study on HER2-positive breast cancer patients undergoing concurrent trastuzumab and adjuvant radiotherapy, Cao et al., reported the role of diastolic dysfunction [79]. Particularly, they found that changes in LVEF, compared with modifications in LV diastolic function (LVDF), are more sensitive for early detection of cardiotoxicity. In patients with left-sided breast cancer treated concurrently with trastuzumab, the dose-volume of the heart contributes significantly to the risk of LVDF. For high-dose irradiation alone there may be a restrictive cardiomyopathy, often coexisting with some degree of constrictive pericardial disease. The restrictive feature is due to reduced ventricular compliance induced by microvascular damage and subsequent ischemia with reparative fibrosis. On the other hand, the cardiac irradiation associated with anthracycline chemotherapy results in a dilated cardiomyopathy.

In patients with end-stage HF, orthotopic heart transplantation could be technically possible. Nevertheless, postsurgery complications, high perioperative mortality, and substantial risk of subsequent malignancy must be considered [80].

In patients under RT, subclinical abnormalities of diastolic function predict an increased risk of late cardiac events [77]. Even if there is a lack of conclusive evidence, it can be assessed that the use of β-blockers causes benefit in patients who have clinical HF with preserved systolic function [81]. This evidence can be relevant for patients with radiation-induced diastolic dysfunction. Up to now there is no evidence of benefit for the treatment of asymptomatic diastolic dysfunction. Moreover, it has been suggested that drugs which block the renin–angiotensin–aldosterone system may reduce mortality [82].

CONCLUSIONS

In the past few decades, novel anticancer drugs have been developed that effectively induce tumor regression, thus prolonging patient survival. However, cardiovascular side effects of these new drugs can lead to therapy-related

HF. New targeted drug therapies are continuously launched in the market, raising side effects that have to be further studied and distant prognosis after biologic therapy is misunderstood because longer follow-up trials are needed. Also, radiotherapy can provoke collateral cardiovascular effects during and after treatment. Sometimes, cardiotoxicity can occur even after several years. Only an effective collaboration between cardiologist and oncologist can contribute to minimize cardiotoxicity related to anthracyclines, target therapy, and RT.

REFERENCES

[1] Darby SC, Ewertz M, McGale P, et al. Risk of ischemic heart disease in women after radiotherapy for breast cancer. N Engl J Med 2013;368:987–98.

[2] Vejpongsa P, Yeh ET. Prevention of anthracycline-induced cardiotoxicity: challenges and opportunities. J Am Coll Cardiol 2014;64(9):938–45.

[3] Van Dam RM, Li T, Spiegelman D, et al. Combined impact of lifestyle factors on mortality: prospective cohort study in US women. BMJ 2008;337–440.

[4] McCullough ML, Patel AV, Kushi LH, et al. Following cancer prevention guidelines reduces risk of cancer, cardiovascular disease, and all-cause mortality. Cancer Epidemiol Biomarkers Prev 2011;20:1089–97.

[5] Mulrooney DA, Yeazel MW, Kawashima T, et al. Cardiac outcomes in a cohort of adult survivors of childhood and adolescent cancer: retrospective analysis of the Childhood Cancer Survivor Study cohort. BMJ 2009;339:b4606.

[6] De Santis CE, Lin CC, Mariotto AB, et al. Cancer treatment and survivorship statistics, 2014. CA Cancer J Clin 2014;64(4):252–71.

[7] Ewer SM, Ewer MS. Cardiotoxicity profile of trastuzumab. Drug Saf 2008;31:459–67.

[8] Suter Thomas M, Ewer Michael S. Cancer drugs and the heart: importance and management. Eur Heart J 2013;34:1102–11.

[9] Tocchetti CG, Ragone G, Coppola C, et al. Detection, monitoring, and management of trastuzumab-induced left ventricular dysfunction: an actual challenge. Eur J Heart Failure 2012;14:130.

[10] Maurea N, Coppola C, Ragone G, et al. Women survive breast cancer but fall victim to heart failure: the shadows and lights of targeted therapy. J Cardiovascular Med 2010; 11:861–8.

[11] ElZarrad MK, Mukhopadhyay P, Mohan N, et al. Trastuzumab alters the expression of genes essential for cardiac function and induces ultrastructural changes of cardiomyocytes in mice. PloS One 2013;8:e79543.

[12] Riccio G, Esposito G, Leoncini E, et al. Cardiotoxic effects, or lack thereof, of anti-ErbB2 immunoagents. Faseb J 2009;23:3171–8.

[13] Wells QS, Lenihan DJ. Reversibility of left ventricular dysfunction resulting from chemotherapy: can this be expected? Progress Cardiovascu Dis 2010;53:140–8.

[14] Cardinale D, Colombo A, Bacchiani G, et al. Early detection of anthracycline cardiotoxicity and improvement with heart failure therapy. Circulation 2015;131:1981–8.

[15] Riccio G, Coppola C, Piscopo G, et al. Trastuzumab and target-therapy side effects: is still valid to differentiate anthracycline Type I from Type II cardiomyopathies? Hum Vaccin Immunother 2016;12(5):1124–31.

[16] Fedele C, Riccio G, Coppola C, et al. Comparison of preclinical cardiotoxic effects of different ErbB2 inhibitors. Breast Cancer Res Treatment 2012;133:511–21.

[17] Jassal DS, Han SY, Hans C, et al. Utility of tissue Doppler and strain rate imaging in the early detection of trastuzumab and anthracycline mediated cardiomyopathy. J Am Society Echocardiogr 2009;22:418–24.

[18] Tarantini L, Gori S, Faggiano P, et al. Adjuvant trastuzumab cardiotoxicity in patients over 60 years of age with early breast cancer: a multicenter cohort analysis. Ann Oncol 2012;23(12):3058–63.

[19] Bowles EJ, Wellman R, Feigelson HS, et al. Risk of heart failure in breast cancer patients after anthracycline and trastuzumab treatment: a retrospective cohort study. J Natl Cancer Inst 2012;104:1293–305.

[20] Serrano C, Cortes J, De Mattos-Arruda L, et al. Trastuzumab-related cardiotoxicity in the elderly: a role for cardiovascular risk factors. Annals Oncol 2012;23:897–902.

[21] Doroshow JH. Effect of anthracycline antibiotics on oxygen radical formation in rat heart. Cancer Res 1983;43:460–72.

[22] Lipshultz SE, Cochran TR, Franco VI, Miller TL. Treatment-related cardiotoxicity in survivors of childhood cancer. Nat Rev Clin Oncol 2013;10(12):697–710.

[23] Link G, Tirosh R, Pinson A, et al. Role of iron in the potentiation of anthracycline cardiotoxicity: identification of heart cell mitochondria as a major site of iron-anthracycline interaction. J Lab Clin Med 1996;127:272–8.

[24] Zhang S, Liu X, Bawa-Khalfe T, et al. Identification of the molecular basis of doxorubicin induced cardiotoxicity. Nat Med 2012;18:1639–42.

[25] Liu LF, Wang JC. Supercoiling of the DNA template during transcription. Proc Natl Acad Sci USA 1987;84:7024–7.

[26] Drake FH, Zimmerman JP, McCabe FL, et al. Purification of topoisomerase II from amsacrine-resistant P388 leukemia cells. Evidence for two forms of the enzyme. J Biol Chem 1987;262:16739–47.

[27] Tewey KM, Rowe TC, Yang L, et al. Adriamycin induced DNA damage mediated by mammalian DNA topoisomerase II. Science 1984;226:466–8.

[28] Capranico G, Tinelli S, Austin CA, et al. Different patterns of gene expression of topoisomerase II isoforms in differentiated tissues during murine development. Biochim Biophys Acta 1992;1132:43–8.

[29] Zhu W, Soonpaa MH, Chen H, et al. Acute doxorubicin cardiotoxicity is associated with p53-induced inhibition of the mammalian target of rapamycin pathway. Circulation 2009; 119:99–106.

[30] Tocchetti CG, Carpi A, Coppola C, et al. Ranolazine protects from doxorubicin-induced oxidative stress and cardiac dysfunction. Eur J Heart Fail 2014;16(4):358–66.

[31] Maurea N, Coppola C, Piscopo G, et al. Ranolazine administered after doxorubicin treatment, prevents cardiotoxicity in mice. Eur J Heart Failure Abstracts Supplement 2014;16 (Suppl. 2):109–19.

[32] Abu-Khalaf MM, Harris L. Anthracycline-induced cardiotoxicity: risk assessment and management. Oncology 2009;23:239, 244, 252.

[33] Franco VI, Henkel JM, Miller TL, Lipshultz SE. Cardiovascular effects in childhood cancer survivors treated with anthracyclines. Cardiol Res Pract 2011; 134679.

[34] Swain SM, Whaley FS, Ewer MS. Congestive heart failure in patients treated with doxorubicin: a retrospective analysis of three trials. Cancer 2003;97:2869–79.

[35] Ewer MS, Ewer SM. Cardiotoxicity of anticancer treatments. Nat Rev Cardiol 2015;12 (9):547–58.

[36] Cardinale D, Colombo A, Torrisi R, et al. Trastuzumab-induced cardiotoxicity: clinical and prognostic implications of troponin I evaluation. J Clin Oncol 2010;28(25):3910–16.

[37] Mendes-Ferreira P, De Keulenaer GW, Leite-Moreira AF, Bras-Silva C. Therapeutic potential of neuregulin-1 in cardiovascular disease. Drug Discovery Today 2013;18(17/18).

[38] Coppola C, Piscopo G, Galletta F, et al. Trastuzumab cardiomyopathy is prevented by the administration of Ranolazine at the end of antineoplastic treatment in model mouse. Circulation 2014;130(A18766):9.

[39] Maurea N, Coppola C, Piscopo G, et al. Ranolazine prevents trastuzumab-cardiotoxicity in experimental models. Global Heart 2014;9(1, Suppl.):e145–6.

[40] De Azambuja E, Bedard PL, Suter T, Piccart-Gebhart M. Cardiac toxicity with anti-HER-2 therapies: what have we learned so far?. Target Oncol 2009;4(2):77–88.

[41] Tocchetti CG, Coppola C, Arra C, Maurea N. Early identification of left ventricular dysfunction induced by trastuzumab. J Am Coll Cardiol 2011;58(25):2698–9.

[42] Freedman NJ, Ginsburg GS. Novel and "neu" therapeutic possibilities for heart failure. JACC 2006;48(7):33.

[43] Cardinale D, Sandri MT, Colombo A. Prognostic value of troponin I in cardiac risk stratification of cancer patients undergoing high-dose chemotherapy. Circulation 2004;109 (22):2749–54.

[44] Cardinale D, Lamantia G, Cipolla CM, Troponin I. And cardiovascular risk stratification in patients with testicular cancer. J Clin Oncol 2006;24(21):3508.

[45] Fallah-Rad N, Walker JR, Wassef A, et al. The utility of cardiac biomarkers, tissue velocity and strain imaging, and cardiac magnetic resonance imaging in predicting early left ventricular dysfunction in patients with human epidermal growth factor receptor II-positive breast cancer treated with adjuvant trastuzumab therapy. J Am Coll Cardiol 2011;57(22):2263–70.

[46] Guarneri V, Lenihan DJ, Valero V, et al. Long-term cardiac tolerability of trastuzumab in metastatic breast cancer: the M.D. Anderson Cancer Center experience. J Clin Oncol 2006;24(25):4107–15.

[47] Oliva S, Cioffi G, Frattini S, et al. Administration of angiotensin-converting enzyme inhibitors and β-blockers during adjuvant trastuzumab chemotherapy for non-metastatic breast cancer: marker of risk or cardioprotection in the real world? Oncologist 2012;17(7): 917–24.

[48] Baselga J, Cortes J, Kim SB, et al. Pertuzumab plus trastuzumab plus docetaxel for metastatic breast cancer. N Engl J Med 2012;366:109–19.

[49] Danese MD, Masaquel A, Santos E, et al. Estimated life-years saved in women with HER2-positive metastatic breast cancer receiving first-line trastuzumab and pertuzumab in the United States. Value Health 2015;18(6):876–83.

[50] Lenihan D, Suter T, Brammer M, et al. Pooled analysis of cardiac safety in patients with cancer treated with pertuzumab. Ann Oncol 2012;23(3):791–800.

[51] Perez EA, Koehler M, Byrne J, et al. Cardiac safety of lapatinib: pooled analysis of 3689 patients enrolled in clinical trials. Mayo Clin Proc 2008;83(6):679–86.

[52] Azim H, Azim Jr HA, Escudier B. Trastuzumab versus lapatinib: the cardiac side of the story. Cancer Treat Rev 2009;35:633–8.

[53] Lorenzen S, Riera Knorrenschild J, Haag GM, et al. Lapatinib versus lapatinib plus capecitabine as second-line treatment in human epidermal growth factor receptor 2-amplified metastatic gastro-oesophageal cancer: a randomised phase II trial of the Arbeitsgemeinschaft Internistische Onkologie. Eur J Cancer 2015;51(5):569–76.

[54] Monsuez JJ, Charniot JC, Vignat N, Artigou JY. Cardiac side-effects of cancer chemotherapy. Int J Cardiol 2010;144:3–15.

[55] Richardson PG, Sonneveld P, Schuster MW, et al. Bortezomib or high-dose dexamethasone for relapsed multiple myeloma. N Engl J Med 2005;352:2487–98.

[56] Folkman J. Tumor angiogenesis: therapeutic implications. N Engl J Med 1971;285: 1182–6.

[57] Cheng H, Force T. Molecular mechanisms of cardiovascular toxicity of targeted cancer therapeutics. Circ Res 2010;106:21–34.

[58] Izumiya Y, Shiojima I, Sato K, et al. Vascular endothelial growth factor blockade promotes the transition from compensatory cardiac hypertrophy to failure in response to pressure overload. Hypertension 2006;47:887–93.

[59] Levy BI. Microvascular plasticity and experimental heart failure. Hypertension 2006;47: 827–9.

[60] Zentilin L, Puligadda U, Lionetti V, et al. Cardiomyocyte VEGFR-1 activation by VEGF-B induces compensatory hypertrophy and preserves cardiac function after myocardial infarction. FASEB J 2010;24:1467–78.

[61] Force T, Krause DS, Van Etten RA. Molecular mechanisms of cardiotoxicity of tyrosine kinase inhibition. Nat Rev Cancer 2007;7:332–44.

[62] Chintalgattu V, Ai D, Langley RR, et al. Cardiomyocyte PDGFR-beta signaling is an essential component of the mouse cardiac response to load-induced stress. J Clin Invest 2010;120:472–84.

[63] Rainer PP, Doleschal B, Kirk JA, et al. Sunitinib causes dose-dependent negative functional effects on myocardium and cardiomyocytes. BJU Int 2012;110:1455–62.

[64] Yamaguchi O, Watanabe T, Nishida K, et al. Cardiac-specific disruption of the c-raf-1 gene induces cardiac dysfunction and apoptosis. J Clin Invest 2004;114:937–43.

[65] Yeh ET, Tong AT, Lenihan DJ, et al. Cardiovascular complications of cancer therapy: diagnosis, pathogenesis, and management. Circulation 2004;109:3122–31.

[66] Chu TF, Rupnick MA, Kerkela R, et al. Cardiotoxicity associated with tyrosine kinase inhibitor sunitinib. Lancet 2007;370(9604):2011–19.

[67] Escudier B, Eisen T, Stadler WM, et al. Sorafenib in advanced clear-cell renal-cell carcinoma. N Engl J Med 2007;356(2):125–34.

[68] Motzer RJ, Hutson TE, Tomczak P, et al. Sunitinib versus interferon alfa in metastatic renal-cell carcinoma. N Engl J Med 2007;356(2):115–24.

[69] Hutson TE, Figlin RA, Kuhn JG, Motzer RJ. Targeted therapies for metastatic renal cell carcinoma: an overview of toxicity and dosing strategies. Oncologist 2008;13(10): 1084–96.

[70] Chen ZI, Ai DI. Cardiotoxicity associated with targeted cancer therapies. Mol Clin Oncol 2016;4:675–81.

[71] Hasinoff BB, Patel D, O'Hara KA. Mechanisms of myocyte cytotoxicity induced by the multiple receptor tyrosine kinase inhibitor sunitinib. Mol Pharmacol 2008;74(6): 1722–8.

[72] Kerkela R, Woulfe KC, Durand JB, et al. Sunitinib-induced cardiotoxicity is mediated by off-target inhibition of AMP-activated protein kinase. Clin Transl Sci 2009;2(1):15–25.

[73] Cheng H, Kari G, Dicker AP, et al. A novel preclinical strategy for identifying cardiotoxic kinase inhibitors and mechanisms of cardiotoxicity. Circ Res 2011;109(12):1401–9.

[74] Kerkela R, Grazette L, Yacobi R, et al. Cardiotoxicity of the cancer therapeutic agent imatinib mesylate. Nat Med 2016;12:908–16.

[75] Yang EH, Watson KE, Herrmann J. Should vascular effects of newer treatments be addressed more completely? Future Oncol 2015;11(14):1995–8.

[76] Ewer MS, Lippman SM. Type II chemotherapy-related cardiac dysfunction: time to recognize a new entity. J ClinOncol 2005;23(13):2900–2.

[77] Heidenreich PA, Hancock SL, Vagelos RH, et al. Diastolic dysfunction after mediastinal irradiation. Am Heart J 2005;150(5):977–82.

[78] Adams MJ, Lipsitz SR, Colan SD, et al. Cardiovascular status in long-term survivors of Hodgkin's disease treated with chest radiotherapy. J Clin Oncol 2004;22(15):3139–48.

[79] Cao L, Cai G, Chang C, et al. Diastolic dysfunction occurs early in HER2-positive breast cancer patients treated concurrently with radiation therapy and trastuzumab. Oncologist 2015;20(6):605–14.

[80] Uriel N, Vainrib A, Jorde UP, et al. Mediastinal radiation and adverse outcomes after heart transplantation. J Heart Lung Transpl 2010;29(3):378–81.

[81] Van Veldhuisen DJ, Cohen-Solal A, Böhm M, et al. Beta-blockade with nebivolol in elderly heart failure patients with impaired and preserved left ventricular ejection fraction: Data From SENIORS (Study of Effects of Nebivolol Intervention on Outcomes and Rehospitalization in Seniors With Heart Failure). J Am Coll Cardiol 2009;53(23):2150–8.

[82] Sciarretta S, Paneni F, Palano F, et al. Role of the renin-angiotensin-aldosterone system and inflammatory processes in the development and progression of diastolic dysfunction. Clin Sci (Lond) 2009;116(6):467–77.

Chapter 9

Alteration of Heart Valves

N. Maurea, A. Rienzo and C. Coppola

Chapter Outline

INTRODUCTION

Radiation therapy (RT), along with new antineoplastic agents, has revolutionized cancer prognosis over the past decades. However, if on one hand chest radiotherapy is very effective, on the other hand it can lead to secondary effects, as the irradiation field could not be bound only to the unhealthy tissue [1]. In particular, in breast cancer, radiation subsequent to conservative surgery, determines a reduction of 50% of disease recurrence and a reduction of 17% of death [2]. A dose–response relationship for radiation-related ischemic heart disease has been, recently, demonstrated in breast cancer patients. Moreover, mediastinal irradiation also increases valvular heart disease [3]. In the treatment of Hodgkin lymphoma (HL) and breast cancer, radiation can affect pericardium, myocardium, valves, coronary arteries, and conduction system, giving rise to a variety of cardiovascular complications. In fact, the third most common cause of death in patients with HL is cardiovascular disease. It occurs long term after RT, with a range of mortality between 12% and 16% [4]. Moreover, a recent screening of HL survivors pointed out that 32% of those treated with mediastinal RT developed asymptomatic valvular defects after 6 years, whilst after 20 years 42% had experienced valvular dysfunction [3]. Finally, it has been recently demonstrated that, in childhood cancer survivors, the association of radiotherapy and antineoplastic drugs promotes the development of congestive heart failure [5].

Anticancer Treatments and Cardiotoxicity. DOI: http://dx.doi.org/10.1016/B978-0-12-802509-3.00009-1

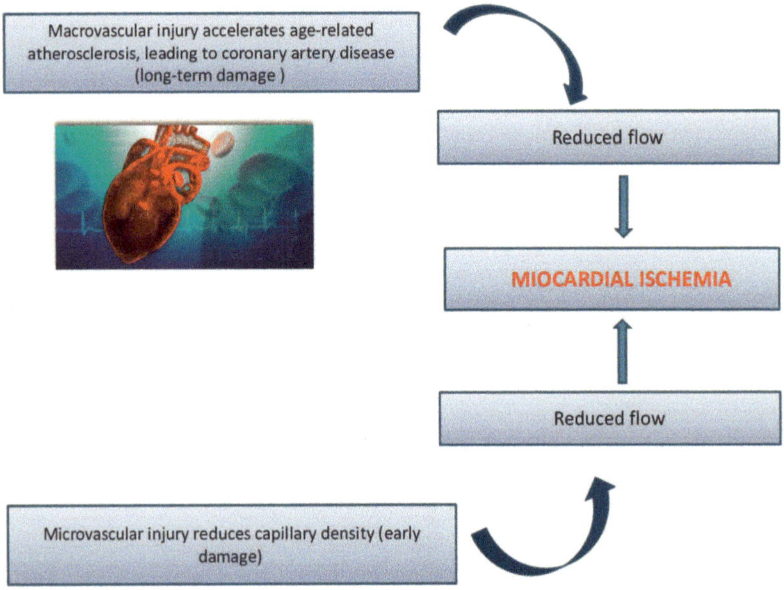

FIGURE 9.1 Physiopathology of myocardial ischemia induced by RT.

PATHOLOGY OF RADIATION-INDUCED VALVULAR DISEASE

The lack of vasculature preserves the valvular tissue from ischemia, a possible consequence of radiation-induced valvulopathy [6] (Fig. 9.1). When grown in culture and exposed to 10 Gy of radiation, aortic valve interstitial cells show an increased expression of alkaline phosphatase, bone morphogenetic protein 2, and osteopontin, typical of osteoblast-like cell phenotypes [7]. This could be a possible route for the development of calcific aortic stenosis.

Diffuse fibrosis is often present in all four valves [8–10]. In up to 75% of patients treated with radiotherapy, valve thickening was observed even after two decades. Even though most patients are asymptomatic, 60% present with mild aortic regurgitation, 16% aortic stenosis, and 52% mitral regurgitation. Moreover, the great majority (90%) have calcification of the aortic or mitral valves [9–13]. Although after radiotherapy, mitral regurgitation occurs more commonly than mitral stenosis, the latter is more likely to be clinically relevant [9–13]. Furthermore, the tricuspid valve and the pulmonary valve are less commonly affected [9,11], whereas a radiation dose greater than 25 or 30 Gy of the left atrium, to either ventricles, increases the risk for valvular disease [14]. Symptoms of heart failure appear with average of 22 years after radiation exposure, depending on the valve involved [11–13,15,16].

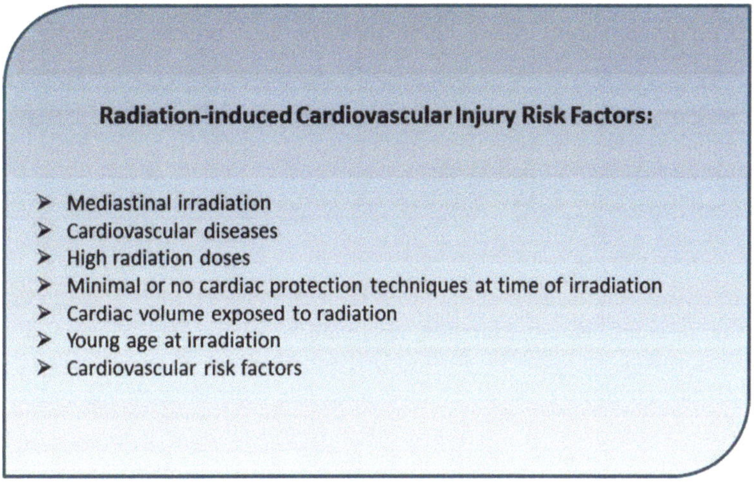

FIGURE 9.2 Radiation-induced heart disease (RIHD) risk factors.

RISK FACTORS AND CLINICAL MANIFESTATIONS

Radiation-induced heart disease (RIHD) must be assigned to several factors (Fig. 9.2), such as irradiated heart volume, radiation technique and, mainly, radiation cumulative dose, which is a function of the number of treatments and dose for treatment [17].

The threshold dose value of approximately 30 Gy defines the upper limit of late RIHD and the lower limit of early RIHD. In fact, below 30 Gy the risk of RIHD can occur more than a decade after RT, whereas at doses above 30 Gy, RIHD can appear within a few years from exposure.

Moreover, higher doses associated with younger age and conventional risk factors may dramatically increase the risk of heart disease. On the other hand, the risk of RIHD associated with lower doses is not yet completely understood and it is not yet clear whether there is a threshold dose below which there is no risk [18].

Radiation-induced valvular disease (RIVD) is another common side effect of RT. According to Darby et al., the left side of the heart has a higher incidence of RIVD due to the greater hemodynamic stressed imposed by the high-pressure left [18]. Moreover, since earlier mediastinal RT was less homogeneous in delivering radiation dose to the patients, it is likely that the left-sided valves have historically received greater radiation doses than those on the right [19].

Basically, in the attempt to reduce toxicity to the esophagus and spinal cord, these earlier regimens predisposed to cardiovascular toxicity. In this regard, contemporary RT approaches have reduced the incidence of cardiac complications, even though the exact cardiotoxicity degree remains unknown [20].

In young patients, up to 20 years old, as well as in children, in whom the heart is not yet totally developed, RIVD is most severe. The dose–response relationship for RIVD is, however, still unknown. Recently, Cutter et al. conducted a useful study to estimate the dose–response relationship for RIVD and to evaluate other possible factors of RIVD risk, in patients with HL unearthing that radiation doses above 30 Gy to the heart valves can increase the risk for RIVD. However, for patients with mediastinal involvement treated today with 20 or 30 Gy, the 30-year risk will be increased by only about 1.4% [3].

Moreover, this study confirms that the main risk factor for the development of valvular disease, following treatment for HL, is the radiation dose to the heart valves. In addition, for the first time a dose–response relationship can be translated into clinical practice, assessing the risk of RIVD and assisting in guiding the appropriate follow-up of HL survivors [3].

Cutter et al.'s findings were supported by three other recent studies on the relationship between valvular disease and RT for HL [3].

In the first study, RIVD was diagnosed in 3% of 1132 HL survivors after 19.5 years follow-up [22]. For doses of 20 Gy none of the patients developed valvular disease, while for doses of 25, 30, and 36 Gy, the 25-year cumulative risks among individuals were 2%, 1%, and 16%, respectively.

In the second study, a pool of 56 HL survivors was screened to assess the presence or not of valvular disease, after a median follow-up of 70.5 months. The screened survivors had a probability of develop a valvular disease of 32% [14]. The risk of valvular defects increased with maximum heart dose, while the risk of left-sided defects increased with the volume of the left cardiac chambers receiving 30 Gy or more [23]. In the third study a group of 143 HL survivors, treated with a mid-mediastinal dose of 40.3 Gy, was screened with cardiovascular magnetic resonance (CMR) imaging, after a median follow-up of 24 years [24]. The study reported that 42% of selected survivors suffered from RIVD. The high percentage could be due to different asymptomatic defects visible by CMR imaging but almost undetectable with echocardiography.

In childhood cancer as well as in breast cancer, RIVD has a statistically significant increase following mean cardiac doses of 15–34 Gy and 35 Gy [25,26].

Taken together, all these studies suggest that for doses greater than or equal to 30 Gy the risk of valvular disease increases, while for doses less than 30 Gy the increase per Gy is smaller.

Aortic arch calcifications are another dramatic consequence of RT. In a study conducted on 1804 survivors of the atomic bombing in Hiroshima, Yamada et al. reported that the prevalence of mild aortic arch calcification was 26.1% for men and 31.9% for women and that of severe calcification was 8.8% for men and 19.1% for women. The use of tangential windows allows to minimize cardiac and aortic damage and makes current radiotherapy techniques much more safe, especially in the treatment of breast cancer [27].

Severe valvulopathy can be treated with valve replacement [28]. The perioperative (30-day) mortality rate is 12% and the 5-year survival rate is 66% [4,29].

The highest independent predictor of perioperative mortality rate was the presence of constrictive pericarditis, with a 30-day mortality rate of 40%.

The high mortality rate can be attributed to fibrosis of the mediastinum [4,16,29,30], whereby transcatheter aortic valve replacement may be the preferred surgical choice [31]. Moreover, in high-risk patients the pulmonary stenosis can be treated with transcatheter pulmonary valve replacement [32]. Echocardiographic screening should be suggested at 10 years after radiotherapy to evaluate valvular disease [10].

MONITORING, DIAGNOSIS, AND MANAGEMENT OF RIVD

Transthoracic echo is the modality of choice for screening RIVD, as it provides real-time noninvasive imaging of cardiac anatomy and function. To identify newly valvular lesions, such investigation should be started 10 years after radiotherapy, and at 5-yearly intervals [33].

In Fig. 9.3 is shown the echo of a 37-year-old male HL survivor treated 13 years before with RT and chemotherapy. Risk factors were high blood pressure and dyslipidemia. The patient presented a fibrosis of

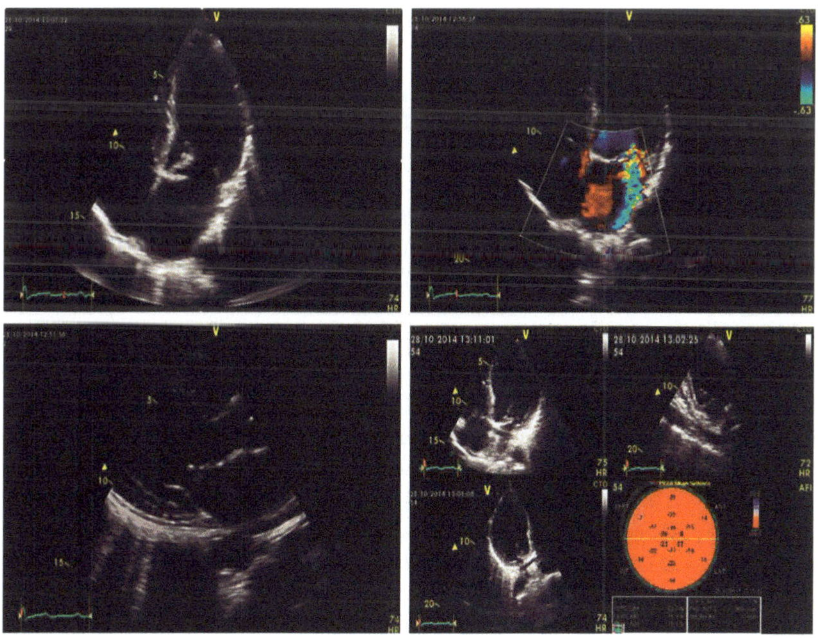

FIGURE 9.3 Echo of a 37-year-old male HL survivor treated 13 years before with RT and chemotherapy.

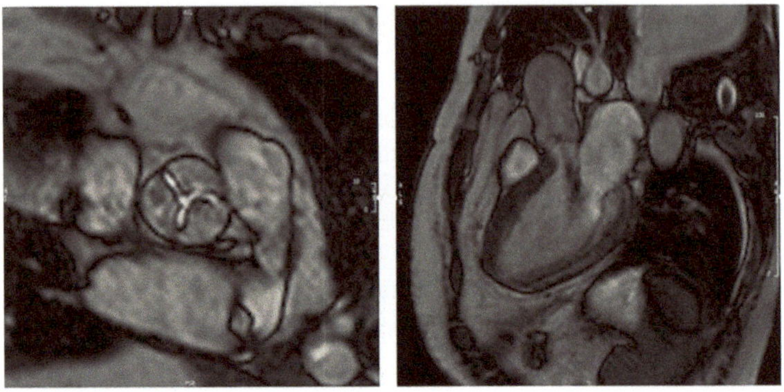

FIGURE 9.4 MRI of a 59-year-old female HL survivor, after a left mastectomy for breast cancer, treated 20 years before with RT and chemotherapy.

mitral valve with important mitral regurgitation, and the involvement of the aortic valve. The global longitudinal strain and ejection fraction were normal [34].

The study of valvular structure, especially the mitral valve, as well as a transesophageal study could be better performed with the three-dimensional (3D) echo. When the quality of echo studies is insufficient, magnetic resonance imaging (MRI) could be the more useful choice.

In Fig. 9.4 is shown the MRI of a 59-year-old female HL survivor, after a left mastectomy for breast cancer, treated 20 years before with RT and chemotherapy. Aortic stenosis and regurgitation are clearly visible in the figure. In this case the echo was of poor quality and insufficient for the diagnosis, because of the impairment of the echographic acoustic window caused by silicone implant due to breast reconstruction technique after mastectomy [34].

We recommend that echo surveillance starts at 5 years after radiotherapy and is undertaken at 5-yearly intervals (Fig. 9.5).

CONCLUSIONS

Antineoplastic treatment-induced valvular disease is primarily related to RT, especially when it does not dependent on the dilated cardiomyopathy subsequent to drug treatment (especially anthracyclines). Currently, there is strong evidence indicating that cancer survivors, treated with RT, have an increased risk of mortality, most likely due to irradiation of the heart and great vessels.

The long latency period between radiation exposure and onset of cardiovascular disease makes instances of RIVD not completely known and most probably underestimated.

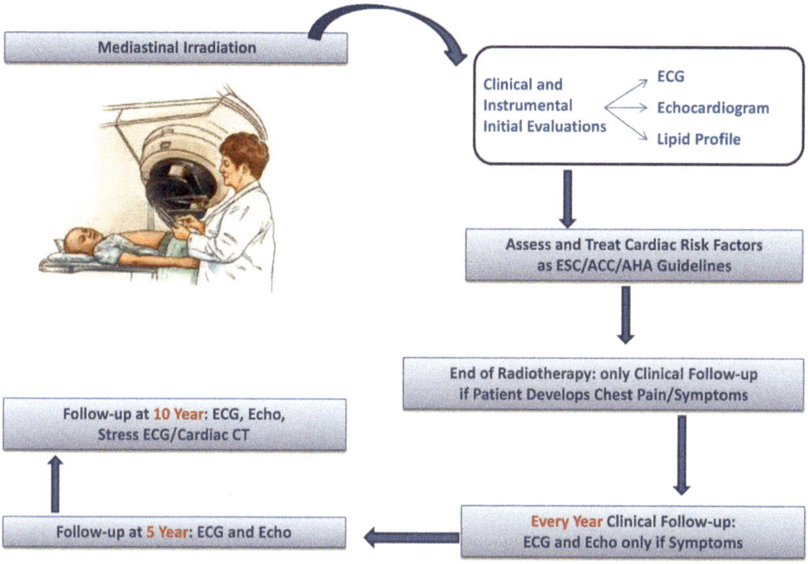

FIGURE 9.5 Algorithm of patient management after radiation.

REFERENCES

[1] Jacob S, Pathak A, Franck D, et al. Early detection and prediction of cardiotoxicity after radiation therapy for breast cancer: the BACCARAT prospective cohort study. Radiat Oncol 2016;11(1):54.

[2] Early Breast Cancer Trialists' Collaborative Group (EBCTCG). Effect of radiotherapy after breast-conserving surgery on 10-year recurrence and 15-year breast cancer death: meta-analysis of individual patient data for 10,801 women in 17 randomised trials. Lancet 2011;378(9804):1707–16.

[3] Cutter DJ, Schaapveld M, Darby SC, et al. Risk of valvular heart disease after treatment for Hodgkin lymphoma. J Natl Cancer Inst 2015;107(4).

[4] Lee MS, Finch W, Mahmud E. Cardiovascular complications of radiotherapy. Am J Cardiol 2013;112:1688–96.

[5] Armenian SH, Hudson MM, Mulder RL, et al. Recommendations for cardiomyopathy surveillance for survivors of childhood cancer: a report from the International Late Effects of Childhood Cancer Guideline Harmonization Group. Lancet Oncol 2015;16(3):e123–36.

[6] Stewart FA. Mechanisms and dose-response relationships for radiation induced cardiovascular disease. Ann ICRP 2012;41(3–4):72–9.

[7] Nadlonek NA, Weyant MJ, Yu JA. Radiation induces osteogenesis in human aortic valve interstitial cells. J Thorac Cardiovasc Surg 2012;144:1466–70.

[8] Brosius FC, Waller BF, Roberts WC. Radiation heart disease. Analysis of 16 young (aged 15 to 33 years) necropsy patients who received over 3,500 rads to the heart. Am J Med 1981;70:519–30.

[9] Veinot JP, Edwards WD. Pathology of radiation-induced heart disease: a surgical and autopsy study of 27 cases. Hum Pathol 1996;27:766–73.

[10] Heidenreich PA, Hancock SL, Lee BK, et al. Asymptomatic cardiac disease following mediastinal irradiation. J Am Coll Cardiol 2003;42:743–9.
[11] Darby SC, Ewertz M, McGale P. Risk of ischemic heart disease in women after radiotherapy for breast cancer. N Engl J Med 2013;368:987–98.
[12] Adabag AS, Dykoski R, Ward H, Anand IS. Critical stenosis of aortic and mitral valves after mediastinal irradiation. Catheter Cardiovasc Interv 2004;63(2):247–50.
[13] Carlson RG, Mayfield WR, Normann S, Alexander JA. Radiation-associated valvular disease. Chest 1991;99(3):538–45.
[14] Cella L, Liuzzi R, Conson M, et al. Dosimetric predictors of asymptomatic heart valvular dysfunction following mediastinal irradiation for Hodgkin's lymphoma. Radiother Oncol 2011;101(2):316–21.
[15] Bruhl SR, Sheikh M, Adlakha S, et al. Endovascular therapy for radiation-induced pulmonary artery stenosis: a case report and review of the literature. Heart Lung 2012;41:87–9.
[16] Janelle GM, Mnookin SC, Thomas JJ, et al. Surgical approach for a patient with aortic stenosis and a frozen mediastinum. J Cardiothorac Vasc Anesth 2003;17:770–2.
[17] Lancellotti P, Nkomo VT, Badano LP, et al. Expert consensus for multimodality imaging evaluation of cardiovascular complications of radiotherapy in adults: a report from the European Association of Cardiovascular Imaging and the American Society of Echocardiography. Eur Heart J Cardiovasc Imaging 2013;14:721–40.
[18] Darby SC, Cutter DJ, Boerma M, et al. Radiation-related heart disease: current knowledge and future prospects. Int J Radiat Oncol Biol Phys 2010;76(3):656–65.
[19] Ewer MS, Yeh ETH. Chapter 7 Cancer and heart. USA: People's Medical Publishing House; 2013.
[20] Groarke JD, Nguyen PL, Nohria A, et al. Cardiovascular complications of radiation therapy for thoracic malignancies: the role for non-invasive imaging for detection of cardiovascular disease. Eur Heart J 2014;35(10):612–23.
[21] Deleted in Review.
[22] Schellong G, Riepenhausen M, Bruch C, et al. Late valvular and other cardiac diseases after different doses of mediastinal radiotherapy for Hodgkin disease in children and adolescents: Report from the longitudinal GPOH follow-up project of the German-Austrian DAL-HD studies. Pediatr Blood Cancer 2010;55(6):1145–52.
[23] Cella L, Liuzzi R, Conson M, et al. Multivariate normal tissue complication probability modeling of heart valve dysfunction in Hodgkin lymphoma survivors. Int J Radiat Oncol Biol Phys 2013;87(2):304–10.
[24] Machann W, Beer M, Breunig M, et al. Cardiac magnetic resonance imaging findings in 20-year survivors of mediastinal radiotherapy for Hodgkin's disease. Int J Radiat Oncol Biol Phys 2010;79(4):1117–23.
[25] Mulrooney DA, Yeazel MW, Kawashima T, et al. Cardiac outcomes in a cohort of adult survivors of childhood and adolescent cancer: retrospective analysis of the Childhood Cancer Survivor Study cohort. BMJ 2009;339:b4606.
[26] McGale P, Darby SC, Hall P, et al. Incidence of heart disease in 35,000 women treated with radiotherapy for breast cancer in Denmark and Sweden. Radiother Oncol 2011; 100(2):167–75.
[27] Yamada M, Naito K, Kasagi F, et al. Prevalence of atherosclerosis in relation to atomic bomb radiation exposure: an RERF Adult Health Study. Int J Radiat Biol 2005;81:821–6.
[28] Handa N, McGregor CG, Danielson GK, et al. Valvular heart operation in patients with previous mediastinal radiation therapy. Ann Thorac Surg 2001;71:1880–4.

[29] Crestanello JA, McGregor CG, Danielson GK, et al. Mitral and tricuspid valve repair in patients with previous mediastinal radiation therapy. Ann Thorac Surg 2004;78:826–31.
[30] Veeragandham RS, Goldin MD. Surgical management of radiation induced heart disease. Ann Thorac Surg 1998;65:1014–19.
[31] Latib A, Montorfano M, Figini F, et al. Percutaneous valve replacement in a young adult for radiation-induced aortic stenosis. J Cardiovasc Med 2012;13:397e398.
[32] Bruhl SR, Sheikh M, Adlakha S, et al. Therapy for radiation-induced pulmonary artery stenosis: a case report and review of the literature. Heart Lung 2012;41:87e89.
[33] Gillette EL, McChesney SL, Hoopes PJ. Isoeffect curves for radiation-induced cardiomyopathy in the dog. Int J Radiat Oncol Biol Phys 1985;11:2091–7.
[34] Heckmann M, Douwes K, Peter R, et al. Vascular activation of adhesion molecule mRNA and cell surface expression by ionizing radiation. Exp Cell Res 1998;238:148–54.

Chapter 10

Pericardial Damage

B. Cosyns

Chapter Outline

In autopsy specimens of radiation-induced heart disease (RIHD), pericardial disease was noted in up to 70% of cases [1]. Pericardial tissue fibrosis is a common finding, leading to a loss of compliance, thickening, adherence, and at a more advance stage to the development of calcification.

In the pericardium, parietal surfaces are more severely damaged, with dense collagen and fibrin deposition on the mesothelial surfaces [2]. Microscopically, fibrosis is often focal in distribution and associated with an interstitial fibrin network for many years after exposure, evidence of continuing microvascular injury (Fig. 10.1).

Despite the power of animal models, including genetic systems, in vitro and in vivo models do not necessarily reflect contemporary radiotherapy treatment strategies, neither in dosage nor in timing of irradiation [3].

Processes deregulated after radiotherapy lead to abnormal remodeling of extracellular matrix (ECM) with pathological fibrosis [4]. Interstitial ECM comprises a mixture of proteins (collagens and elastin), glycoproteins and proteoglycans (fibronectin, laminin, and tenascin), and glycosaminoglycans (heparin and chondroitin sulfates) lying in a hyaluronic acid gel composed of long polysaccharide chains [5].

Oxidative stress, hypoxia, and microvascular damage are potential factors stimulating fibrosis in the context of radiotherapy. Among others, secreted factors driving fibrosis, transforming growth factor beta 1 (TGF-β1) are produced by a wide range of inflammatory, mesenchymal, and epithelial cells that convert fibroblasts and other cell types into matrix-producing myofibroblasts [6].

Anticancer Treatments and Cardiotoxicity. DOI: http://dx.doi.org/10.1016/B978-0-12-802509-3.00010-8

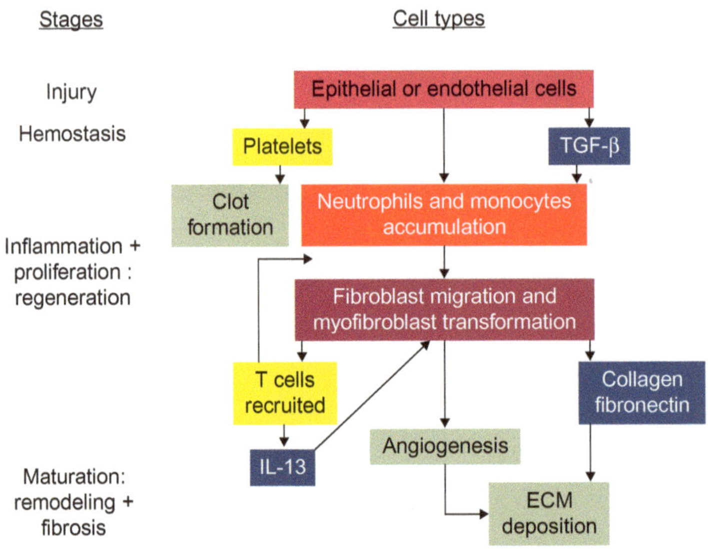

FIGURE 10.1 Basic mechanisms of radio-induced pericardial damage.

The relevance of very early events, from inflammatory responses in blood vessels to fibrosis, remains uncertain. Observations on the timing of changes in humans are limited by tissue availability (autopsy or surgery), but light microscopy describes vascular changes within a few weeks of exposure, including narrowing and obliteration of capillaries by endothelial swelling, fibrin plugs, and endothelial hyperplasia.

Even if required for the initiation of fibrosis, inflammation and the continued stimulus of TGF-β1 may not be needed to maintain it.

Myofibroblasts are active biosynthetic cells with characteristic α-smooth muscle stress fibers anchored to ECM via strong focal adhesion sites and to neighboring myofibroblasts. In animal models of fibrosis, myofibroblasts originate from several different progenitor cell types, not just resident fibroblasts. Most, if not all, of these progenitor cell types are likely to contribute to human fibrotic states, including radiation fibrosis [7].

After myofibroblast activation, collagen production can be perpetuated independently of TGF-β1 by autocrine induction of a cytokine called connective tissue growth factor. The lack of a prominent cellular inflammatory response, described as a general feature of delayed radiation injury, questions the role of adaptive immune responses [8].

Finally, radiation is also a potent stimulator of procalcifying factors and may explain the frequent occurrence of pericardial calcifications at later stages [9].

REFERENCES

[1] Veinot JP, Edwards WD. Pathology of radiation-induced heart disease: a surgical and autopsy study of 27 cases. Human Pathol 1996;27(8):766–73.

[2] Stewart JR, Fajardo LF. Radiation-induced heart disease: an update. Prog Cardiovasc Dis 1984;27(3):173–94.

[3] Heidenreich PA, Kapoor JR. Radiation induced heart disease: systemic disorders in heart disease. Heart 2009;95(3):252–8.

[4] Schultz-Hector S, Trott KR. Radiation-induced cardiovascular diseases: is the epidemiologic evidence compatible with the radiobiologic data? Int J Radiat Oncol Biol Phys 2007;67(1):10–18.

[5] Alberts B, Johnson A, Lewis J, Raff M, Roberts K, Walter P. Molecular biology of the cell. New York, NY: Garland Science, Taylor and Francis Group; 2008.

[6] Barcellos-Hoff MH. How do tissues respond to damage at the cellular level? The role of cytokines in irradiated tissues. Radiat Res 1998;150:S109–20.

[7] Desmouliere A, Redard M, Darby I, Gabbiani G. Apoptosis mediates the decrease in cellularity during the transition between granulation tissue and scar. Am J Pathol 1995;146: 56–66.

[8] Fajardo L-G. Morphological patterns of radiation injury. Basel: Karger; 1989.

[9] Nadlonek NA, Weyant MJ, Yu JA, Cleveland Jr JC, Reece TB, Meng X, et al. Radiation induces osteogenesis in human aortic valve interstitial cells. J Thorac Cardiovasc Surg 2012;144(6):1466–70.

Chapter 11

Effects of Radiotherapy on Vessels and Coronary Arteries

F. Rigo

Chapter Outline

PATHOPHYSIOLOGY AND HISTOPATHOLOGY

Radiation therapy is used in the treatment of many types of cancer [1]. Radiation-induced cardiac disease encompasses a spectrum of deleterious effects on the heart from preclinical histopathologic findings to symptomatic clinical disease. Multiple studies have shown that these patients have an increased risk of coronary artery disease (CAD), congestive heart failure, valvular heart disease, pericardial disease, and sudden death [1,2].

Irradiation can damage all cells, both cancer cells and healthy cells, and can affect blood vessels of all sizes. Radiation therapy causes an increase in capillary wall permeability, with dilation of vessels leading to the characteristic radiation erythema. Radiation treatment causes direct damage to blood vessels by the generation of reactive oxygen species that disrupt DNA strands leading to an inflammatory cascade [1,2]. The same process occurs in the vasculature of the heart. This inflammatory cell infiltrate disturbs the filtration properties of the endothelium, and the membrane of the capillary wall thickens as a result of collagen deposition and fibrosis [1]. Endothelial dysfunction is believed to be a precipitating factor in the development of cardiac sequelae [3] and is most likely a combination of impaired endothelial function, stimulation of growth factors, and eventual fibrosis [4]. Analogous to atheromatous plaques, however differing in their microvascular location, there is progressive hypoperfusion with microvascular thrombosis and ischemia, with eventual small-vessel occlusion and cell death.

Anticancer Treatments and Cardiotoxicity. DOI: http://dx.doi.org/10.1016/B978-0-12-802509-3.00011-X

CORONARY ARTERY DISEASE

The pathohistologic hallmarks include diffuse fibrosis of the interstitium of the myocardium and arterial lumen narrowing [4]. Pathologically, vascular radiation injury is accompanied by an increase in capillary wall permeability, the generation of reactive oxygen species, and activation of an inflammatory cascade [3]. This subsequently leads to intimal proliferation with collagen deposition and fibrosis [1]. As such, initial endothelial dysfunction is believed to be a key factor in the development of cardiac sequelae [3].

In the case of CAD, the stenoses might be due to intimal proliferation, damage to the intima, or atherosclerotic lesions [5]. This initiates a cascade of events that is typical of atherosclerosis, including replacement of damaged cells with myofibroblasts along with platelet deposition. In vitro studies have also revealed the prothrombotic effect of radiation associated with higher release of von Willebrand factor which can provoke and contribute to coronary thrombosis [6–8]. Ultimately, the mechanism involved in plaque formation is thought to mirror spontaneous atherosclerosis; however, plaques in irradiated patients have been found to be more fibrous with a decreased lipid component [4–8]. Coronary artery ostial stenoses are typical in cases of radiation-induced lesions [8].

Vascular injury from radiation therapy can be silent; approximately 50% of asymptomatic patients develop new myocardial perfusion defects [8]. Clinically, most patients present with angina, dyspnea, or heart failure, although sudden death has been reported. Sudden death in patients subjected to radiation therapy is thought to result from diffuse intimal hyperplasia of all coronary arteries or from significant left main stenosis. The mean interval for developing CAD after radiation therapy is about 80 months [9].

Macroscopically, there is a significantly higher incidence of severe left main disease, followed by ostial right coronary artery and left anterior descending artery stenoses correlating with the anatomic location of radiation treatment [3]. In general, the lesions are consistently longer, more proximal, smoother, concentric, and tubular [10]. The incidence of radiation-induced CAD is increased by the standard cardiac risk factors. A study on patients after therapy for Hodgkin's lymphoma found that 10.4% of patients developed significant CAD (defined as having history of myocardial infarction/coronary artery bypass graft/ > 75% luminal stenosis on angiography or autopsy) at a median of 9 years of follow-up [11].

REFERENCES

[1] Gaya AM, Ashford RF. Cardiac complications of radiation therapy. Clin Oncol (R Coll Radiol) 2005;17:153–9.

[2] Hatoum OA, Otterson MF, Kopelman D, et al. Radiation induces endothelial dysfunction in murine intestinal arterioles via enhanced production of reactive oxygen species. Arterioscler Thromb Vasc Biol 2006;26:287–94.

[3] Paris F, Fuks Z, Kang A, et al. Endothelial apoptosis as the primary lesion initiating intestinal radiation damage in mice. Science 2001;293:293–7.

[4] Darby SC, Cutter DJ, Boerma M, et al. Radiation-related heart disease: current knowledge and future prospects. Int J Radiat Oncol Biol Phys 2010;76:656–65.

[5] McEniery PT, Dorosti K, Schiavone WA, Pedrick TJ, Sheldon WC. Clinical and angiographic features of coronary artery disease after chest irradiation. Am J Cardiol 1987;60:1020–4.

[6] Sebag-Montefiore D, Hope-Stone H. Radiation induced coronary heart disease. Br Heart J 1993;69:481–2.

[7] Boerma M, Kruse JJ, van Loenen M, et al. Increased deposition of von Willebrand factor in the rat heart after local ionizing irradiation. Strahlenther Onkol 2004;180:109–16.

[8] Veinot JP, Edwards WD. Pathology of radiation-induced heart disease: a surgical and autopsy study of 27 cases. Hum Pathol 1996;27:766–73.

[9] Basavaraju SR, Easterly CE. Pathophysiological effects of radiation on atherosclerosis development and progression, and the incidence of cardiovascular complications. Med Phys 2002;29:2391–403.

[10] Brosius III FC, Waller BF, Roberts WC. Radiation heart disease. Analysis of 16 young (aged 15 to 33 years) necropsy patients who received over 3,500 rads to the heart. Am J Med 1981;70:519–30.

[11] Hull MC, Morris CG, Pepine CJ, Mendenhall NP. Valvular dysfunction and carotid, subclavian, and coronary artery disease in survivors of Hodgkin lymphoma treated with radiation therapy. JAMA 2003;290:2831–7.

Chapter 12

Cardiac Conduction Disturbances

F. Rigo

Chapter Outline

PHYSIOPATHOLOGIC MECHANISMS

The conduction system is the least commonly involved of all the cardiac structures and its true incidence is not known. ECG changes after irradiation range from nonspecific ST-T changes to low-voltage and right bundle branch block (RBBB) [1].

RBBB is commonly associated with mediastinal irradiation because the right bundle lies close to the endocardium on the right side [1]. Injury to the bundle may occur either directly from radiation or indirectly from associated myocardial fibrosis and ischemia. One of the common serious manifestations is complete atrioventricular (AV) block [2]. Dual-chamber pacing has been found to be somewhat more efficacious in symptom improvement in such patients [2]. A postmortem study in a 20-year-old man with Hodgkin's disease and previous radiation who had earlier developed heart block revealed marked arteriosclerosis with fibrosis of the epicardium, myocardium, and endocardium. Examination of the conduction system revealed extensive arteriolosclerosis of the sinoatrial node and its approaches. In addition, there was marked fibrosis of the approaches to the AV node, the AV bundle, and both bundle branches [1]. Complete heart block has been reported to occur at an interval of less than 1 year from radiation to 23 years after completion of radiation therapy [2].

Diffuse interstitial fibrosis occurs after relatively low doses of radiation through microvascular insufficiency and ischemia, involving damage to the capillary endothelial cells [1]. Most patients with myocardial involvement have some degree of interstitial fibrosis [2], typically developing at radiation doses above 30 Gy.

Anticancer Treatments and Cardiotoxicity. DOI: http://dx.doi.org/10.1016/B978-0-12-802509-3.00012-1

CLINICAL MANIFESTATIONS

Abnormalities along the entire conduction system have been described in the setting of radiotherapy, including varying degrees of AV block, sick sinus syndrome, prolonged QT, supraventricular arrhythmias, and ventricular tachycardia [3,4]. RBBB is more commonly observed than left bundle branch block postradiotherapy, likely due to higher radiation exposure of the right ventricle due to its anterior location. Ventricular ectopy might occur in up to 50% of patients exposed to mediastinal irradiation, often secondary to ventricular fibrosis [3–7]. A high postoperative prevalence of conduction disease after valvular surgery has also been found in this patient cohort, with 27% of patients requiring permanent pacemaker placement [8]. Dysfunction of the autonomic nervous system, leading to persistent tachycardia, loss of circadian heart rhythm, and respiratory phasic heart rate variability has also been described after irradiation [9]. The latter clinical picture is similar to heart transplant patients who have a denervated heart [9]. Persisting tachycardia might further increase the patient risk of developing a tachycardia-mediated cardiomyopathy. Complete heart block has been reported to occur at an interval of less than 1 year from radiation to 23 years after completion of radiation therapy [9].

REFERENCES

[1] Brosius 3rd FC, Waller BF, Roberts WC. Radiation heart disease. Analysis of 16 young (aged 15 to 33 years) necropsy patients who received over 3,500 rads to the heart. Am J Med 1981;70(3):519–30.

[2] Slama MS, Le Guludec D, Sebag C, et al. Complete atrioventricular block following mediastinal irradiation: areport of six cases. Pacing Clin Electrophysiol 1991;14(7):1112–18.

[3] Heidenreich PA, Kapoor JR. Radiation induced heart disease: systemic disorders in heart disease. Heart 2009;95:252–8.

[4] Nellessen U, Zingel M, Hecker H, Bahnsen J, Borschke D. Effects of radiation therapy on myocardial cell integrity and pump function: which role for cardiac biomarkers? Chemotherapy 2010;56:147–52.

[5] Veinot JP, Edwards WD. Pathology of radiation-induced heart disease: a surgical and autopsy study of 27 cases. Hum Pathol 1996;27:766–73.

[6] Heidenreich PA, Hancock SL, Vagelos RH, Lee BK, Schnittger I. Diastolic dysfunction after mediastinal irradiation. Am Heart J 2005;150:977–82.

[7] Larsen RL, Jakacki RI, Vetter VL, Meadows AT, Silber JH, Barber G. Electrocardiographic changes and arrhythmias after cancer therapy in children and young adults. Am J Cardiol 1992;70:73–7.

[8] Crestanello JA, McGregor CG, Danielson GK, et al. Mitral and tricuspid valve repair in patients with previous mediastinal radiationtherapy. Ann Thorac Surg 2004;78:826–31.

[9] Adams MJ, Lipshultz SE, Schwartz C, Fajardo LF, Coen V, Constine LS. Radiation-associated cardiovascular disease: manifestations and management. Semin Radiat Oncol 2003;13:346–56.

Section III

Cardiovascular Complications of Cancer Treatments

Chapter 13

Cardiac Rhythm Disturbances

C.R. Manrique, N. Tiwari and J.C. Plana

Chapter Outline

INTRODUCTION

Advancements in the early detection and effective treatment of cancer have led to a significant decline in mortality among cancer patients [1]. The resultant improvement in survival brings new challenges such as the recognition and management of arrhythmias as a result of the neoplasia or its treatment [2–4]. The exact prevalence and incidence of cancer-related arrhythmia are unknown. There could be several plausible explanations for it, such as the absence of cardiac monitoring as part of the old chemotherapy trials, exclusion of cancer patients in cardiology trials, the exclusion of patients at higher risk of developing cardiotoxicity from oncology trials, and the combination of different chemotherapy regimens or chemotherapy along with radiation. In this chapter, we discuss the various cardiac rhythm disturbances arising from cancer as well as secondary to chemotherapy or radiotherapy.

RHYTHM DISTURBANCES ASSOCIATED WITH NEOPLASMS

The underlying pathophysiology of cardiac arrhythmias in the cancer patient is still poorly understood. However, it can be attributed to either a direct effect of the neoplastic process on the heart or as an indirect effect occurring from changes in cardiac structure and function, generating an arrhythmogenic substrate that might lead to different rhythm or conduction disturbances.

Anticancer Treatments and Cardiotoxicity. DOI: http://dx.doi.org/10.1016/B978-0-12-802509-3.00013-3

Cardiac amyloidosis, in addition to primary cardiac tumors, though rare can affect the cardiac conduction system. In the same way, noncardiac malignancies, by direct extension or by metastasis, may cause local damage via hemorrhagic pericardial effusion, invasion of the ventricular structures causing outflow or inflow obstruction with arrhythmias, or involvement of the conduction system producing variable blocks of the electrical pathways. On the other hand, an elevated state of inflammation, increased sympathetic drive, and altered metabolic milieu due to cancer may also create a proarrhythmic environment [5].

RHYTHM DISTURBANCES SECONDARY TO CANCER THERAPEUTICS

Risk factors for development of cardiac arrhythmias with cancer therapeutics include patient's age (> 70 years), female sex, preexisting arterial hypertension, diabetes, chronic kidney disease, coronary artery disease (CAD), and heart failure. In addition, cancer therapeutics-related factors, such as use of high doses and continuous infusion schedules [6,7], prior mediastinal radiation, or previous treatment with anthracyclines, have been identified [2,3,8–10].

Cancer therapeutics may cause a wide spectrum of bradyarrythmias, supraventricular, and ventricular tachyarrythmias.

Bradyarrhythmias

The two important classes of agents that may cause bradycardia are taxanes (i.e., paclitaxel) and the angiogenesis inhibitor, thalidomide. Asymptomatic sinus bradycardia is the most common rhythm that has been associated with the administration of antineoplastic medications (0.1–31%). On the other hand, atrioventricular conduction disorders and bundle branch block are seen infrequently (about 3% of patients) especially after administration of paclitaxel. They usually occur within the first 24 h after initiation of the infusion (range 2.5 h to 6 days), resolving spontaneously over the next 48–72 h [11,12]. Direct effect of paclitaxel on the Purkinje system and extracardiac autonomic system, along with histamine release induced by Cremophor EL, the vehicle used for its formulation, have been hypothesized to potentiate negative chronotropic effects. Thalidomide, a tumor necrosis factor-α inhibitor, currently being used in the treatment of multiple myeloma, Kaposi's sarcoma, malignant melanoma, myelodysplastic syndrome, and some solid tumors causes mild sinus bradycardia in about 55% of patients, but severe sinus bradycardia is seen in 1–3% of the cases [13–17]. The exact mechanism of this effect is not totally understood, but it is likely secondary to uninhibited vagus nerve discharges, thereby mimicking parasympathetic surge [14]. In addition, patients on thalidomide are prone to development of hypothyroidism which, in turn, is also associated with bradycardia [3,14,16].

Patients undergoing treatment with taxanes or thalidomide should be monitored for symptoms of bradycardia such as fatigue, lightheadedness, dizziness, or syncope. Continuous electrocardiogram (EKG) monitoring is recommended only in patients with symptomatic bradycardia or progressive conduction abnormalities. Pretreatment with antihistamines and corticosteroids to prevent the release of histamine, as well as avoidance of concomitant use of AV nodal blocking agents may reduce the likelihood of bradyarrythmias. In symptomatic patients, discontinuation of these agents should be considered. A permanent pacemaker implantation may be needed depending on the severity of symptoms, hemodynamic status of the patient, and the need to continue these therapeutic agents as part of the treatment [3,18].

Tachyarrythmias

A wide range of tachyarrythmias including supraventricular tachycardia (SVT), ventricular ectopy (VE), ventricular tachycardia (VT), and ventricular fibrillation (VF) have been reported with the use of cancer therapeutics. Alkylating agents (i.e., cisplatin, cyclophosphamide, ifosfamide, and melphalan) may induce coronary vasospasm, damage to cardiomyocytes and endothelial injury by formation of intracapillary microthrombi [19]. Intrapericardial use of cisplatin has been associated with high incidence of paroxysmal SVT [20] and atrial fibrillation (AF) [21]. Approximately 8–10% of patients receiving a high dose of cyclophosphamide develop atrial and ventricular tachyarrhythmias in the 24–72 h following its administration, but usually resolve spontaneously within a week [19,22–24]. Similarly, in about one-third of patients pretreated with CHOP therapy (cyclophosphamide, doxorubicin, vincristine, and prednisone) and whole-body radiation for bone marrow transplantation (BMT), cardiac arrhythmias (SVT, paroxysmal AF, premature ventricular contractions (PVC), and VT) and QT interval prolongation are seen [19,23]. Melphalan administered before BMT is associated with AF or flutter in 6.6–11% of patients; however, AF is not observed in patients receiving BMT alone [25–28].

LV systolic dysfunction is the most common mechanism of anthracycline-induced arrhythmias, especially AF. Also, an increased incidence of premature ventricular complexes has been reported acutely after doxorubicin infusion (3% in the first hour and 24% in the first 24 h) without any long-term consequences [29]. Myocardial ischemia is a well-recognized arrhythmogenic stimulus. 5-Fluorouracil may induce coronary vasospasm with direct cytotoxic effects on the myocardium giving rise to AF, polymorphic PVC, VT, and VF [30,31]. Similarly, interleukin-2, used in the treatment of metastatic renal carcinoma and malignant melanoma, may induce myocardial ischemia due to coronary vasospasm and myocarditis. These deleterious effects potentially induce arrhythmias, mostly SVT (9.7–17%), AF (5–8%), and VT (<1%). Also, in 10% of the patients, it may cause SVT or

VT due to capillary leak syndrome [3,32]. Finally, methotrexate use has been infrequently associated with premature atrial contractions (PACs), PVCs, VT, VF, and junctional escape beats [33].

RHYTHM DISTURBANCES SECONDARY TO RADIOTHERAPY

Radiotherapy, either adjunctive or primary, has been the mainstay of treatment for patients with cancer within malignancies such as Hodgkin's lymphoma, breast, lung, and esophageal cancer. It has been commonly associated with a variety of cardiovascular complications involving the pericardium, myocardium, valves, coronary arteries, and the conduction system.

These complications are related to the total dose of radiation received and the fractioning of the doses. Higher radiotherapy dose, younger age at treatment, and the presence of conventional risk factors for CAD increase the risk of cardiac injury. The underlying mechanism is multifactorial and likely involves radiation-induced myocardial fibrosis, endothelial damage of the microvasculature and coronary arteries, and liberation of multiple inflammatory and profibrotic cytokines [34]. Repolarization abnormalities and PVCs, both asymptomatic, are seen in up to 50% of patients exposed to mediastinal radiation [35]. Right bundle branch block is more common than left bundle branch block due to its anterior location, thereby receiving a higher radiation dose. Complete heart block, syncope, and sudden death are rare but can occur even 10 years after mediastinal radiation. Autonomic nervous system dysfunction with a loss of circadian rhythm, inappropriate vasogenic compensatory mechanisms, and inappropriate sinus tachycardia are also seen [36]. Permanent pacemaker implantation is usually indicated for high-degree AV blocks [37].

QT PROLONGATION IN THE CANCER PATIENT

Prolonged QT interval raises concern of life-threatening cardiac arrhythmias, such as Torsades de pointes (TdP) and sudden cardiac death. Arsenic trioxide, used for the treatment of acute promyelocytic leukemia, is notorious for causing QT prolongation [38,39]. However, even with a high incidence of QT prolongation, the risk of TdP remains low due to simultaneous action on current channels $I_{\text{Kr or Ks (inhibition) and}}$ $I_{\text{K-ATP}}$ (activation) which promotes normal repolarization and thus mitigates its arrhythmogenicity [40]. Blockade of hERG channel is another important mechanism of action for QT prolongation from arsenic trioxide and tyrosine kinase inhibitors [41]. Recently, it has been shown that inhibition of tyrosine kinase downregulates phosphatidylinositol 3-kinase (PI3K) signaling, which prolongs the QT interval by affecting multiple ion channels [42]. Imatinib, a tyrosine kinase inhibitor, inhibits hepatic drug metabolism performed by the CYP3A4, CYP1A2, CYP2D6, CYP2C9, and CYP2C19 systems. The concurrent use of imatinib

TABLE 13.1 Chemotherapeutic Agents With High Incidence of QT Prolongation

QT Prolongation	**Tyrosine Kinase Inhibitors**	**Rituximab, Dasatinib, Lapatinib, Nilotinib, Ponatinib, Sorafenib, Sunitinib, Vandetanib**
	Anthracyclines	Daunorubicin, doxorubicin
	Antimetabolites	Capecitabine
	Histone deacetylase inhibitors	Dacinostat, panobinostat, romidepsin, vorinostat
	Miscellaneous	Arsenic trioxide, amasacrine
Torsades de pointes		Arsenic trioxide, dacinostat, daunorubicin, HDAC inhibitors, vorinostat

and other drugs, such as ketoconazole, phenothiazines, or quinolones, might result in progressive QT interval prolongation directly related to impaired hepatic metabolism of these other agents [35,36]. Careful attention to potential drug–drug interactions is required with the use of imatinib.

The most common risk factors such as older age, female gender, structural heart disease, myocardial ischemia or infarction, heart failure, and family history of long QT syndrome should be explored in all patients prior to starting chemotherapeutic agents with a high incidence of QT prolongation. Table 13.1 summarizes the most important cancer therapeutics agents associated with QT prolongation.

Serial EKG monitoring is advocated by some in patients receiving arsenic trioxide [39]. If a patient develops QT of >500 ms or reports symptoms such as palpitations or syncope, he/she should be promptly hospitalized under cardiac telemetry and the offending agent should be held temporarily, and repeated EKGs obtained to reassess QT [43]. Administration of intravenous magnesium sulfate and prompt correction of electrolyte abnormalities are recommended. Concomitant use of multiple QT prolonging medications or drugs interfering with their metabolism should be avoided.

INTERACTION BETWEEN SUPPORTIVE THERAPY AND ANTIARRHYTHMIC MEDICATION

Class IA antiarrhythmic agents (i.e., quinidine and procainamide) and class III antiarrhythmic agents (i.e., amiodarone and sotalol) prolong QT as a part of their mechanism of action [44]. In the same way, supporting medications like antiemetics, such as ondansetron and droperidol, are known to cause QT prolongation greater than 500 ms [31]. Similarly, methadone, a synthetic opioid used to treat chronic pain, is frequently associated with significant prolongation of the QT interval duration. It has a significantly increased risk of TdP when used in high doses [45]. Special attention to the potential pharmacological interaction between methadone and antineoplastic agents is recommended because it may decrease the metabolism of chemotherapeutic drugs, especially arsenic trioxide and tyrosine kinase inhibitors. Additionally, tricyclic antidepressants, specifically amitriptyline, doxepin, desipramine, and clomipramine, cause QT prolongation and confer a greater risk of TdP [46]. Hence, caution should be taken when using these drugs concomitantly with other chemotherapeutic and antiarrhythmic agents.

CONCLUSION

The existing guidelines for arrhythmias and cancer do not specifically address screening or early monitoring and treatment of various conduction disorders in patients undergoing treatment for cancer [47–53]. There is a dire need for a better understanding of the arrhythmogenic mechanisms associated with cancer therapy, evidence-based cardiac monitoring guidelines, and development of newer cancer therapeutics with lower arrhythmogenic potential.

Close collaboration between cardiologists and oncologists is prudent to provide optimal care to this unique patient population and for better understanding the relationship between cardiac arrhythmias and cancer therapies.

REFERENCES

[1] Suter TM, Ewer MS. Cancer drugs and the heart: importance and management. Eur Heart J Apr 2013;34(15):1102–11.

[2] Guglin M, Aljayeh M, Saiyad S, Ali R, Curtis AB. Introducing a new entity: chemotherapy-induced arrhythmia. Europace Dec 2009;11(12):1579–86.

[3] Yeh ET, Bickford CL. Cardiovascular complications of cancer therapy: incidence, pathogenesis, diagnosis, and management. J Am Coll Cardiol Jun 16 2009;53(24):2231–47.

[4] Tamargo J, Caballero R, Delpon E. Cancer chemotherapy and cardiac arrhythmias: a review. Drug Saf Feb 2015;38(2):129–52.

[5] Medenwald D, Kors JA, Loppnow H, et al. Inflammation and prolonged QT time: results from the Cardiovascular Disease, Living and Ageing in Halle (CARLA) study. PLoS One 2014;9(4):e95994.

[6] de Forni M, Malet-Martino MC, Jaillais P, et al. Cardiotoxicity of high-dose continuous infusion fluorouracil: a prospective clinical study. J Clin Oncol Nov 1992;10(11):1795–801.

[7] Kosmas C, Kallistratos MS, Kopterides P, et al. Cardiotoxicity of fluoropyrimidines in different schedules of administration: a prospective study. J Cancer Res Clin Oncol Jan 2008;134(1):75–82.

[8] Floyd JD, Nguyen DT, Lobins RL, Bashir Q, Doll DC, Perry MC. Cardiotoxicity of cancer therapy. J Clin Oncol Oct 20 2005;23(30):7685–96.

[9] Morandi P, Ruffini PA, Benvenuto GM, Raimondi R, Fosser V. Cardiac toxicity of high-dose chemotherapy. Bone Marrow Transplant Feb 2005;35(4):323–34.

[10] Arbel Y, Swartzon M, Justo DQT. Prolongation and Torsades de Pointes in patients previously treated with anthracyclines. Anticancer drugs Apr 2007;18(4):493–8.
[11] Arbuck SG, Strauss H, Rowinsky E, et al. A reassessment of cardiac toxicity associated with Taxol. J Natl Cancer Inst Monogr 1993;15:117–30.
[12] Rowinsky EK, Eisenhauer EA, Chaudhry V, Arbuck SG, Donehower RC. Clinical toxicities encountered with paclitaxel (Taxol). Semin Oncol Aug 1993;20(4 Suppl. 3):1–15.
[13] Barlogie B, Tricot G, Anaissie E, et al. Thalidomide and hematopoietic-cell transplantation for multiple myeloma. N Engl J Med Mar 9 2006;354(10):1021–30.
[14] Fahdi IE, Gaddam V, Saucedo JF, et al. Bradycardia during therapy for multiple myeloma with thalidomide. Am J Cardiol Apr 15 2004;93(8):1052–5.
[15] Rajkumar SV, Blood E, Vesole D, Fonseca R, Greipp PR. Phase III clinical trial of thalidomide plus dexamethasone compared with dexamethasone alone in newly diagnosed multiple myeloma: a clinical trial coordinated by the Eastern Cooperative Oncology Group. J Clin Oncol Jan 20 2006;24(3):431–6.
[16] Kaur A, Yu SS, Lee AJ, Chiao TB. Thalidomide-induced sinus bradycardia. Ann Pharmacother Jul-Aug 2003;37(7–8):1040–3.
[17] Palumbo A, Facon T, Sonneveld P, et al. Thalidomide for treatment of multiple myeloma: 10 years later. Blood Apr 15 2008;111(8):3968–77.
[18] Kietpeerakool C, Tiyayon J, Suprasert P, Kanjanavanit R, Srisomboon J. Benefit of electrocardiography during front-line combination paclitaxel and carboplatin chemotherapy for epithelial ovarian cancer. J Med Assoc Thai Nov 2006;89(11):1805–10.
[19] Kupari M, Volin L, Suokas A, Timonen T, Hekali P, Ruutu T. Cardiac involvement in bone marrow transplantation: electrocardiographic changes, arrhythmias, heart failure and autopsy findings. Bone Marrow Transplant Feb 1990;5(2):91–8.
[20] Canobbio L, Fassio T, Gasparini G, et al. Cardiac arrhythmia: possible complication from treatment with cisplatin. Tumori Apr 30 1986;72(2):201–4.
[21] Lara Jr. PN, Mack PC, Synold T, et al. The cyclin-dependent kinase inhibitor UCN-01 plus cisplatin in advanced solid tumors: a California cancer consortium phase I pharmacokinetic and molecular correlative trial. Clin Can Res Jun 15 2005;11(12):4444–50.
[22] Cazin B, Gorin NC, Laporte JP, et al. Cardiac complications after bone marrow transplantation. A report on a series of 63 consecutive transplantations. Cancer May 15 1986;57 (10):2061–9.
[23] Gottdiener JS, Appelbaum FR, Ferrans VJ, Deisseroth A, Ziegler J. Cardiotoxicity associated with high-dose cyclophosphamide therapy. Arch Intern Med May 1981;141(6):758–63.
[24] Ando M, Yokozawa T, Sawada J, et al. Cardiac conduction abnormalities in patients with breast cancer undergoing high-dose chemotherapy and stem cell transplantation. Bone Marrow Transplant Jan 2000;25(2):185–9.
[25] Olivieri A, Corvatta L, Montanari M, et al. Paroxysmal atrial fibrillation after high-dose melphalan in five patients autotransplanted with blood progenitor cells. Bone Marrow Transplant May 1998;21(10):1049–53.
[26] Moreau P, Milpied N, Mahe B, et al. Melphalan 220 mg/m^2 followed by peripheral blood stem cell transplantation in 27 patients with advanced multiple myeloma. Bone Marrow Transplant May 1999;23(10):1003–6.
[27] Phillips GL, Meisenberg B, Reece DE, et al. Amifostine and autologous hematopoietic stem cell support of escalating-dose melphalan: a phase I study. Biol Blood Marrow Transplant Jul 2004;10(7):473–83.
[28] Feliz V, Saiyad S, Ramarao SM, Khan H, Leonelli F, Guglin M. Melphalan-induced supraventricular tachycardia: incidence and risk factors. Clin Cardiol Jun 2011;34(6):356–9.

[29] Steinberg JS, Cohen AJ, Wasserman AG, Cohen P, Ross AM. Acute arrhythmogenicity of doxorubicin administration. Cancer Sep 15 1987;60(6):1213–18.

[30] Hrovatin E, Viel E, Lestuzzi C, et al. Severe ventricular dysrhythmias and silent ischemia during infusion of the antimetabolite 5-fluorouracil and cis-platin. J Cardiovasc Med (Hagerstown) Aug 2006;7(8):637–40.

[31] Keefe DL. The cardiotoxic potential of the 5-HT(3) receptor antagonist antiemetics: is there cause for concern? Oncologist 2002;7(1):65–72.

[32] Lee RE, Lotze MT, Skibber JM, et al. Cardiorespiratory effects of immunotherapy with interleukin-2. J Clin Oncol Jan 1989;7(1):7–20.

[33] Perez-Verdia A, Angulo F, Hardwicke FL, Nugent KM. Acute cardiac toxicity associated with high-dose intravenous methotrexate therapy: case report and review of the literature. Pharmacotherapy Sep 2005;25(9):1271–6.

[34] Lee MS, Finch W, Mahmud E. Cardiovascular complications of radiotherapy. Am J Cardiol Nov 15 2013;112(10):1688–96.

[35] Wittig A, Engenhart-Cabillic R. Cardiac side effects of conventional and particle radiotherapy in cancer patients. Herz Jun 2011;36(4):311–24.

[36] Adams MJ, Lipsitz SR, Colan SD, et al. Cardiovascular status in long-term survivors of Hodgkin's disease treated with chest radiotherapy. J Clin Oncol Aug 1 2004;22 (15):3139–48.

[37] Slama MS, Le Guludec D, Sebag C, et al. Complete atrioventricular block following mediastinal irradiation: a report of six cases. Pacing Clin Electrophysiol Jul 1991;14(7):1112–18.

[38] Barbey JT, Pezzullo JC, Soignet SL. Effect of arsenic trioxide on QT interval in patients with advanced malignancies. J Clin Oncol Oct 1 2003;21(19):3609–15.

[39] Ohnishi K, Yoshida H, Shigeno K, et al. Prolongation of the QT interval and ventricular tachycardia in patients treated with arsenic trioxide for acute promyelocytic leukemia. Ann Intern Med Dec 5 2000;133(11):881–5.

[40] Drolet B, Simard C, Roden DM. Unusual effects of a QT-prolonging drug, arsenic trioxide, on cardiac potassium currents. Circulation Jan 6 2004;109(1):26–9.

[41] Kim TD, le Coutre P, Schwarz M, et al. Clinical cardiac safety profile of nilotinib. Haematologica Jun 2012;97(6):883–9.

[42] Lu Z, Wu CY, Jiang YP, et al. Suppression of phosphoinositide 3-kinase signaling and alteration of multiple ion currents in drug-induced long QT syndrome. Sci Translat Med Apr 25 2012;4(131):131ra150.

[43] Unnikrishnan D, Dutcher JP, Garl S, Varshneya N, Lucariello R, Wiernik PH. Cardiac monitoring of patients receiving arsenic trioxide therapy. Br J Haematol Mar 2004;124 (5):610–17.

[44] Vaughan Williams EM. A classification of antiarrhythmic actions reassessed after a decade of new drugs. J Clin Pharmacol Apr 1984;24(4):129–47.

[45] Krantz MJ, Lowery CM, Martell BA, Gourevitch MN, Arnsten JH. Effects of methadone on QT-interval dispersion. Pharmacotherapy Nov 2005;25(11):1523–9.

[46] Vieweg WV, Wood MA. Tricyclic antidepressants, QT interval prolongation, and torsade de pointes. Psychosomatics Sep-Oct 2004;45(5):371–7.

[47] Hensley ML, Hagerty KL, Kewalramani T, et al. American Society of Clinical Oncology 2008 clinical practice guideline update: use of chemotherapy and radiation therapy protectants. J Clin Oncol Jan 1 2009;27(1):127–45.

[48] Carver JR, Shapiro CL, Ng A, et al. American Society of Clinical Oncology clinical evidence review on the ongoing care of adult cancer survivors: cardiac and pulmonary late effects. J Clin Oncol Sep 1 2007;25(25):3991–4008.

[49] American Society of Clinical O. European Society for Medical O. ASCO-ESMO consensus statement on quality cancer care. Ann Oncol Jul 2006;17(7):1063–4.

[50] Task Force M, Priori SG, Blomstrom-Lundqvist C, et al. ESC Guidelines for the management of patients with ventricular arrhythmias and the prevention of sudden cardiac death: The Task Force for the Management of Patients with Ventricular Arrhythmias and the Prevention of Sudden Cardiac Death of the European Society of Cardiology (ESC) Endorsed by: Association for European Paediatric and Congenital Cardiology (AEPC). Eur Heart J 2015;17(11):1601–87.

[51] European Heart Rhythm A, Heart Rhythm S, Zipes DP, et al. ACC/AHA/ESC 2006 guidelines for management of patients with ventricular arrhythmias and the prevention of sudden cardiac death: a report of the American College of Cardiology/American Heart Association Task Force and the European Society of Cardiology Committee for Practice Guidelines (Writing Committee to Develop Guidelines for Management of Patients With Ventricular Arrhythmias and the Prevention of Sudden Cardiac Death). J Am Coll Cardiol Sep 5 2006;48(5):e247–346.

[52] January CT, Wann LS, Alpert JS, et al. AHA/ACC/HRS guideline for the management of patients with atrial fibrillation: executive summary: a report of the American College of Cardiology/American Heart Association Task Force on practice guidelines and the Heart Rhythm Society. Circulation 2014;130(23):2071–104.

[53] Page RL, Joglar JA, Caldwell MA, et al. ACC/AHA/HRS Guideline for the Management of Adult Patients With Supraventricular Tachycardia: A Report of the American College of Cardiology/American Heart Association Task Force on Clinical Practice Guidelines and the Heart Rhythm Society. Circulation 2015;67(13):e27–e115.

Chapter 14

Acute and Chronic Heart Failure

J. Brown and J.C. Plana

Chapter Outline

INTRODUCTION

Cancer therapeutics-related cardiac dysfunction (CTRCD) is a major cause of morbidity and mortality in cancer survivors. Anthracyclines continue to be the key chemotherapeutic agent in the treatment of breast cancer, sarcomas, lymphomas, and leukemias; and as a result remain the most common cause of CTRCD [1]. Newer medications, such as trastuzumab, have shown cardiotoxic potential, and serve as additional culprits for CTRCD when given sequentially after anthracyclines, or alone in high-risk patients.

ETIOLOGY, DEMOGRAPHICS, AND PROGNOSIS

Anthracycline-induced CTRCD occurs in a cumulative dose-dependent fashion through the generation of reactive oxygen species. The expression of damage is related to preexisting disease, the state of cardiac reserve at the time of administration, coexisting damage, and individual variability [2]. CTRCD has been reported in up to 10% of cancer survivors, and more than 50% of all patients exposed to anthracyclines will show some degree of cardiac dysfunction 10–20 years after chemotherapy; 5% of individuals treated with a cumulative dose of 400 mg/m^2 will develop overt heart failure (HF) [1,3–5]. Breast cancer patients are at the highest risk of CTRCD and HF, as doxorubicin and tratuzumab are both frequently used in the treatment of advanced disease. Up to 27% of these patients may develop CTRCD and could potentially progress to HF [3,6,7]. One study noted that in patients

Anticancer Treatments and Cardiotoxicity. DOI: http://dx.doi.org/10.1016/B978-0-12-802509-3.00014-5

undergoing orthotopic heart transplantation (OHT), hematologic malignancies were the most common prior malignancy in CTRCD patients, followed by breast and sarcoma. More than 70% of CTRCD patients undergoing OHT had malignancies for which anthracyclines were the mainstay of treatment [3].

Patients who develop CTRCD are most commonly female. While this group includes a high proportion of breast cancer survivors, this gender gap raises the question of whether women are more susceptible to developing cardiomyopathy after chemotherapy and more likely to progress to end-stage HF.

The underlying cause of HF is independently associated with survival among patients with certain types of cardiomyopathy. Patients with cardiomyopathy due to doxorubicin therapy have an especially poor prognosis, with 2-year mortality rate of up to 60% [8]. Despite the fact that patients with CTRCD have fewer comorbidities when compared to patients with ischemic and nonischemic cardiomyopathy (NICMP), they are known to have a worse prognosis [9]. Multiple studies have shown that the key to mitigating this risk is early detection and treatment with accepted HF therapies including ACE-inhibitors and β-blockers.

IMPORTANCE OF EARLY DETECTION AND TREATMENT

Cardinale et al. have substantiated the principle of early detection and treatment in patients with anthracycline-induced CTRCD. When detected early it has been shown to respond well to contemporary HF medical therapy, with the possibility of complete left ventricular (LV) recovery [1].

Left ventricular ejection fraction (LVEF) recovery and cardiac event reduction were demonstrated with early detection of cardiac dysfunction and prompt initiation of modern HF treatment. In this cohort, the percentage of patients who responded to medical therapy progressively decreased as the time from the end of chemotherapy to the start of HF treatment increased. Responders had CTRCD detected at an earlier stage, with less advanced NYHA functional class. In fact, prolonged (greater than 6 months) time-to-HF treatment and advanced NYHA functional class were the only independent predictors of a lack of complete LVEF recovery. Furthermore, after 12 months, the possibility of obtaining even partial LVEF improvement was exceedingly small. This study emphasized the crucial point that monitoring patients exclusively based on symptom evaluation squanders the opportunity to detect cardiotoxicity early (at a stage where it could still be potentially reversible), and underscores the importance of standard HF medical therapy in CTRCD patients.

Given the poor prognosis and proven benefit of early therapy, timely detection of LV dysfunction following chemotherapy is imperative. Several studies have demonstrated that changes in myocardial mechanics detected with strain echocardiography precede significant changes in LVEF [10], giving us the opportunity of identifying and rapidly treating the patient with early evidence of subclinical LV dysfunction.

ADVANCED HF THERAPY

Delayed detection, specifically with advanced NHYA functional class, eliminates the chances of meaningful LV recovery [1], and often necessitates advanced therapies including mechanical circulatory support (MCS) or OHT.

Mechanical Circulatory Support

As the population of patients with CTRCD grows, so does the proportion of patients with end-stage HF. MCS has increasingly become a viable option for these patient for whom transplant may not be immediately acceptable due to concerns for recurrent malignancy.

A recent report of CTRCD patients treated with MCS revealed that while the overall survival of CTRCD patients who received LVAD support was equivalent to that of other MCS patients, CTRCD patients had a significantly higher risk of right ventricular (RV) failure and need for right ventricular assist device (RVAD) support [3]. In this study, almost one in five patients with CTRCD had RV failure requiring a RVAD. As seen in previous reports of patients needing biventricular support, CTRCD patients who received biventricular assist device support fared significantly worse than those who only received an LVAD.

The finding of such a high rate of RV failure in CTRCD patients is critical, in that in the preponderance of cardiomyopathies, the left ventricle is the only one affected, and thus a significant majority of MCS patients are successfully treated with only an LVAD [9,11]. This finding suggests that the RV is more frequently and severely involved by the cardiomyopathic process in CTRCD patients than in those with other forms of NICMP [3], and that CTRCD patients (especially those with anthracycline-induced CTRCD) undergoing evaluation for MCS must be thoroughly assessed in light of their increased risk of RV failure. Preoperative preparation should therefore include the availability and feasibility of biventricular support.

Orthotopic Heart Transplantation

OHT has been shown to be an effective definitive therapy for patients with CTRCD and end-stage HF [3,4]. While the optimal interval of remission prior to heart transplantation has not been conclusively established, CTRCD patients who undergo OHT have similar short- and long-term posttransplant survival as other NICMP patients. This is despite the fact that, as noted above, CTRCD patients are twice as likely as other NICMP patients to require RVAD before OHT. Compared with other NICMP patients, CTRCD patients also have significantly longer ischemic times, and have been shown to have higher rates of post-OHT infection and malignancies (unrelated to their previous malignancy), though none of these factors affected survival. This finding, in conjunction with the discovery that CTRCD patients have lower rates of post-OHT rejection, supports the theory of continued impairment of the recipient immune system after chemotherapy. As with preoperative MCS evaluation, clinicians caring for CTRCD patients undergoing OHT must keep these factors in mind for procedural planning and post-OHT immunosuppression. As a whole, CTRCD patients have favorable outcomes following transplantation, and thus OHT should be an integral part in the discussion of care for CTRCD patients with end-stage HF.

CONCLUSION

The increasing number of cancer survivors treated with cardiotoxic agents combined with the rising recognition of cardiotoxicity of new chemotherapeutic agents is certain to expand the population of patients with CTRCD. The importance of early detection and implementation of standard HF medical therapy to improve or even reverse LV dysfunction cannot be overemphasized. If left untreated, a significant proportion of these patients will progress to end-stage HF requiring advanced therapies. This population, while overwhelmingly female, younger, and with fewer comorbidities than their NICMP and ICMP counterparts, has a significantly higher incidence of concomitant RV dysfunction and overall much worse prognosis. If deemed appropriate for MCS, HF specialists must be prepared to offer biventricular support. Heart transplantation is also a viable option for CTRCD patients, with overall lower rates of rejection, and short- and long-term survival comparable to patients who receive allografts for other cardiomyopathies. Special attention should be paid to post-OHT care given the increased frequency of infection and malignancy, though without impact on survival.

REFERENCES

[1] Cardinale D, et al. Anthracycline-induced cardiomyopathy: clinical relevance and response to pharmacologic therapy. J Am Coll Cardiol 2010;55(3):213–20.

[2] Plana JC, et al. Expert consensus for multimodality imaging evaluation of adult patients during and after cancer therapy: a report from the American Society of Echocardiography and the European Association of Cardiovascular Imaging. J Am Soc Echocardiogr 2014;27(9):911–39.

[3] Oliveira GH, et al. Characteristics and survival of patients with chemotherapy-induced cardiomyopathy undergoing heart transplantation. J Heart Lung Transplant 2012;31(8):805–10.

[4] Lenneman AJ, et al. Heart transplant survival outcomes for adriamycin-dilated cardiomyopathy. Am J Cardiol 2013;111(4):609–12.

[5] Steinherz LJ, et al. Cardiac toxicity 4 to 20 years after completing anthracycline therapy. JAMA 1991;266(12):1672–7.

[6] Harbeck N, et al. Cardiovascular complications of conventional and targeted adjuvant breast cancer therapy. Ann Oncol 2011;22(6):1250–8.

[7] Buzdar AU, et al. Neoadjuvant therapy with paclitaxel followed by 5-fluorouracil, epirubicin, and cyclophosphamide chemotherapy and concurrent trastuzumab in human epidermal growth factor receptor 2-positive operable breast cancer: an update of the initial randomized study population and data of additional patients treated with the same regimen. Clin Cancer Res 2007;13(1):228–33.

[8] Felker GM, et al. Underlying causes and long-term survival in patients with initially unexplained cardiomyopathy. N Engl J Med 2000;342(15):1077–84.

[9] Oliveira GH, et al. Increased need for right ventricular support in patients with chemotherapy-induced cardiomyopathy undergoing mechanical circulatory support: outcomes from the INTERMACS Registry (Interagency Registry for Mechanically Assisted Circulatory Support). J Am Coll Cardiol 2014;63(3):240–8.

[10] Thavendiranathan P, et al. Use of myocardial strain imaging by echocardiography for the early detection of cardiotoxicity in patients during and after cancer chemotherapy: a systematic review. J Am Coll Cardiol 2014;63(25 Pt A):2751–68.

[11] Cleveland Jr. JC, et al. Survival after biventricular assist device implantation: an analysis of the Interagency Registry for Mechanically Assisted Circulatory Support database. J Heart Lung Transplant 2011;30(8):862–9.

Chapter 15

Coronary Artery Disease

B. Ayach and J.C. Plana

Chapter Outline

Cardiovascular disease and cancer are the two most prevalent diseases around the world. As they coexist, it would be ideal to have an assessment of cardiovascular risk factors in every patient prior to initiation of cancer treatment [1–4]. If not feasible in every patient, it is recommended in the patient who has known coronary artery disease (CAD) or equivalence (peripheral artery disease, cerebral vascular disease, aneurysmal dilatations, or end-stage renal disease), age >60 years old, or prior mediastinal radiation. The objective of the assessment is to risk-stratify the patient and work on reducing modifiable risk factors prior to and during cancer treatment. This includes, but is not limited to, blood pressure control, cholesterol lowering, smoking cessation, and tight blood glucose control [3–5]. This is particularly important when using chemotherapy agents that may affect the coronary vessels, or radiation therapy that may accelerate CAD.

A baseline history, physical examination and electrocardiogram (EKG) are recommended for the initial evaluation of the patient. If the patient has underlying symptoms or known CAD, a stress test prior to the initiation of treatment is also recommended [3–5]. While undergoing cancer treatment, attention should be paid to new or worsening symptoms. Chest discomfort, shortness of breath, or other atypical chest pain presentations should prompt evaluation and treatment in the same way it is done for the noncancer patient [3–8]. In the case of an acute coronary syndrome the risks and benefits of a percutaneous coronary intervention need to be weighed, especially in the

Anticancer Treatments and Cardiotoxicity. DOI: http://dx.doi.org/10.1016/B978-0-12-802509-3.00015-7

thrombocytopenic patient or the one with metastatic disease. A 10-year outcome evaluation of cancer patients has demonstrated that bare metal stents are twice as likely to be used over drug-eluting stents in cancer patients presenting with either non-ST elevation myocardial infarction (NSTEMI) or ST elevation myocardial infarction (STEMI) [6]. This may be secondary to the duration of recommended dual antiplatelet therapy (6 weeks vs 1 year with drug-eluting stents) and the risk of bleeding.

In addition to the care of the patient with acute or chronic CAD while on treatment, it is important to recognize the direct toxicity of some cancer therapeutic agents.

CANCER THERAPEUTICS

As mentioned above, there are cancer therapeutic agents that are associated with coronary artery thrombosis, arteritis, or spasm.

Antimetabolites (Fluorouracil and Capecitabine)

Fluorouracil (5-FU) is a synthetic pyrimidine agent that is commonly used for different solid malignancies such as adenocarcinomas and squamous cell cancers, including those of the gastrointestinal, urinary tract, breast, cervical, and neck cancers [9,10]. Common side effects of 5-FU include myelosuppression, diarrhea, stomatitis, alopecia, as well as nausea and vomiting [11]. However, more severe cardiotoxic side effects, that occur at a rate of 0.5–7.6% of treated patients, include vasospastic angina, coronary thrombosis, myocardial infarction (MI), coronary dissection, supraventricular or ventricular arrhythmias, congestive heart failure, cardiogenic shock, or sudden death [9–12]. Cardiotoxic effects are more common to occur acutely within 12–48 h of the first treatment cycle, but can also occur as late as 7 days. They are more common with doses greater than 600–1000 mg/m^2 per day infusion [13–15], in patients concurrently receiving radiation therapy, or in patients with underlying CAD (complicated by vasospasm or an acute coronary syndrome) [9,16]. Different mechanisms have been proposed for the cardiotoxicity, including nitric oxide (NO) synthase or protein kinase C defect leading to coronary artery spasm, thrombus formation causing perfusion defects, or direct myocyte damage leading to cardiomyopathy [9,10]. Retrospective and prospective studies have observed symptomatic or nonsymptomatic EKG changes in up to 88% of patients receiving 5-FU, and 22–35% may actually have suffered an acute MI. Cardiac emergencies are treated as mandated by American College of Cardiology/American Heart Association guidelines [7,8]. If the patient is suspected of experiencing 5-FU cardiotoxicity, treatment should be stopped immediately and nitrates or calcium channel blockers should be initiated for vasodilator therapy [10]. However, if chest pain and dynamic ECG changes persist, angiographic evaluation should be considered urgently. Benefits and risks of cancer treatment as well as risks of cardiac toxicity should be discussed with the patient prior to starting treatment.

Antimicrotubule Agents (Paclitaxel/Docetaxel)

These agents are better known for their higher incidence of bradycardia and high degree of atrioventricular blocks [17], however there have also been reported cases of ischemia and infarction associated with paclitaxel administration. Rowinsky et al. reviewed the cardiac events in four trials and reported that manifestations of cardiac ischemia were observed in 5% of patients [18], while MI was reported in less than 0.5% of cases [17]. However, it is unclear whether these effects are secondary to drug–drug interactions or underlying risk factors or CAD. Overall, in the review of the cancer therapy evaluation program's adverse drug reaction database, the overall incidence of grades 4 and 5 cardiac events was 0.29% [17,18].

The only information about docetaxel toxicity comes from its package insert. The insert quotes the study by Vermorken et al., where myocardial ischemia was reported in 1.7% when compared to 0.6% in the placebo arm [19]. A recent multicenter study on the use of docetaxel in combination with other chemotherapeutic agents also reported that one of the 83 participants experienced a MI [20].

Monoclonal Antibodies (Bevacizumab)

Bevacizumab, a novel antiangiogenic agents and recombinant humanized monoclonal antibody agent against vascular endothelial growth factor (VEGF) targeting new vessel formation, is widely used in cancer treatment and has shown a significant survival benefit in colorectal, renal, and breast cancers [21,22]. However, there have been reported incidents of cardiac ischemia [23], with events varying between 0.52% and 1.7% in randomized control trials [24,25]. A meta-analysis by Chen et al., demonstrated a summary incidence of ischemic heart disease to be between 0.6% and 1.4%, at both low and high doses, with an increase in relative risk of 2.14 and 2.49, respectively [26]. It is believed that bevacizumab interferes with VEGF levels in endothelial cells, leading to a decrease in NO, increase in platelet activation and adhesion, and an increase of proinflammatory cytokines, resulting in an increase in ischemic events [26,27]. For that reason it is important for oncologists and cardiologists to be aware of the risks and monitor for ischemic events while using bevacizumab [28].

Small-Molecule Tyrosine Kinase Inhibitors (Erlotinib/Ponatinib/Nilotinib)

Advancement of small molecular targeting inhibitors, such as erlotinib and tyrosine kinase inhibitors (TKI), has significantly improved treatment and outcomes for cancer patients. Erlotinib is an epidermal growth factor receptor (EGFR) and tyrosine TKI, which has demonstrated significant survival benefits in patients with non small-cell lung cancer, especially those with EGFR-sensitizing mutations [29]. Originally believed to target only cancer cells, clinical trials and case reports have reported that erlotinib and other TKIs may also induced heart failure, cardiomyopathy, QT prolongation, and acute coronary syndromes [30–32]. Two studies demonstrated that the combination of gemcitabine and erlotinib together increased the rate of myocardial ischemia and infarction compared to those treated with gemcitabine alone [33,34]. As a result cardiac ischemia and MI have been added to the drug label warning for TKIs [31]. However, a recent population based on a cohort study from Ontario, Canada, evaluated 1642 cancer patients receiving TKIs, of which 64% were on erlotinib, and found that the rate of cardiovascular events was similar to age- and gender-matched individuals without cancer [31].

Up to 7.1% of cardiovascular events were reported in a phase II (PACE) trial of ponatinib in patients with chronic myelogenous leukemia (CML) or Philadelphia-positive acute lymphoblastic leukemia with the major predisposing factor for an event being preexisting cardiovascular comorbidities [35]. A meta-analysis in patients with CML treated with TKIs was done by Chai-Adisakopha et al., demonstrating that the rate of major arterial events was also increased in nilotinib- or ponatinib-treated patients [32]. With more patients receiving small molecular targeting inhibitors more data will emerge regarding cardiac safety, mechanisms, and risk factors that may increase the risk of ischemia or infarction.

RADIATION-INDUCED ACCELERATED CAD

Radiation therapy is a common treatment modality for various types of cancers. Most concerning are radiation treatments that involve thoracic and mediastinal regions as they cause direct injury to the heart. Studies of long-term survivors of radiation treatment of various childhood and adult patients (breast cancer) demonstrate a dose-related effect with a resultant increase in cardiovascular morbidity and mortality. Cardiac injury postradiation may include pericardial disease, myocardial fibrosis, valvular injury, conduction delay, cardiomyopathy, and accelerated CAD [36,37].

The relative risk of cardiovascular death secondary to radiation treatment ranged from 1.2 to 25 depending on the radiation dose. A dose greater than 15 Gy increased the relative risk to 25, whereas 5–15 Gy increased relative risk to 12.5, and <5 Gy had no significant relative risk increase [38]. The MI hazard ratio ranged from 1.2 to 4.9 with radiation doses greater than 15 Gy, when compared to nonradiated cancer survivors [39,40]. Women receiving left-sided breast and internal mammary radiation received a range of 3–17 Gy of radiation to the heart and even more so to the left anterior coronary artery (> 20 Gy) in some cases, which significantly increased coronary artery risks [41–43]. Darby et al., reported that the rate of major coronary event in patients receiving breast cancer treatment increased linearly by 7.4% per Gy received (CI 2.9–14.5) [44]. Even though arteritis of the endothelium of the coronary arteries can cause premature CAD and atherosclerosis over 10–15 years, functional imaging suggested myocardial perfusion defects, following the radiation field, may occur 6 months after radiation for breast cancer treatment [45,46]. Newer radiation techniques seem to decrease the risk of accelerated cardiac disease but longer follow-up is needed.

Patients at the highest risk of radiotherapy-induced complications are those previously treated in childhood or young adulthood cancers, as Hodgkin's lymphoma, with outdated doses of greater than 30 Gy of radiation to the mediastinum [47]. This is especially concerning as up to 50% of vascular injury with myocardial perfusion defects may be silent [48]. Clinically symptomatic patients present with angina, dyspnea, heart failure, or sudden death [36,49,50]. These patients should be followed closely and if they present with early signs or symptoms of CAD, treatment should be initiated. This would include risk reduction treatment, medical or interventional therapy (percutaneous stunting or coronary artery bypass).

REFERENCES

[1] Nguyen KL, et al. The crossroads of geriatric cardiology and cardio-oncology. Curr Geriatr Rep 2015;4(4):327–37.

[2] Accordino MK, Neugut AI, Hershman DL. Cardiac effects of anticancer therapy in the elderly. J Clin Oncol 2014;32(24):2654–61.

[3] Higgins AY, O'Halloran TD, Chang JD. Chemotherapy-induced cardiomyopathy. Heart Fail Rev 2015;20(6):721–30.

[4] Khakoo AY, Yeh ET. Therapy insight: management of cardiovascular disease in patients with cancer and cardiac complications of cancer therapy. Nat Clin Pract Oncol 2008;5(11):655–67.

[5] Curigliano G, et al. Cardiovascular toxicity induced by chemotherapy, targeted agents and radiotherapy: ESMO Clinical Practice Guidelines. Ann Oncol 2012;23(Suppl. 7): vii155–66.

[6] Guddati AK, Joy PS, Kumar G. Analysis of outcomes of percutaneous coronary intervention in metastatic cancer patients with acute coronary syndrome over a 10-year period. J Cancer Res Clin Oncol 2016;142(2):471–9.

[7] Levine GN, et al. 2015 ACC/AHA/SCAI focused update on primary percutaneous coronary intervention for patients with ST-elevation myocardial infarction: an update of the 2011 ACCF/AHA/SCAI guideline for percutaneous coronary intervention and the 2013 ACCF/AHA guideline for the management of ST-Elevation myocardial infarction: a report of the American College of Cardiology/American Heart Association task force on clinical practice guidelines and the society for cardiovascular angiography and interventions. J Am Coll Cardiol 2016;133(11):1135–47.

[8] Amsterdam EA, et al. 2014 AHA/ACC guideline for the management of patients with non-ST-elevation acute coronary syndromes: a report of the American College of Cardiology/American Heart Association task force on practice guidelines. J Am Coll Cardiol 2014;64(24):e139–228.

[9] Alter P, et al. Cardiotoxicity of 5-fluorouracil. Cardiovasc Hematol Agents Med Chem 2006;4(1):1–5.

[10] Sorrentino MF, et al. 5-Fluorouracil induced cardiotoxicity: review of the literature. Cardiol J 2012;19(5):453–8.

[11] Shoemaker LK, Arora U, Lima CM Rocha. 5-Fluorouracil-induced coronary vasospasm. Cancer Control 2004;11(1):46–9.

[12] Keefe DL, Roistacher N, Pierri MK. Clinical cardiotoxicity of 5-fluorouracil. J Clin Pharmacol 1993;33(11):1060–70.

[13] Saif MW, Shah MM, Shah AR. Fluoropyrimidine-associated cardiotoxicity: revisited. Expert Opin Drug Saf 2009;8(2):191–202.

[14] Meydan N, et al. Cardiotoxicity of de Gramont's regimen: incidence, clinical characteristics and long-term follow-up. Jpn J Clin Oncol 2005;35(5):265–70.

[15] de Forni M, et al. Cardiotoxicity of high-dose continuous infusion fluorouracil: a prospective clinical study. J Clin Oncol 1992;10(11):1795–801.

[16] Rezkalla S, et al. Continuous ambulatory ECG monitoring during fluorouracil therapy: a prospective study. J Clin Oncol 1989;7(4):509–14.

[17] Arbuck SG, et al. A reassessment of cardiac toxicity associated with Taxol. J Natl Cancer Inst Monogr 1993;15:117–30.

[18] Rowinsky EK, et al. Cardiac disturbances during the administration of taxol. J Clin Oncol 1991;9(9):1704–12.

[19] Vermorken JB, et al. Cisplatin, fluorouracil, and docetaxel in unresectable head and neck cancer. N Engl J Med 2007;357(17):1695–704.

[20] Tryfonidis K, et al. A multicenter phase I-II study of docetaxel plus epirubicin plus bevacizumab as first-line treatment in women with HER2-negative metastatic breast cancer. Breast 2013;22(6):1171–7.

[21] Motzer RJ, Bukowski RM. Targeted therapy for metastatic renal cell carcinoma. J Clin Oncol 2006;24(35):5601–8.

[22] Su Y, et al. Effect of angiogenesis inhibitor bevacizumab on survival in patients with cancer: a meta-analysis of the published literature. PLoS One 2012;7(4):e35629.

[23] Ranpura V, et al. Risk of cardiac ischemia and arterial thromboembolic events with the angiogenesis inhibitor bevacizumab in cancer patients: a meta-analysis of randomized controlled trials. Acta Oncol 2010;49(3):287–97.

[24] Giantonio BJ, et al. Bevacizumab in combination with oxaliplatin, fluorouracil, and leucovorin (FOLFOX4) for previously treated metastatic colorectal cancer: results from the Eastern Cooperative Oncology Group Study E3200. J Clin Oncol 2007;25(12):1539–44.

[25] Price TJ, et al. Bevacizumab is equally effective and no more toxic in elderly patients with advanced colorectal cancer: a subgroup analysis from the AGITG MAX trial: an international randomised controlled trial of Capecitabine, Bevacizumab and Mitomycin C. Ann Oncol 2012;23(6):1531–6.

[26] Chen XL, et al. Angiogenesis inhibitor bevacizumab increases the risk of ischemic heart disease associated with chemotherapy: a meta-analysis. PLoS One 2013;8(6):e66721.

[27] Gonzalez-Pacheco FR, et al. Mechanisms of endothelial response to oxidative aggression: protective role of autologous VEGF and induction of VEGFR2 by H2O2. Am J Physiol Heart Circ Physiol 2006;291(3):H1395–401.

[28] Senkus E, Jassem J. Cardiovascular effects of systemic cancer treatment. Cancer Treat Rev 2011;37(4):300–11.

[29] Minguet J, Smith KH, Bramlage P. Targeted therapies for treatment of non-small cell lung cancer-recent advances and future perspectives. Int J Cancer 2015.

[30] Force T, Krause DS, Van Etten RA. Molecular mechanisms of cardiotoxicity of tyrosine kinase inhibition. Nat Rev Cancer 2007;7(5):332–44.

[31] Srikanthan A, et al. Cardiovascular toxicity of multi-tyrosine kinase inhibitors in advanced solid tumors: a population-based observational study. PLoS One 2015;10(3):e0122735.

[32] Chai-Adisaksopha C, Lam W, Hillis C. Major arterial events in patients with chronic myeloid leukemia treated with tyrosine kinase inhibitors: a meta-analysis. Leuk Lymphoma 2015;1–11.

[33] Monsuez JJ, et al. Cardiac side-effects of cancer chemotherapy. Int J Cardiol 2010;144 (1):3–15.

[34] Senderowicz AM, et al. Erlotinib/gemcitabine for first-line treatment of locally advanced or metastatic adenocarcinoma of the pancreas. Oncology (Williston Park) 2007;21 (14):1696–706 discussion 1706–1709, 1712, 1715.

[35] Cortes JE, et al. A phase 2 trial of ponatinib in Philadelphia chromosome-positive leukemias. N Engl J Med 2013;369(19):1783–96.

[36] Orzan F, et al. Severe coronary artery disease after radiation therapy of the chest and mediastinum: clinical presentation and treatment. Br Heart J 1993;69(6):496–500.

[37] Lancellotti P, et al. Expert consensus for multi-modality imaging evaluation of cardiovascular complications of radiotherapy in adults: a report from the European Association of Cardiovascular Imaging and the American Society of Echocardiography. Eur Heart J Cardiovasc Imaging 2013;14(8):721–40.

[38] Stewart FA, et al. Understanding radiation-induced cardiovascular damage and strategies for intervention. Clin Oncol (R Coll Radiol) 2013;25(10):617–24.

[39] Tukenova M, et al. Role of cancer treatment in long-term overall and cardiovascular mortality after childhood cancer. J Clin Oncol 2010;28(8):1308–15.

[40] Mulrooney DA, et al. Cardiac outcomes in a cohort of adult survivors of childhood and adolescent cancer: retrospective analysis of the Childhood Cancer Survivor Study cohort. BMJ 2009;339:b4606.

[41] Hooning MJ, et al. Long-term risk of cardiovascular disease in 10-year survivors of breast cancer. J Natl Cancer Inst 2007;99(5):365–75.

[42] Borst GR, et al. Clinical results of image-guided deep inspiration breath hold breast irradiation. Int J Radiat Oncol Biol Phys 2010;78(5):1345–51.

[43] Clarke M, et al. Effects of radiotherapy and of differences in the extent of surgery for early breast cancer on local recurrence and 15-year survival: an overview of the randomised trials. Lancet 2005;366(9503):2087–106.

[44] Darby SC, et al. Risk of ischemic heart disease in women after radiotherapy for breast cancer. N Engl J Med 2013;368(11):987–98.

[45] Marks LB, et al. The incidence and functional consequences of RT-associated cardiac perfusion defects. Int J Radiat Oncol Biol Phys 2005;63(1):214–23.

[46] Seddon B, et al. Detection of defects in myocardial perfusion imaging in patients with early breast cancer treated with radiotherapy. Radiother Oncol 2002;64(1):53–63.

[47] Bovelli D, et al. Cardiotoxicity of chemotherapeutic agents and radiotherapy-related heart disease: ESMO Clinical Practice Guidelines. Ann Oncol 2010;21(Suppl. 5):v277–82.

[48] Gyenes G, et al. Detection of radiation-induced myocardial damage by technetium-99m sestamibi scintigraphy. Eur J Nucl Med 1997;24(3):286–92.

[49] Brosius 3rd FC, Waller BF, Roberts WC. Radiation heart disease. Analysis of 16 young (aged 15 to 33 years) necropsy patients who received over 3,500 rads to the heart. Am J Med 1981;70(3):519–30.
[50] Yeh ET, et al. Cardiovascular complications of cancer therapy: diagnosis, pathogenesis, and management. Circulation 2004;109(25):3122–31.

Chapter 16

Pericardial Effusion and Pericarditis

B. Cosyns

Chapter Outline

RADIOTHERAPY

Acute Pericarditis During Radiation

Acute pericarditis is uncommon, and most of the time occurs due to necrosis or from inflammation of large tumors contiguous to the heart. It is not usually related to a direct effect of irradiation of the pericardium. The clinical presentation is similar to acute nonspecific presentation and resolves rapidly even if radiation is sustained. It is important to note that it generally does not lead to significant subsequent pericardial damage and has little consequence regarding the outcome. Therefore, the treatment should not be interrupted because of it [1].

Delayed Pericarditis After Radiation

Most cases occur within the first 12 months, but it may range from 4 months to several years after radiation [2–6]. The clinical presentation is comparable to acute pericarditis of any cause. It is often associated with pleural effusion. Some patients will develop clinical signs of tamponade, confirmed by imaging, and could further require a pericardiocentesis. Some others will evolve to chronic effusion.

Anticancer Treatments and Cardiotoxicity. DOI: http://dx.doi.org/10.1016/B978-0-12-802509-3.00016-9

Patients with chronic effusion are often asymptomatic and effusion is an incidental finding.

Except patients with tamponade, the majority of the effusions will resolve spontaneously with only supportive treatment in many cases. In about 20% of cases, constriction may develop requiring further pericardiotomy [7].

In some rare cases, radiation may induce effusive constrictive pericarditis. In these patients requiring a pericardiocentesis for a moderate or large amount of pericardial effusion and/or a clinical tamponade, the removal of the fluid will lead to a physiology of constriction [8].

Pancarditis

The combination of pericarditis with myocardial fibrosis is the most severe form of radiation-induced heart disease (RIHD). The prognosis of patients with pancarditis is very poor [9] compared to radiation-induced myocardial fibrosis or isolated pericarditis occurring [10]. The clinical presentation is often very close to congestive heart failure not responding to classical treatment. In some patients, the signs and symptoms of constriction are dominant. The diagnosis may be challenging with echocardiography or catheterization. The classical signs (i.e., respiratory variation of mitral inflow seen in typical constrictive pericarditis) may be absent. The evaluation of filling pressures by echocardiography may also be disturbed, depending on the underlying degree

TABLE 16.1 Chemo Agents That Could Potentially Be a Source of Pericarditis

Agent	References
Anthracyclines	[15–18]
Cyclophosphamide	[19–24]
Cytrabine	[25–29]
Imatinib mesylate	[30,31]
Dasatinib	[32,33]
Interferon-α	[34–38]
Retinoic acid	[39,40]
Busulfan	[41]
Methotrexate	[42–45]
Arsenic trioxide	[46,47]
5-Fluorouracil	[48]
Docetaxel	[49]

of myocardial fibrosis [11]. In the past, the diagnosis was often made at necropsy, by transarterial endomyocardial biopsy or biopsy during pericardiotomy. Nowadays, cardiovascular magnetic resonance (CMR) offers the possibility to evaluate both myocardial fibrosis and pericarditis [12]. The use of deformation imaging can also be useful in that perspective [13]. CMR is particularly recommended in patients scheduled for a pericardiotomy. If the concomitant degree of myocardial fibrosis is too severe, the prognosis of pericardiotomy is usually very poor and heart transplantation should be discuss.

CHEMOTHERAPY

Pericarditis may be observed during or after chemotherapy. Myocarditis and pleural effusion may accompany the pericardial disease.

Table 16.1 summarizes the agents that could potentially be a source of pericarditis.

Constrictive pericarditis may also be seen with high doses of some agents [14].

REFERENCES

[1] Jones A, Wedgwood J. Effects of radiation on the heart. Br J Radiol 1960;33:138–58.

[2] Cohn KE, Stewart JR, Fajardo LF, et al. Heart disease following radiation. Medicine 1967;46:281–98.

[3] Stewart JR, Cohn KE, Fajardo LF, et al. Radiation induced heart disease. A study of twenty-five patients. Radiology 1967;89:302–10.

[4] Fajardo LF, Stewart JR, Cohn KE. Morphology of radiation-induced heart disease. Arch Pathol 1968;86(5):512–19.

[5] Morton DL, Glancy DL, Joseph WL, et al. Management of patients with radiation-induced pericarditis with effusion: a note on the development of aortic regurgitation in two of them. Chest 1973;64:291–7.

[6] Byhardt R, Brace K, Ruckdeschel J, et al. Dose and treatment factors in radiation-related pericardial effusion associated with the mantle technique for Hodgkin's disease. Cancer 1975;35:795–802.

[7] Fajardo LF, Stewart JR. Radiation-induced heart disease. Human and experimental observations. In: Bristow MR, editor. Drug-induced heart disease. Amsterdam: Elsevier, North-Holland Biomedical Press; 1980. p. 241–60.

[8] Sagristà-Sauleda J, Angel J, Sánchez A, Permanyer-Miralda G, Soler-Soler J. Effusive-constrictive pericarditis. N Engl J Med 2004;350(5):469–75.

[9] Ling LH, Oh JK, Schaff HV, et al. Constrictive pericarditis in the modern era: evolving clinical spectrum and impact on outcome after pericardiectomy. Circulation 1999;100 (13):1380–6.

[10] Yamada H, Tabata T, Jaffer SJ, Drinko JK, Jasper SE, Lauer MS, et al. Clinical features of mixed physiology of constriction and restriction: echocardiographic characteristics and clinical outcome. Eur J Echocardiogr 2007;8(3):185–94.

[11] Chhabra L, Spodick DH. Annulus paradoxus and constrictive pericarditis: a need for revisiting the association! Am J Cardiol 2015;115(4):554.

[12] Cosyns B, Plein S, Nihoyanopoulos P, Smiseth O, Achenbach S, Andrade MJ, et al. European Association of Cardiovascular Imaging (EACVI); European Society of Cardiology Working Group (ESC WG) on Myocardial and Pericardial diseases. European Association of Cardiovascular Imaging (EACVI) position paper: multimodality imaging in pericardial disease. Eur Heart J Cardiovasc Imaging 2015;16(1):12–31.
[13] Skiles J, Rajagopalan N, Klein A. Role of tissue Doppler imaging and color M-mode in the characterization of mixed constriction/restriction. J Am Coll Cardiol 1999;33:433A.
[14] Tulleken JE, Kooiman CG, van der Werf TS, Zijlstra JG, de Vries EG. Constrictive pericarditis after high-dose chemotherapy. Lancet 1997;350:1601.
[15] Krupicka J, Markova J, Pohlreich D, Kozak T, Linkova H, Diehl V, et al. Echocardiographic evaluation of acute cardiotoxicity in the treatment of Hodgkin disease according to the German Hodgkin's Lymphoma Study Group. Leuk Lymphoma 2002;43: 2325–9.
[16] Tohda S, Kobayashi H, Suzuki T, Koyama T, Kamiyama T, Nakamura Y, et al. Acute pericarditis caused by daunorubicin in acute myelocytic leukemia. Rinsho Ketsueki 1988;29:874–8.
[17] Casey DJ, Kim AY, Olszewski AJ. Progressive pericardial effusion during chemotherapy for advanced Hodgkin lymphoma. Am J Hematol 2012;87:521–4.
[18] Dazzi H, Kaufmann K, Follath F. Anthracycline-induced acute cardiotoxicity in adults treated for leukaemia. Analysis of the clinico-pathological aspects of documented acute anthracycline-induced cardiotoxicity in patients treated for acute leukaemia at the University Hospital of Zurich, Switzerland, between 1990 and 1996. Ann Oncol 2001;12:963–6.
[19] Katayama M, Imai Y, Hashimoto H, Kurata M, Nagai K, Tamita K, et al. Fulminant fatal cardiotoxicity following cyclophosphamide therapy. J Cardiol 2009;54:330–4.
[20] Santos GW, Sensenbrenner LL, Burke PJ, Colvin M, Owens Jr. AH, Bias WB, et al. Marrow transplanation in man following cyclophosphamide. Transplant Proc 1971;3:400–4.
[21] Gottdiener JS, Appelbaum FR, Ferrans VJ, Deisseroth A, Ziegler J. Cardiotoxicity associated with high-dose cyclophosphamide therapy. Arch Intern Med 1981;141:758–63.
[22] Goldberg MA, Antin JH, Guinan EC, Rappeport JM. Cyclophosphamide cardiotoxicity: an analysis of dosing as a risk factor. Blood 1986;68:1114–18. Abstract/FREE Full Text
[23] Yamamoto R, Kanda Y, Matsuyama T, Oshima K, Nannya Y, Suguro M, et al. Myopericarditis caused by cyclophosphamide used to mobilize peripheral blood stem cells in a myeloma patient with renal failure. Bone Marrow Transplant 2000;26:685–8.
[24] Braverman AC, Antin JH, Plappert MT, Cook EF, Lee RT. Cyclophosphamide cardiotoxicity in bone marrow transplantation: a prospective evaluation of new dosing regimens. J Clin Oncol 1991;9:1215–23.
[25] Gahler A, Hitz F, Hess U, Cerny T. Acute pericarditis and pleural effusion complicating cytarabine chemotherapy. Onkologie 2003;26:348–50. CrossRefMedlineWeb of Science
[26] Reykdal S, Sham R, Kouides P. Cytarabine-induced pericarditis: a case report and review of the literature of the cardio-pulmonary complications of cytarabine therapy. Leuk Res 1995;19:141–4.
[27] Yamada T, Tsurumi H, Hara T, Sawada M, Oyama M, Moriwaki H. Cytarabine-induced pericarditis. Rinsho Ketsueki 1998;39:1115–20.
[28] Hermans C, Straetmans N, Michaux JL, Ferrant A. Pericarditis induced by high-dose cytosine arabinoside chemotherapy. Ann Hematol 1997;75:55–7.
[29] Vaickus L, Letendre L. Pericarditis induced by high-dose cytarabine therapy. Arch Intern Med 1984;144:1868–9.

[30] Barton JC, Jones SC, Lamberth WC, Reymann MT, Scott VC. Cardiac tamponade associated with imatinib mesylate therapy of chronic myelogenous leukemia. Am J Hematol 2002;71:139–40.

[31] Breccia M, D'Elia GM, D'Andrea M, Latagliata R, Alimena G. Pleural-pericardic effusion as uncommon complication in CML patients treated with Imatinib. Eur J Haematol 2005;74:89–90.

[32] Breccia M, Alimena G. Pleural/pericardic effusions during dasatinib treatment: incidence, management and risk factors associated to their development. Expert Opin Drug Saf 2010;9:713–21.

[33] Krauth MT, Herndlhofer S, Schmook MT, Mitterbauer-Hohendanner G, Schlogl E, Valent P. Extensive pleural and pericardial effusion in chronic myeloid leukemia during treatment with dasatinib at 100 mg or 50 mg daily. Haematologica 2011;96:163–6.

[34] Rauw J, Ahmed S, Petrella T. Pericardial effusion and tamponade following interferon alpha treatment for locally advanced melanoma. Med Oncol 2012;29:1304–7.

[35] Cervera Miguel JI, Vallalta M, Iranzo E, Navarro Ibanez V. Pericardial effusion associated with interferon therapy. Med Clin (Barc) 2004;122:636–7.

[36] Velasco J, Orinuela I, Sanjuan AZ, Ortiz de Zarate Z. Pericardial effusion associated to interferon in an immunocompetent patient. Enferm Infecc Microbiol Clin 2010;28:749–50.

[37] Wisniewski B, Denis J, Fischer D, Labayle D. Pericarditis secondary to interferon alpha in chronic hepatitis C. Gastroenterol Clin Biol 2004;28:315–16. CrossRefMedline

[38] Popescu C, Arama V, Gliga S. Acute pericarditis due to pegylated interferon alpha therapy for chronic HCV hepatitis—case report. BMC Gastroenterol 2011;11:30–230. X-11-30

[39] Tallman MS, Andersen JW, Schiffer CA, Appelbaum FR, Feusner JH, Ogden A, et al. All-trans-retinoic acid in acute promyelocytic leukemia. N Engl J Med 1997;337:1021–8.

[40] Frankel SR, Eardley A, Lauwers G, Weiss M, Warrell Jr. RP. The "retinoic acid syndrome" in acute promyelocytic leukemia. Ann Intern Med 1992;117:292–6.

[41] Terpstra W, de Maat CE. Pericardial fibrosis following busulfan treatment. Neth J Med 1989;35:249–52.

[42] Forbat LN, Hancock BW, Gershlick AH. Methotrexate-induced pericarditis and pericardial effusion; first reported case. Postgrad Med J 1995;71:244–5.

[43] Savoia F, Gaddoni G, Casadio C, Patrizi A, Spadola G, Bassi P, et al. A case of aseptic pleuropericarditis in a patient with chronic plaque psoriasis under methotrexate therapy. Dermatol Online J 2010;16:13.

[44] Mohyuddin T, Elyan M, Kushner I. Pericarditis: a rare complication of methotrexate therapy. Clin Rheumatol 2007;26:2157–8.

[45] Palungwachira P, Palungwachira P, Laohathai P. Methotrexate induced pericarditis and pericardial effusion in psoriatic patient. J Med Assoc Thai 1998;81:141–5.

[46] Huang SY, Chang CS, Tang JL, Tien HF, Kuo TL, Huang SF, et al. Acute and chronic arsenic poisoning associated with treatment of acute promyelocytic leukaemia. Br J Haematol 1998;103:1092–5.

[47] Ueda K, Nagai S, Miyashita SI, Kaise T, Ichikawa M, Kumano K, et al. Arsenic-induced pericardial and pleural effusion without acute promyelocytic leukemia differentiation syndrome. Leuk Res 2010;34:e25–6.

[48] Calik AN, Celiker E, Velibey Y, Cagdas M, Guzelburc O. Initial dose effect of 5-fluorouracil: rapidly improving severe, acute toxic myopericarditis. Am J Emerg Med 2012;30:257.e1–3.

[49] Vincenzi B, Santini D, Frezza AM, Rocci L, Tonini G. Docetaxel induced pericardial effusion. J Exp Clin Cancer Res 2007;26:417–20.

Chapter 17

Radiation-Induced Carotid Atherosclerosis

F. Rigo

Chapter Outline

The association of neck radiotherapy and higher risks of asymptomatic or symptomatic carotid atherosclerosis has been currently well demonstrated. The risk of radiation-induced carotid atherosclerosis increases with the time interval from radiotherapy, with routine ultrasound screening proposed in patients who had received radiotherapy more than 5 years previously [1]. The disease is limited to the irradiated area, less likely associated with risk factors of the classical atherosclerotic process and dependent on radiotherapy dose [1]. Increased intima-medial thickness and higher grade of abnormality in the bulb wall were observed at doses higher than 35 Gy [2]. The relative risk of stroke has been reported to be as high as 5.6 in patients treated for head and neck cancer compared with a more modest relative risk of 1.12 in breast cancer patients and 2.3 in patients treated with $>$ 40 Gy for nonHodgkin's lymphoma [3].

The diagnostic and grading of radiation-induced carotid atherosclerosis using duplex ultrasound is based on the same principles as atherosclerotic carotid artery stenosis grading and plaque morphologic description [3].

Carotid intima-medial thickness may be an early and accurate means of evaluation of radiation-induced carotid atherosclerosis. Indeed, neck irradiation has been demonstrated to significantly increase the thickness of the carotid wall during the first year after treatment, on average 21 times more than in epidemiologically matched control volunteers [4]. In patients with Hodgkin's disease, when compared to controls, the irradiated cases had a greater intima-media thickness in the carotid artery distribution [5]. During a

Anticancer Treatments and Cardiotoxicity. DOI: http://dx.doi.org/10.1016/B978-0-12-802509-3.00017-0

3-year follow-up, it was noted that despite improvement in intima-media thickness at 3 years, there was persistently reduced flow-mediated dilatation in the irradiated carotid artery, suggesting that early endothelial damage persists [6].

Radiation-induced carotid disease differs from traditional carotid disease. Radiotherapy often produces carotid lesions that are more extensive than the traditional bifurcation stenosis, often involving atypical areas such as long segments of carotid artery [7]. Three possible mechanisms of chronic postradiation effects on medium and large arteries have been identified: (1) fibrosis due to a damaged vasa-vasorum; (2) adventitial fibrosis producing obstruction; and (3) accelerated atherosclerosis [8].

The treatment of radiation-induced carotid disease is similar to those in the general population with both percutaneous intervention and surgery used in selective cases [9].

REFERENCES

[1] Cheng SW, Wu LL, Ting AC, Lau H, Lam LK, Wei WI. Irradiation-induced extracranial carotid stenosis in patients with head and neck malignancies. Am J Surg 1999;178:323–8.

[2] Martin JD, Buckley AR, Graeb D, Walman B, Salvian A, Hay JH. Carotid artery stenosis in asymptomatic patients who have received unilateral head-and-neck irradiation. Int J Radiat Oncol Biol Phys 2005;63:1197–205.

[3] Gujral DM, Shah BN, Chahal NS, Senior R, Harrington KJ, Nutting CM. Clinical features of radiation-induced carotid atherosclerosis. Clin Oncol (R Coll Radiol) 2014;26:94–102.

[4] Muzaffar K, Collins SL, Labropoulos N, Baker WH. A prospective study of the effects of irradiation on the carotid artery. Laryngoscope 2000;110:1811–14.

[5] Bilora F, Pietrogrande F, Petrobelli F, Polato G, Pomerri F, Muzzio PC. Is radiation a risk factor for atherosclerosis? An echo-color Doppler study on Hodgkin and non-Hodgkin patients. Tumori 2006;92(4):295–8.

[6] Bilora F, Pietrogrande F, Campagnolo E, et al. Are Hodgkin and non-Hodgkin patients at a greater risk of atherosclerosis? A follow-up of 3 years. Eur J Cancer Care 2010;19(3): 417–19.

[7] Cheng SWK, Ting ACW, Lam LK, Wei WI. Carotid stenosis after radio therapy for nasopharyngeal carcinoma. Archives of Otolaryngology—Head and Neck Surgery 2000;126 (4):517–21.

[8] Carmody BJ, Arora S, Avena R, Curry KM, Simpkins J, Cosby K, et al. Accelerated carotid artery disease after high-dose head and neck radiotherapy: is there a role for routine carotid surveillance? J Vasc Surg 1999;30:1045–51.

[9] Lam WW, Leung SF, So NM, et al. Incidence of carotid stenosis in nasopharyngeal carcinoma patients after radiotherapy. Cancer 2001;92(9):2357–63.

Chapter 18

Valvular Heart Disease

J.C. Plana

Chapter Outline

Cancer therapeutics do not affect the cardiac valves directly. However, valvular heart disease may manifest in the oncologic patient for a number of other reasons: (1) preexisting valvular heart disease; (2) as a result of the malignancy itself; (3) due to concomitant or previous radiation therapy; (4) due to endocarditis in the setting of immune suppression as a complication of chemotherapy; or (5) as a result of left ventricular (LV) remodeling in the setting of cancer therapeutics-related cardiac dysfunction (CTRCD).

PREEXISTING LESIONS

Valve disease is highly prevalent in the general population with both mitral valve prolapse (MVP) and bicuspid aortic valve (BAV) each occurring in up to 2% of the population [1,2]. Additionally, degenerative disease, particularly of the aortic valve, is highly prevalent in older individuals.

VALVE DISEASE AS A RESULT OF THE MALIGNANCY

Valve disease is an uncommon complication of primary neoplastic disease. Primary or secondary cardiac tumors may impact valve function by their local extension.

Anticancer Treatments and Cardiotoxicity. DOI: http://dx.doi.org/10.1016/B978-0-12-802509-3.00018-2

However, what is more common is the development of nonthrombotic or marantic endocarditis. This condition is particularly prevalent in patients with lung, prostate, pancreas, or colon cancer. They most commonly occur in the left-sided valves and may result in thromboembolism. The valve lesions may vary in size from microscopic to large bulky lesions easily identifiable on transthoracic echocardiography. The lesions consist of a network of fibrin and platelets and may be associated with disseminated intravascular coagulopathy. The lesions may lead to impaired valve coaptation and regurgitation, which may evolve to be severe in nature. Rarely, the lesions are sufficiently bulky to give rise to significant stenosis. However, it is thromboembolism from these lesions that are most consequential to the patient, rather than their hemodynamic impact. Anticoagulation may lead to their resolution or at least a reduction in their size.

VALVE DISEASE DUE TO RADIATION THERAPY

Valve disease may occur secondary to previous or concomitant radiation therapy [3–5]. The pathological effects of radiation on valve tissue usually are not manifest acutely but rather develop over decades. Both valvular stenosis and regurgitation may occur, with regurgitation being somewhat more frequent. Left-sided valves are more commonly affected and radiation often leads to calcification of the valve and the subvalvular apparatus. The mitroaortic intervalvular fibrosa is particularly prone. As radiation may cause or exacerbate already existing coronary artery disease, ischemic valve lesions may also occur.

VALVE DISEASE RELATED TO INFECTIOUS COMPLICATIONS OF CHEMOTHERAPY

Cancer therapeutics may lead to pancytopenia which can be complicated by the development of bacteremia and endocarditis [6,7]. This is more likely to occur in those with predisposing valve lesions (i.e., MVP and BAV) but may occur even with normal valves in the setting of overwhelming bacteremia. Patients may develop endocarditis associated with the presence of bacteremia in the setting of a central venous catheter placed for vascular access during chemotherapeutic regimens.

VALVE DISEASE RELATED TO CARDIOTOXIC EFFECTS OF CHEMOTHERAPY

Valve disease may occur as a consequence of CTRCD. This usually manifests as mitral regurgitation from annular dilation or apical tethering in the setting of LV dysfunction and compensatory LV remodeling. Secondary tricuspid regurgitation may also occur due to right ventricular dysfunction or increased pulmonary arterial pressure in the setting of LV dysfunction. Both secondary mitral and tricuspid regurgitation occur later in the course of CTRCD, usually once significant dysfunction and geometric ventricular remodeling have occurred.

EVALUATION OF VALVULAR DISEASE IN PATIENTS WITH POTENTIAL CARDIOTOXICITY FROM CANCER CHEMOTHERAPEUTIC AGENTS

Echocardiography is the technique of choice in the evaluation of valvular disease in patients being screened for suspected cardiotoxicity from cancer chetherapeutics. Given the high prevalence of preexisting valve lesions and their impact on potential chemotherapeutic regimens, a careful echocardiographic examination of valve structure and function should be carried out before the initiation of cancer therapeutics, even in the absence of significant physical examination findings. Although physical examination may yield evidence of significant valve disease, milder lesions may not be audible and lesions associated with increased risk of endocarditis, for instance BAV, may not be apparent. Careful evaluation of the structure of each of the valves should be performed, paying careful attention to the presence of mobile echodensities suggestive of endocarditis or of calcification of the valve. Assessment of the severity of valvular stenosis or regurgitation should be performed based on the current ASE and EAE recommendations [8–11]. Although a complete transthoracic Doppler echocardiographic evaluation is often sufficient to evaluate the valve pathology and the hemodynamic consequences of valve dysfunction, transesophageal echocardiography may be of incremental value in the setting of suspected endocarditis, when transthoracic echo images are suboptimal or when there is concern for tumor involvement of valve tissue. Both CT scanning and MRI are not usually required in the routine evaluation of valve disease in oncologic patients but may have a role in assessing tumor infiltration of valvular structures or when radiation induced constriction or restrictive cardiomyopathy. Cardiac MRI may also be valuable in following ventricular volumes and function in patients with significant valve regurgitation.

Patients receiving chemotherapy with potential cardiotoxicity should have a careful reevaluation of valve structure and function on subsequent echocardiograms throughout the course of their treatment and subsequently. Patients with significant or changing valvular findings need to be evaluated more frequently and the relationship of the various therapeutic treatments to these structural and hemodynamic derangements assessed at each visit. The indications for follow-up and interventions on specific valve lesions should be based on the guidelines published by the American Heart Association/American College of Cardiology and the European Society of Cardiology [12,13], though these need to be adjusted to the individual prognosis and clinical situation of the patient.

REFERENCES

[1] Freed LA, Levy D, Levine RA, Larson MG, Evans JC, Fuller DL, et al. New prevalence and clinical outcome of mitral-valve prolapse. N Engl J Med 1999;341:1−347.

[2] Roberts WC. The congenitally bicuspid aortic valve. A study of 85 autopsy cases. Am J Cardiol 1970;26:72−83.

[3] Hamza A, Tunick PA, Kronzon I. Echocardiographic manifestations of complications of radiation therapy. Echocardiography 2009;26:724−8.

[4] Heidenreich PA, Kapoor JR. Radiation induced heart disease: systemic disorders in heart disease. Heart 2009;95:252−8.

[5] Heidenreich PA, Hancock SL, Lee BK, Mariscal CS, Schnittger I. Asymptomatic cardiac disease following mediastinal irradiation. J Am Coll Cardiol 2003;42:743−9.

[6] Edoute Y, Haim N, Rinkevich D, Brenner B, Reisner SA. Cardiac valvular vegetations in cancer patients: a prospective echocardiographic study of 200 patients. Am J Med 1997; 102:252−8.

[7] Eiken P, Edwards W, Tazelaar H, McBane R, Zehr K. Surgical pathology of nonbacterial thrombotic endocarditis in 30 patients, 1985−2000. Mayo Clinic Proc 2001;76:1204−12.

[8] Baumgartner H, Hung J, Bermejo J, Chambers JB, Evangelista A, Griffin BP, et al. EAE/ASE. Echocardiographic assessment of valve stenosis: EAE/ASE recommendations for clinical practice. Eur J Echocardiogr 2009;10:1−25.

[9] Lancellotti P, Tribouilloy C, Hagendorff A, Moura L, Popescu BA, Agricola E, et al. European Association of Echocardiography. European Association of Echocardiography recommendations for the assessment of valvular regurgitation. Part 1: aortic and pulmonary regurgitation (native valve disease). Eur J Echocardiogr 2010;11:223−44.

[10] Lancellotti P, Moura L, Pierard LA, Agricola E, Popescu BA, Tribouilloy C, et al. European Association of Echocardiography. European Association of Echocardiography recommendations for the assessment of valvular regurgitation. Part 2: mitral and tricuspid regurgitation (native valve disease). Eur J Echocardiogr 2010;11:307−32.

[11] Zoghbi WA, Enriquez-Sarano M, Foster E, Grayburn PA, Kraft CD, Levine RA, et al. American Society of Echocardiography. Recommendations for evaluation of the severity of native valvular regurgitation with two-dimensional and Doppler echocardiography. J Am Soc Echocardiogr 2003;16:777−802.

[12] Bonow RO, Carabello BA, Chatterjee K, de Leon Jr AC, Faxon DP, Freed MD, et al. 2008 focused update incorporated into the ACC/AHA 2006 guidelines for the management of patients with valvular heart disease: a report of the American College of Cardiology/American Heart Association Task Force on Practice Guidelines (Writing Committee to revise the 1998 guidelines for the management of patients with valvular heart disease). Endorsed by the Society of Cardiovascular Anesthesiologists, Society for Cardiovascular Angiography and Interventions, and Society of Thoracic Surgeons. J Am Coll Cardiol 2008;52:e1−142.

[13] Vahanian A, Alfieri O, Andreotti F, Antunes MJ, Barón-Esquivias G, Baumgartner H, et al. Guidelines on the management of valvular heart disease (version 2012): The Joint Task Force on the Management of Valvular Heart Disease of the European Society of Cardiology (ESC) and the European Association for Cardio-Thoracic Surgery (EACTS). Eur Heart J 2012;33:2451−96.

[14] Hering D, Faber L, Horstkotte D. Echocardiographic features of radiation-associated valvular disease. Am J Cardiol 2003;92:226−30.

Chapter 19

Atrial Fibrillation and Stroke in Cancer Patients

C.R. Manrique and J.C. Plana

Chapter Outline

INTRODUCTION

Atrial fibrillation (AF) has a significant impact on our society. Currently, this disease is considered a growing epidemic in the world with an estimated 33.5 million cases worldwide in 2010, and the expectation for the number of cases to rise by at least 5% per year [1]. In the same way, the number of patients with AF in the United States is expected to grow from 2.3 million in 2001 to 5.6–6.3 million in 2050 [2]. An epidemiological study conducted by Colilla et al. shows an incidence of 1.2 million cases in 2010, with a statistical projection to 2.6 million in 2030 [3]. Similar data have been reported in Europe with an estimated prevalence of AF in the general population of approximately 1.5–2% with an elevated economic cost for the healthcare systems [4]. However, the dimension of the real problem could be underestimated in the light of subclinical disease.

AF has been associated with major cardiovascular events including stroke, progressive heart failure, and sudden cardiac death, with the resultant disability and elevated mortality [5–7]. Stroke, the most feared complication of AF, has a high burden on society. European epidemiological reports consider it the leading cause of disability, morbidity, and mortality, and one of the most frequent etiologies of dementia, seizure disorders, and depression in the elderly [8]. According to the 2015 Heart Disease and Stroke Report from the American Heart Association (AHA), approximately 795,000 strokes are reported each year in the United States. One occurs every 40 s, and causes the death of an American every 4 min [9].

Anticancer Treatments and Cardiotoxicity. DOI: http://dx.doi.org/10.1016/B978-0-12-802509-3.00019-4

It is estimated that AF confers a fivefold increase in the likelihood of cerebrovascular events in all ages and accounts for 15% of all strokes [5]. This has special impact on the elderly. But other populations identified with an elevated risk are females, patients with hypertension, diabetes mellitus, heart failure, vascular disease, and anyone with a history of cerebrovascular disease. In addition, elevation of cardiac biomarker including N-terminal pro-B-type natriuretic peptide and troponin I in patients affected by this entity have been related to an increase in the risk for thromboembolic events and death [10].

CANCER AND ATRIAL FIBRILLATION

Although several chronic conditions including valvular heart disease (especially mitral valve pathology), hypertension, cardiomyopathies, and coronary artery disease, as well as alcohol consumption and hyperthyroidism, are traditionally related to the development of AF in the general population [11], malignancy is not considered part of the clinical entities that confer predisposition for it. Cancer is not part of the pathological states that are taken into account in the different clinical scores developed to predict the risk of thromboembolic events in patients with AF (i.e., CHADS2, CHA2DS2-VASc, and ATRIA scores) [12–14]. However, malignancy has been incorporated in some (HEMORR2HAGES, RIETE) [15] but not in all of bleeding risk scores used in the guidance of antithrombotic therapy in patients with AF (i.e., HAS-BLED, ATRIA scores) [16–17].

Despite this, there has been a growing body of scientific evidence establishing the association of malignant disease and AF over recent decades. Large epidemiological studies have found an increased association between cancer and elevated prevalence of AF compared to the general population [18–19]. Additionally, several groups have described an increased frequency of AF in the cancer population, especially in patients undergoing surgical intervention as part of their treatment. An incidence of up to 28% of postoperative AF has been reported for lung, esophageal, and colorectal cancer, incidence that is elevated when compared to similar populations undergoing surgery for nonneoplastic conditions [20–22]. Moreover, increased postoperative mortality, critical care unit admission rates, longer hospitalization, and higher rates of death from cardiovascular diseases have been described in patients with AF after oncologic surgery [23]. It has also been suggested as a predictor of poor long-term mortality among 5-year survivors, although the current evidence in this regard is controversial. Finally, a retrospective study comparing cardiovascular outcomes reported a greater tendency to thromboembolic events in patients with AF undergoing treatment for colorectal, breast, head and neck, and cervical cancers [18].

The underlying mechanism responsible for the association between AF and malignancy is not well understood. The cancer population is usually affected by other comorbidities that may predispose to the development of AF. Furthermore, the amplified inflammatory response seen in patients affected by neoplastic processes, the hyperadrenergic state with the characteristic autonomic nervous system imbalance, and the frequent metabolic and electrolyte derangements typical of this patients have been proposed as the perfect substrate for electrical disturbances of the cardiovascular system [24]. Additionally, AF may be induced by chemotherapeutic agents and/or associated with surgical protocols that are usually required for the effective treatment of the disease [25–26]. Finally, a direct contribution of the tumor due to primary or metastatic involvement of the cardiac structures or adjacent organs, as well as paraneoplastic syndromes have been postulated as associated factors to this arrhythmia.

AF SECONDARY TO CANCER TREATMENT

It is known that initiation of AF requires a trigger event and a well-defined substrate for its perpetuation through reentrant circuits. As previously discussed, the burden of cardiovascular comorbidities in patients with cancer is elevated, promoting atrial and pulmonary vein dilatation and atrial fibrosis, pathophysiological conditions considered to be the substrate required for the maintenance of conduction disorders [27]. Some of the cancer therapeutics have been related to induction of AF, most likely through generation of ectopic activity or due to their effect on the electrical properties of the atrial tissue.

Delayed after-depolarizations is the most important mechanism associated with ectopic atrial activity, which in the setting of the described electrical and structural changes, is the most common trigger seen in AF generation. Additionally, activation of the autonomic nervous system (parasympathetic and sympathetic) has been associated with changes in the action potential, refractoriness, and repolarization of the atrial tissue leading to proarrhythmic activity.

Drug-induced AF related to antineoplastic agents have been reported in small studies, especially for antimicrotubule agents (paclitaxel and docetaxel) in 1% of the patients [28], interleukin-2 (4–8%) [29–30], alkylating agents (cisplatin, cyclophosphamide), antimetabolites (5-fluorouracil), and anthracyclines (doxorubicin and mitoxantrone) in 10.3% of patients; paroxysmal AF manifested early after infusion has been the most frequent form reported [31]. In the same way, corticosteroids, predominantly high-dose methylprednisolone, have been reported in clinical trials to be associated with AF, but evidence is conflicting and equivocal.

On the other hand, causality of a single agent has been difficult to establish. Multiantineoplastic regimens used as part of the therapeutic approach against malignant disease, the presence of medical conditions in most of the patients that are predisposed to cardiac events, the significant systemic inflammation, and the elevated psychosocial stress are factors that are present most of the time in patients undergoing cancer therapy. Additionally, prediction of AF events secondary to chemotherapy is challenging due to the lack of biochemical or electrocardiographic markers for drug-induced AF.

MANAGEMENT AND STROKE PREVENTION

Current guidelines contain well-defined recommendations for the treatment of AF in the general population, including antithrombotic guidance for stroke prevention. However, these strategies have to be applied with caution in cancer patients, for whom the decision-making process can be challenging due to several factors that should be considered throughout the clinical evaluation.

Medications recommended for rate control including β-blockers, nondihydropyridynes calcium channel blockers, and digoxin. They should be used taking into consideration the individual clinical presentation, patient comorbidities, volume status, and hemodynamic condition. Potential interactions with concomitant antineoplastic agents should be evaluated to avoid side effects. Commonly, QT interval prolongation is seen as a result of antiarrhythmic therapy (i.e., amiodarone, sotalol), as well as therapies for cancer or antiemetics (frequently used as supportive treatment during chemotherapy). For those reasons, special attention to electrocardiographic changes should be encouraged when therapeutic plans include the use of medications that cause QT prolongation, including histone deacetylase inhibitors (i.e., vorinostat), tyrosine kinase inhibitors (i.e., dasatinib, lapatinib, sunitinib), the BRAF inhibitor vemurafenib, and arsenic trioxide, although no formal recommendations have been made [32].

Nevertheless, one of the most challenging aspects of AF treatment in the cancer patient is the prevention of cardioembolic events and stroke. As previously discussed, malignant disease confers a hypercoagulable state increasing the risk of thromboembolic complications in patients with AF, favoring the implementation of antithrombotic therapy. But at the same time, frequently the cancer patients have predisposition to hemorrhagic complications, especially in individuals with hematological malignancies (including myeloproliferative or myelodysplastic disorders), profound thrombocytopenia related to cancer or secondary to cancer treatment, and intracranial tumors. In this context, a judicious evaluation of the particular clinical situation is necessary to determine the risk–benefit relationship of anticoagulation or antiplatelet medications as part of a tailored therapeutic approach.

Although the current guidelines for AF management (AHA, American College of Cardiology (ACC), and the European Society of Cardiology (ESC)) [4–33] recommend the use of CHA2DS2-VASc score for prediction of stroke, none of the tools used in daily clinical practice (CHADS2, CHA2DS2-VASc, and ATRIA) has been validated in cancer patients [12–14]. In addition, there are some concerns about the reliability of these tools in this special population. This was elucidated in a large epidemiological study that included 24,125 cancer patients in which the CHADS2 score could not predict the incidence of thromboembolism in patients with new-onset AF compared to patients with known AF [18]. Finally, the risk assessment should include the antineoplastic therapy used, especially when medications that have potential thromboembolic complications, such as alkylating agents (i.e., cisplatin) [34], hormonal therapy (i.e., tamoxifen) [35], or angiogenesis inhibitors (i.e., bevacizumab, sunitinib, sorafenib) [36, 37], are required.

Finally, bleeding scores provide an estimation of the bleeding risk, allowing the optimization of the correctable predisposing factors for hemorrhagic events [4]. Although the Canadian Cardiovascular Society Guidelines, the European Heart Rhythm Association (EHRA), and the ESC recommended the use of the HAS-BLED score for bleeding risk assessment in the general population, the HEMORR2HAGES score (which includes malignancy as a risk factor) could be more accurate for the prediction of hemorrhagic complications in patients with cancer. However, this hypothesis needs to be further evaluated in clinical trials.

Selection of the best therapeutic approach for prevention of thromboembolic events in AF is critical. Use of antiplatelet medications (aspirin (ASA) or ASA in combination with clopidogrel) has shown a similar risk of major bleeding or intracranial hemorrhage compared with oral anticoagulants (especially in the elderly), without offering a reliable protection against stroke in patients with AF [38,39]. For those reasons, their use is not recommended by the current AHA/ACC guidelines as part of the therapeutic strategy for stroke prevention in patients with AF [33]. Similarly, in 2012 the ESC recommended antiplatelet therapy only in cases where patients who are at risk of stroke refuse any systemic anticoagulation. Also, ASA monotherapy is recommended only in patients refusing anticoagulation with excessive risk of bleeding [4].

Vitamin K antagonists have been the cornerstone of stroke prevention in high-risk patients during recent decades [40]. However, special attention is required to avoid pharmacological interaction with concomitant cancer therapy that may lead to an unpredictable anticoagulant effect, especially in the setting of frequent gastrointestinal symptoms (diarrhea, vomiting), liver dysfunction, and metabolic disturbances seen in patients with malignant diseases. Close follow-up of the international normalized ratio is required to assure effective protection against stroke, which may be challenging in this population. Some reports have documented elevated risk of hemorrhagic events in patients with cancer (compared to the general population) who received warfarin due to venous thromboembolism [41]. However, no robust data are available at this time for delineation of formal recommendations to address this concern.

Although the novel oral anticoagulants (NOACs) have demonstrated a better safety profile due to less intracranial hemorrhage with noninferior preventive effect as opposed to stroke patients with nonvalvular AF, the experience in cancer patients is limited at this time. Unfortunately, recent clinical trials evaluating the efficacy for stroke prevention of the NOACs including dabigatran (RE-LY) [42], apixiban (ARISTOTLE) [43], and rivaroxaban

(ROCKET AF) [44] excluded patients with cancer. Additionally, the increased risk of bleeding in patients with active malignancy has raised concerns about the safety of NOACs, especially in the setting of potential drug interactions with chemotherapeutic agents metabolized by the CYP3A4 enzyme and/or P-glycoprotein transporter, as well as the frequent metabolic disturbance with changing liver and renal function, and the lack of effective reversal strategies for this group of medications. These medications should be used with caution in patients with active malignancy until solid evidence regarding efficacy and safety is derived from clinical studies. In the same way, there is no clinical experience of the role of left atrial appendage closure devices in cancer populations.

CONCLUSIONS

AF is a frequent entity in patients with cancer. Managing it and preventing stroke are challenging due to the elevated risk of bleeding and thrombosis seen in this population. Development of new clinical tools for assessing the risk of stroke and predicting hemorrhagic complications are required. ASA is not recommended at this time for prevention of thromboembolic events even in low-risk patients. Finally, larger prospective studies are required for evaluation of NOACs and advanced therapies in patients affected with malignant diseases.

REFERENCES

[1] Piccini JP, Hammill BG, Sinner MF, et al. Incidence and prevalence of atrial fibrillation and associated mortality among Medicare beneficiaries, 1993-2007. Circ Cardiovasc Qual Outcomes 2012;5(1):85–93.

[2] Go AS, Hylek EM, Phillips KA, et al. Prevalence of diagnosed atrial fibrillation in adults: national implications for rhythm management and stroke prevention: the AnTicoagulation and Risk Factors in Atrial Fibrillation (ATRIA) Study. Jama 2001;285(18):2370–5.

[3] Colilla S, Crow A, Petkun W, Singer DE, Simon T, Liu X. Estimates of current and future incidence and prevalence of atrial fibrillation in the U.S. adult population. Am J Cardiol 2013;112(8):1142–7.

[4] Camm AJ, Lip GY, De Caterina R, et al. 2012 focused update of the ESC Guidelines for the management of atrial fibrillation: an update of the 2010 ESC Guidelines for the management of atrial fibrillation. Developed with the special contribution of the European Heart Rhythm Association. Eur Heart J 2012;33(21):2719–47.

[5] Wolf PA, Abbott RD, Kannel WB. Atrial fibrillation as an independent risk factor for stroke: the Framingham Study. Stroke 1991;22(8):983–8.

[6] Marijon E, Le Heuzey JY, Connolly S, et al. Causes of death and influencing factors in patients with atrial fibrillation: a competing-risk analysis from the randomized evaluation of long-term anticoagulant therapy study. Circulation 2013;128(20):2192–201.

[7] Gottdiener JS, Arnold AM, Aurigemma GP, et al. Predictors of congestive heart failure in the elderly: the Cardiovascular Health Study. J Am Coll Cardiol 2000;35(6):1628–37.

[8] European Stroke Organisation Executive C, Committee ESOW. Guidelines for management of ischaemic stroke and transient ischaemic attack 2008. Cerebrovasc Dis 2008;25 (5):457–507.

[9] Mozaffarian D, Benjamin EJ, Go AS, et al. Heart disease and stroke statistics–2015 update: a report from the American Heart Association. Circulation 2015;131(4):e29–322.
[10] Hijazi Z, Oldgren J, Andersson U, et al. Cardiac biomarkers are associated with an increased risk of stroke and death in patients with atrial fibrillation: a Randomized Evaluation of Long-term Anticoagulation Therapy (RE-LY) substudy. Circulation 2012;125(13):1605–16.
[11] Page RL. Clinical practice. Newly diagnosed atrial fibrillation. N Engl J Med 2004;351 (23):2408–16.
[12] Gage BF, Waterman AD, Shannon W, Boechler M, Rich MW, Radford MJ. Validation of clinical classification schemes for predicting stroke: results from the National Registry of Atrial Fibrillation. Jama 2001;285(22):2864–70.
[13] Lip GY, Nieuwlaat R, Pisters R, Lane DA, Crijns HJ. Refining clinical risk stratification for predicting stroke and thromboembolism in atrial fibrillation using a novel risk factor-based approach: the euro heart survey on atrial fibrillation. Chest 2010;137(2):263–72.
[14] Singer DE, Chang Y, Borowsky LH, et al. A new risk scheme to predict ischemic stroke and other thromboembolism in atrial fibrillation: the ATRIA study stroke risk score. J Am Heart Assoc 2013;2(3):e000250.
[15] Gage BF, Yan Y, Milligan PE, et al. Clinical classification schemes for predicting hemorrhage: results from the National Registry of Atrial Fibrillation (NRAF). Am Heart J 2006;151(3):713–19.
[16] Pisters R, Lane DA, Nieuwlaat R, de Vos CB, Crijns HJ, Lip GY. A novel user-friendly score (HAS-BLED) to assess 1-year risk of major bleeding in patients with atrial fibrillation: the Euro Heart Survey. Chest 2010;138(5):1093–100.
[17] Fang MC, Go AS, Chang Y, et al. A new risk scheme to predict warfarin-associated hemorrhage: the ATRIA (Anticoagulation and Risk Factors in Atrial Fibrillation) Study. J Am Coll Cardiol 2011;58(4):395–401.
[18] Hu YF, Liu CJ, Chang PM, et al. Incident thromboembolism and heart failure associated with new-onset atrial fibrillation in cancer patients. Int J Cardiol 2013;165(2):355–7.
[19] Erichsen R, Christiansen CF, Mehnert F, Weiss NS, Baron JA, Sorensen HT. Colorectal cancer and risk of atrial fibrillation and flutter: a population-based case-control study. Intern Emerg Med 2012;7(5):431–8.
[20] Onaitis M, D'Amico T, Zhao Y, O'Brien S, Harpole D. Risk factors for atrial fibrillation after lung cancer surgery: analysis of the Society of Thoracic Surgeons general thoracic surgery database. Ann Thorac Surg 2010;90(2):368–74.
[21] Siu CW, Tung HM, Chu KW, Jim MH, Lau CP, Tse HF. Prevalence and predictors of new-onset atrial fibrillation after elective surgery for colorectal cancer. Pacing Clin Electrophysiol 2005;28(Suppl. 1):S120–123.
[22] Nojiri T, Maeda H, Takeuchi Y, et al. Predictive value of B-type natriuretic peptide for postoperative atrial fibrillation following pulmonary resection for lung cancer. Eur J Cardiothorac Surg 2010;37(4):787–91.
[23] Imperatori A, Mariscalco G, Riganti G, Rotolo N, Conti V, Dominioni L. Atrial fibrillation after pulmonary lobectomy for lung cancer affects long-term survival in a prospective single-center study. J Cardiothorac Surg 2012;7:4.
[24] Guo Y, Lip GY, Apostolakis S. Inflammation in atrial fibrillation. J Am Coll Cardiol 2012;60(22):2263–70.
[25] Kaakeh Y, Overholser BR, Lopshire JC, Tisdale JE. Drug-induced atrial fibrillation. Drugs 2012;72(12):1617–30.
[26] van der Hooft CS, Heeringa J, van Herpen G, Kors JA, Kingma JH, Stricker BH. Drug-induced atrial fibrillation. J Am Coll Cardiol 2004;44(11):2117–24.

[27] Wakili R, Voigt N, Kaab S, Dobrev D, Nattel S. Recent advances in the molecular pathophysiology of atrial fibrillation. J Clin Invest 2011;121(8):2955–68.

[28] Kamineni P, Prakasa K, Hasan SP, Akula R, Dawkins F. Cardiotoxicities of paclitaxel in African Americans. J Natl Med Assoc 2003;95(10):977–81.

[29] Margolin KA, Rayner AA, Hawkins MJ, et al. Interleukin-2 and lymphokine-activated killer cell therapy of solid tumors: analysis of toxicity and management guidelines. J Clin Oncol 1989;7(4):486–98.

[30] Lee RE, Lotze MT, Skibber JM, et al. Cardiorespiratory effects of immunotherapy with interleukin-2. J Clin Oncol 1989;7(1):7–20.

[31] Kilickap S, Barista I, Akgul E, Aytemir K, Aksoy S, Tekuzman G. Early and late arrhythmogenic effects of doxorubicin. South Med J 2007;100(3):262–5.

[32] Kim PY, Ewer MS. Chemotherapy and QT prolongation: overview with clinical perspective. Curr Treat Options Cardiovasc Med 2014;16(5):303.

[33] January CT, Wann LS, Alpert JS, et al. 2014 AHA/ACC/HRS guideline for the management of patients with atrial fibrillation: a report of the American College of Cardiology/American Heart Association Task Force on Practice Guidelines and the Heart Rhythm Society. J Am Coll Cardiol 2014;64(21):e1-76.

[34] Moore RA, Adel N, Riedel E, et al. High incidence of thromboembolic events in patients treated with cisplatin-based chemotherapy: a large retrospective analysis. J Clin Oncol 2011;29(25):3466–73.

[35] Freedman AN, Yu B, Gail MH, et al. Benefit/risk assessment for breast cancer chemoprevention with raloxifene or tamoxifen for women age 50 years or older. J Clin Oncol 2011;29(17):2327–33.

[36] Scappaticci FA, Skillings JR, Holden SN, et al. Arterial thromboembolic events in patients with metastatic carcinoma treated with chemotherapy and bevacizumab. J Natl Cancer Inst 2007;99(16):1232–9.

[37] Choueiri TK, Schutz FA, Je Y, Rosenberg JE, Bellmunt J. Risk of arterial thromboembolic events with sunitinib and sorafenib: a systematic review and meta-analysis of clinical trials. J Clin Oncol 2010;28(13):2280–5.

[38] Hart RG, Pearce LA, Aguilar MI. Meta-analysis: antithrombotic therapy to prevent stroke in patients who have nonvalvular atrial fibrillation. Ann Intern Med 2007;146(12):857–67.

[39] Lip GY. The role of aspirin for stroke prevention in atrial fibrillation. Nat Rev Cardiol 2011;8(10):602–6.

[40] Meschia JF, Bushnell C, Boden-Albala B, et al. Guidelines for the primary prevention of stroke: a statement for healthcare professionals from the American Heart Association/American Stroke Association. Stroke 2014;45(12):3754–832.

[41] Hutten BA, Prins MH, Gent M, Ginsberg J, Tijssen JG, Buller HR. Incidence of recurrent thromboembolic and bleeding complications among patients with venous thromboembolism in relation to both malignancy and achieved international normalized ratio: a retrospective analysis. J Clin Oncol 2000;18(17):3078–83.

[42] Connolly SJ, Ezekowitz MD, Yusuf S, et al. Dabigatran versus warfarin in patients with atrial fibrillation. N Engl J Med 2009;361(12):1139–51.

[43] Granger CB, Alexander JH, McMurray JJ, et al. Apixaban versus warfarin in patients with atrial fibrillation. N Engl J Med 2011;365(11):981–92.

[44] Patel MR, Mahaffey KW, Garg J, et al. Rivaroxaban versus warfarin in nonvalvular atrial fibrillation. N Engl J Med 2011;365(10):883–91.

Section IV

Imaging Evaluation of Cardiac Structure and Function in Cancer Patients

Chapter 20

The Role of Echocardiography

Chapter Outline

Anticancer Treatments and Cardiotoxicity. DOI: http://dx.doi.org/10.1016/B978-0-12-802509-3.00020-0

Chapter 20.1

Standard Echo-Doppler Evaluation: LV Systolic and Diastolic Function, Right Ventricular Function, Valvular Heart Disease

M. Galderisi and R. Sorrentino

Among the different cardiac imaging modalities, echocardiography has a key role in the evaluation of cancer patients because of its large availability and feasibility and also the lack of radiation exposure in comparison with other modalities. Echocardiography is therefore particularly suitable for serial assessment of left ventricular (LV) and right ventricular (RV) structure and function as well as for a comprehensive assessment of cardiac valves, aorta, and pericardium. The joint recommendations from the American Society of Echocardiography (ASE) and the European Association of Cardiovascular Imaging (EACVI) have recently described the role of echocardiography in the oncologic setting [1].

LV SYSTOLIC FUNCTION

The exposure to potentially cardiotoxic anticancer agents is a recognized indication for baseline and sequential evaluation of LV systolic function during and after cancer therapy treatment including radiotherapy [2,3]. Table 20.1 summarizes echo parameters of LV structure and systolic function (and their cutoff points of normalcy), which can also be used in the oncologic setting.

The most commonly used parameter for monitoring LV function with echocardiography is *LV ejection fraction* (LVEF). Additional measurements of LV systolic function include *stroke volume* (mL, LV end-diastolic volume−LV end-systolic volume) and *cardiac output* (L/m, stroke volume × heart rate). Accurate assessment of EF by 2D echocardiography should be done at baseline, during, and after cancer treatment and is particularly useful in patients who present cardiac morbidities or clinical findings suggestive of LV systolic dysfunction [4,5]. According to the joint recommendations from The American Society of Echocardiography (ASE) and the European Association of Echocardiography (EAE), the method of choice for LV volume quantitation and LVEF determination (%, LVEDV−LVESV/LVEDV × 100, where EDV is end-diastolic volume and ESV is end-systolic volume) is the modified biplane Simpson's (method of discs) in apical four-chamber and two-chamber views [6]. Fig. 20.1 shows a reduced LVEF (=45%) in a patient with lymphoma undergoing anthracycline treatment. The use of *endocardial*

TABLE 20.1 Main Echo Doppler Parameters of LV and RV Function (and Relative Cutoff Points of Normalcy) to Be Evaluated in Cancer Patients During Time

Echo Doppler Parameter	Cutoff Point of Normalcy in Women	Cutoff Point of Normalcy in Men
LV end-diastolic diameter (mm)	<52.2 mm	<58.4 mm
LV end-systolic diameter (mm)	<34.8 mm	<39.8 mm
LV ejection fraction (%)	<54%	>52%
Septal e′ velocity (cm/s)[a]	>7.6	>7.6
Lateral e′ velocity (cm/s)[a]	>11.5	>11.5
E/e′ ratio (average e′)[a]	<13	<13
RV basal diameter (mm)	<42	<42
TAPSE (mm)	<17	<17
Tricuspid annular s′ velocity (cm/s)[a]	<9.5	<9.5

E, transmitral early velocity; e′, early diastolic velocity; LV, left ventricular; RV, right ventricular; s′, systolic velocity; TAPSE, tricuspid annular systolic excursion.
[a]*Data referring to age range of 41–60 years.*

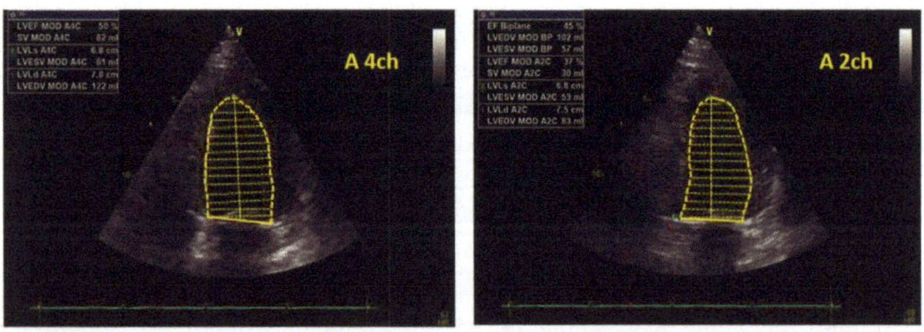

FIGURE 20.1 Calculation of LVEF by 2D echocardiography in a patient with lymphoma undergoing anthracyclines. LVEF is 50% in apical four-chamber view (left panel) and 37% in apical two-chamber view (right panel). The final value of biplane LVEF is 45% (right panel). *LVEDV*, LV end-diastolic volume; *LVEF*, LV ejection fraction; *LVESV*, LV end-systolic volume; *SV*, stroke volume.

fractional shortening (%) by using linear measurements of LV internal diameters ((LV end-diastolic diameter−LV end-systolic diameter)/LV end-diastolic diameter × 100), used in the past and particularly in cancer childhood, should be discouraged because coronary artery disease may occur in patients with cancer and cancer therapy-related cardiac toxicity can even induce regional wall motion abnormalities in LV walls other than anterior septum and posterior wall which are taken into account when calculating endocardial fractional shortening. Since regional wall motion abnormalities often involve only few LV segments or walls without necessarily affecting global LV function, the visual assessment of the wall motion score index should be also reported [7].

LVEF itself and LVEF drop during and after cancer treatment are currently used to define the onset of cardiotoxicity in cancer patients. Different cutoff values of LVEF (e.g., $<50\%$, $<55\%$) have been used to define cardiac toxicity based on LVEF at rest [8,9]. New, normal cutoff points of LVEF ($\geq 52\%$ in men and ≥ 54 in women) have been recently established by 2015 chamber quantification ASE/EACVI paper [6] and should be recommended. Changes in LVEF indicative of LV damage can be more appropriately identified when comparisons are made between baseline and follow-up studies. ASE/EACVI recommendations on the use of cardiac imaging in cancer patients fix the drop of LVEF of at least 10 points to an LVEF $<50\%$ as indicative of cardiotoxicity [1].

Although LVEF drop can also be used to predict the development of subsequent heart failure [10–12], the ability of serial LVEF calculation in the oncologic setting remains controversial [13]. General limitations of 2D echo-derived LVEF include its failure to detect small changes in LV contractility, the possibility of inadequate visualization of true LV apex and the inherent variability of the measurement. In addition, a detectable decrease in LVEF will occur only when a substantial amount of myocardial damage occur. Thus, a decreased posttreatment LVEF is often a marker of already extensive damage. In a study of cancer patients undergoing chemotherapy but free of heart failure symptoms, the upper limit of the confidence interval of 2D LVEF was 10% (range = 9.1–11.8) [14]. Therefore, 2D echo appears to be reliable in the detection of differences of LVEF $\geq 10\%$. Since this magnitude of change is often used to establish the presence of cardiotoxicity, the sensitivity of 2D LVEF appears to be poor for changes during time lower than 10%.

LV DIASTOLIC FUNCTION

In general, heart failure can develop even in the presence of normal EF (heart failure with normal or preserved EF), it being substantially due to LV diastolic dysfunction. Table 20.1 summarizes Doppler diastolic parameters (and their cutoff points of normalcy) which can be used also in the oncologic setting to identify LV diastolic dysfunction. Of interest, Doppler measurements are age-dependent and should therefore be considered in relation to the age of individual patients.

Isolated diastolic abnormalities have been found to be an early sign of anthracycline-induced LV dysfunction [15–19]. Pulsed tissue Doppler (reduction of early diastolic (e′) velocity of LV mitral annulus) is more

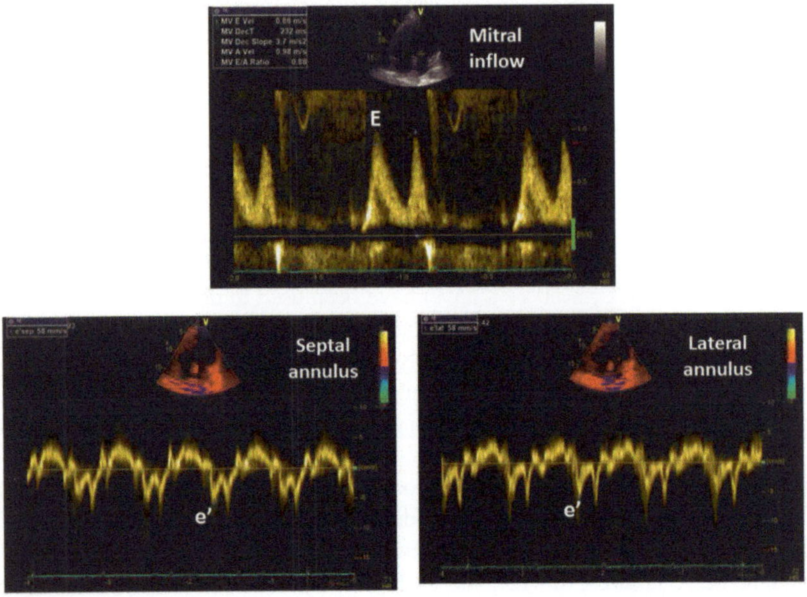

FIGURE 20.2 Elevated estimate of LV filling pressures in a woman with breast cancer, undergoing epirubicine followed by trastuzumab. The E/e′ ratio is 14.83 (normal value <13).

sensitive than standard Doppler-derived mitral inflow to detect LV diastolic dysfunction as a result of chemotherapy [20–23]. A recent position statement from the Heart Failure Association of the European Society of Cardiology on cardiovascular adverse effects of cancer therapies suggests to take attention also on LV diastolic function for detecting cardiotoxicity [5]. A comprehensive assessment of LV diastolic function, including an estimate of LV filling pressure (in particular E/e′ ratio) should be performed according to the joint ASE–EAE recommendations on LV diastolic function [24]. Because of its relative preload independency, e′ velocity can in fact be used to correct for the effect of LV relaxation on mitral E velocity [24]. Fig. 20.2 shows a high E/e′ ratio in a breast cancer woman undergoing anthracycline followed by trastuzumab and referring for dyspnea. However, the use of the E/e′ ratio has been questioned in oncologic patients as variations of e′ velocity amplitude could be the consequence of changes in sudden loading conditions occurring as a result of adverse effects induced by chemotherapy (nausea, vomiting, and diarrhea), more than the result of a real impairment of diastolic performance [1]. Little information is available about other recognized estimates of LV filling pressure such as the time duration difference between pulmonary venous flow atrial reverse velocity (Ar) and transmitral atrial (A) velocity and/or the use of Valsalva maneuver applied to LV mitral inflow. Also, left atrial dilation (left atrial volume index ≥ 34 mL/m^2) has been poorly investigated in the oncologic setting. It is noteworthy, however, that diastolic parameters have not shown any power in predicting subsequent cancer therapy-related cardiotoxicity [1].

RV FUNCTION

RV abnormalities may occur in oncologic patients for a number of reasons: preexisting RV dysfunction, neoplastic involvement (primary or metastatic), or as a result of the cardiotoxic effects of chemotherapy [25]. However, frequency and prognostic value of RV involvement have not been investigated in the oncologic setting [26]. Parameters (and cutoff points of normalcy) to be evaluated are reported in Table 20.1 [6]. An estimate of right ventricular systolic pressure should be provided, in particular in patients treated with dasatinib, a tyrosine kinase inhibitor, as pulmonary arterial hypertension may be a specific complication [27].

HEART VALVE DISEASE

Valvular disease may develop in oncologic patients for several reasons. Primary (malignant) or secondary (metastases) tumors may affect valve function (in particular left valves). They may be due also to concomitant or previous radiation therapy [28,29]. Valve function should be carefully monitored during and after radiotherapy according to standardized ASE/EACVI procedures [30]. Chemotherapy-induced pancytopenia is associated with an increased risk of endocarditis, in particular on predisposing valve lesions (i.e., mitral valve prolapse and bicuspid aortic valve) [31], or on central venous catheters placed for vascular access [32]. Functional mitral regurgitation, due to LV dilation and dysfunction, and/or secondary tricuspid regurgitation, due to RV dysfunction or pulmonary hypertension can also occur as a consequence of cancer-related cardiotoxicity. Although transthoracic echo is often sufficient to evaluate valve dysfunction and its hemodynamic consequences, transesophageal echocardiography may add incremental information.

REFERENCES

[1] Plana JC, Galderisi M, Barac A, Ewer MS, Ky B, Scherrer-Crosbie M, et al. Expert consensus for multimodality imaging evaluation of adult patients during and after cancer therapy: a report from the American Society of Echocardiography and the European Association of Cardiovascular Imaging. Eur Heart J Cardiovasc Imaging 2014;15:1063–93.

[2] Cheitlin MD, Armstrong WF, Aurigemma GP, Beller GA, Bierman FZ, Davis JL, et al. ACC/AHA/ASE 2003 Guideline Update for the Clinical Application of Echocardiography: summary article. A report of the American College of Cardiology/American Heart Association Task Force on Practice Guidelines (ACC/AHA/ASE Committee to Update the 1997 Guidelines for the Clinical Application of Echocardiography). J Am Soc Echocardiogr 2003;16:1091–110.

[3] American College of Cardiology Foundation Appropriate Use Criteria Task Force, American Society of Echocardiography, American Heart Association, American Society of Nuclear Cardiology, Heart Failure Society of America, Heart Rhythm Society, et al. ACCF/ASE/AHA/ASNC/HFSA/HRS/SCAI/SCCM/SCCT/SCMR 2011 Appropriate Use Criteria for Echocardiography. A Report of the American College of Cardiology Foundation Appropriate Use Criteria Task Force, American Society of Echocardiography, American Heart Association, American Society of Nuclear Cardiology, Heart Failure Society of America, Heart Rhythm Society, Society for Cardiovascular Angiography and Interventions, Society of Critical Care Medicine, Society of Cardiovascular Computed Tomography, Society for Cardiovascular Magnetic Resonance American College of Chest Physicians. J Am Soc Echocardiogr 2011;24:229–67.

[4] Steingart RM, Bakris GL, Chen HX, Chen MH, Force T, Ivy SP, et al. Management of cardiac toxicity in patients receiving vascular endothelial growth factor signaling pathway inhibitors. Am Heart J 2012;163:156–63.

[5] Eschenhagen T, Force T, Ewer MS, de Keulenaer GW, Suter TM, Anker SD, et al. Cardiovascular side effects of cancer therapies: a position statement from the Heart Failure Association of the European Society of Cardiology. Eur J Heart Fail 2011;13:1–10.

[6] Lang RM, Badano LP, Mor-Avi V, Afilalo J, Armstrong A, Ernande L, et al. Recommendations for cardiac chamber quantification by echocardiography in adults: an update from the American Society of Echocardiography and the European Association of Cardiovascular Imaging. Eur Heart J Cardiovasc Imaging 2015;16:233–70.

[7] Bountioukos M, Doorduijn JK, Roelandt JR, Vourvouri EC, Bax JJ, Schinkel AF, et al. Repetitive dobutamine stress echocardiography for the prediction of anthracycline cardiotoxicity. Eur J Echocardiogr 2003;4:300–5.

[8] Moja L, Tagliabue L, Balduzzi S, Parmelli E, Pistotti V, Guarneri V, et al. Trastuzumab containing regimens for early breast cancer. Cochrane Database Syst Rev 2012;4:CD006243.

[9] Seidman A, Hudis C, Pierri MK, Shak S, Paton V, Ashby M, et al. Cardiac dysfunction in the trastuzumab clinical trials experience. J Clin Oncol 2002;20:1215–21.

[10] Mitani I, Jain D, Joska TM, Burtness B, Zaret BL. Doxorubicin cardiotoxicity: prevention of congestive heart failure with serial cardiac function monitoring with equilibrium radionuclide angiocardiography in the current era. J Nucl Cardiol 2003;10:132–9.

[11] Jensen BV, Skovsgaard T, Nielsen SL. Functional monitoring of anthracycline cardiotoxicity: a prospective, blinded, long-term observational study of outcome in 120 patients. Ann Oncol 2002;13:699–709.

[12] Steinherz LJ, Steinherz PG, Tan CT, Heller G, Murphy ML. Cardiac toxicity 4 to 20 years after completing anthracycline therapy. JAMA 1991;266:1672–7.

[13] Swain SM, Whaley FS, Ewer MS. Congestive heart failure in patients treated with doxorubicin: a retrospective analysis of three trials. Cancer 2003;97:2869–79.

[14] Thavendiranathan P, Grant AD, Negishi T, Plana JC, Popovic ZB, Marwick TH. Reproducibility of echocardiographic techniques for sequential assessment of left ventricular ejection fraction and volumes: application to patients undergoing cancer chemotherapy. J Am Coll Cardiol 2013;61:77–84.

[15] Stoddard MF, Seeger J, Liddell NE, Hadley TJ, Sullivan DM, Kupersmith J. Prolongation of isovolumetric relaxation time as assessed by Doppler echocardiography predicts doxorubicin-induced systolic dysfunction in humans. J Am Coll Cardiol 1992;20:62–9.

[16] Dorup I, Levitt G, Sullivan I, Sorensen K. Prospective longitudinal assessment of late anthracycline cardiotoxicity after childhood cancer: the role of diastolic function. Heart 2004;90:1214–16.

[17] Cottin Y, Touzery C, Coudert B, Gilles A, Walker P, Massing JL, et al. Impairment of diastolic function during short-term anthracycline chemotherapy. Br Heart J 1995;73:61–4.

[18] Marchandise B, Schroeder E, Bosly A, Doyen C, Weynants P, Kremer R, et al. Early detection of doxorubicin cardiotoxicity: interest of Doppler echocardiographic analysis of left ventricular filling dynamics. Am Heart J 1989;118:92–8.

[19] Tjeerdsma G, Meinardi MT, van Der Graaf WT, van Den Berg MP, Mulder NH, Crijns HJ, et al. Early detection of anthracycline induced cardiotoxicity in asymptomatic patients with normal left ventricular systolic function: autonomic versus echocardiographic variables. Heart 1999;81:419–23.

[20] Tassan-Mangina S, Codorean D, Metivier M, Costa B, Himberlin C, Jouannaud C, et al. Tissue Doppler imaging and conventional echocardiography after anthracycline treatment in adults: early and late alterations of left ventricular function during a prospective study. Eur J Echocardiogr 2006;7:141–6.

[21] Kapusta L, Thijssen JM, Groot-Loonen J, Antonius T, Mulder J, Daniels O. Tissue Doppler imaging in detection of myocardial dysfunction in survivors of childhood cancer treated with anthracyclines. Ultrasound Med Biol 2000;26:1099–108.

[22] Nagy AC, Tolnay E, Nagykalnai T, Forster T. Cardiotoxicity of anthracycline in young breast cancer female patients: the possibility of detection of early cardiotoxicity by TDI. Neoplasma 2006;53:511–17.

[23] Nagy AC, Cserep Z, Tolnay E, Nagykalnai T, Forster T. Early diagnosis of chemotherapy-induced cardiomyopathy: a prospective tissue Doppler imaging study. Pathol Oncol Res 2008;14:69–77.

[24] Nagueh SF, Appleton CP, Gillebert TC, Marino PN, Oh JK, Smiseth OA, et al. Recommendations for the evaluation of left ventricular diastolic function by echocardiography. Eur J Echocardiogr 2009;10:165–93.

[25] Mason JW, Bristow MR, Billingham ME, Daniels JR. Invasive and non invasive methods of assessing Adriamycin cardiotoxic effects in man: superiority of histiopathologic assessment using endomyocardial biopsy. Cancer Treat Rep 1978;62:857–64.

[26] Tanindi A, Demirci U, Tacoy G, Buyukberber S, Alsancak Y, Coskun U, et al. Assessment of right ventricular functions during cancer chemotherapy. Eur J Echocardiogr 2011;12:834–40.

[27] Montani D, Bergot E, Gunther S, Savale L, Bergeron A, Bourdin A, et al. Pulmonary arterial hypertension in patients treated by dasatinib. Circulation 2012;125:2128–37.

[28] Hamza A, Tunick PA, Kronzon I. Echocardiographic manifestations of complications of radiation therapy. Echocardiography 2009;26:724–8.

[29] Heidenreich PA, Kapoor JR. Radiation induced heart disease: systemic disorders in heart disease. Heart 2009;95:252–8.

[30] Lancellotti P, Nkomo VT, Badano LP, Bergler J, Bogaert J, Davin L, et al. Expert consensus for multi-modality imaging evaluation of cardiovascular complications of radiotherapy in adults: a report from the European Association of Cardiovascular Imaging and the American Society of Echocardiography. Eur Heart J Cardiovasc Imaging 2013;14:721–40.

[31] Edoute Y, Haim N, Rinkevich D, Brenner B, Reisner SA. Cardiac valvular vegetations in cancer patients: a prospective echocardiographic study of 200 patients. Am J Med 1997;102:252–8.

[32] Tomlinson D, Mermel LA, Ethier MC, Matlow A, Gillmeister B, Sung L. Defining bloodstream infections related to central venous catheters in patients with cancer: a systematic review. Clin Infect Dis 2011;53:697–710.

Chapter 20.2

Pericardial Disease in Oncologic Patients

M. Galderisi, F. Ilardi and C. Santoro

Pericardial diseases (PDs) may be either isolated disease or part of a systemic disease. The most common cause of PD are infectious, but, among the noninfectious etiologie, neoplastic (primary and secondary), radiation-induced, and drug-related PDs are frequently represented in the clinical setting.

The main PDs encountered in oncologic setting include:

1. Pericarditis (acute, subacute, and chronic);
2. Pericardial effusion and cardiac tamponade;
3. Constrictive pericarditis [1].

An appropriate and timely diagnosis of PD in oncologic patients is very important in order to manage individual treatment and stratify prognosis. Transthoracic echocardiography is the first-line imaging modality in patients with suspected PD, because it is simple and easy to perform, widely available, and repeatable. Echocardiography can be completely satisfactory for diagnosis of pericarditis, pericardial effusion, and cardiac tamponade. Conversely, a multimodality imaging approach—including cardiovascular magnetic resonance (CMR) and cardiac computed tomography (CCT) when needed—is often requested for a comprehensive diagnosis of constrictive pericarditis [2].

ETIOLOGY

PD in oncologic patients is relatively common. It may be secondary to neoplastic disease (primary or secondary) [3], or may be a consequence of radiotherapy [4,5] and/or chemotherapy [6,7].

1. *Primary tumors of pericardium* are 40 times less common than *metastatic tumors*. Among them, mesothelioma is the most frequent. The pericardium is the site of metastases derived from lung cancer, breast cancer, malignant melanoma, lymphomas, and leukemias [3]. Malignant pericardial effusion occurs in up to 21% of cancer patients and it is often accompanied by pleural effusion. In one-half of cases it is the first sign of malignant disease. In the majority of the cases it is not suspected until clinical symptoms or signs are not overt. Slight pericardial effusions, in fact, are frequently asymptomatic, whereas symptomatic effusions often

begin suddenly with cardiac tamponade, which can rapidly lead to cardiovascular collapse or death [8]. Malignancy-related pericardial effusion is associated with significantly decreased patient survival, therefore, early diagnosis and timely treatment may decrease the patient's short-term risk of death [9].

2. *Acute radiation pericarditis* might be one of the earliest cardiac complication of radiotherapy. It can be asymptomatic or present as symptomatic pericarditis. Cardiac tamponade is rare. Spontaneous clearance of this effusion may take up to 2 years. Modern radiotherapy procedures, including lower doses and shielding methods, have reduced the incidence from 20% to 2.5%, it being proportional to dose and treatment volume. Pericarditis is usually self-limiting. However, 10% up to 20% of patients develop a *chronic or constrictive pericarditis*, which becomes overt 5–10 years after treatment. This appears to be dose-dependent and related to the presence of pericardial effusion in the delayed acute phase. *Delayed chronic pericarditis* appears several weeks to years after radiotherapy and might occur even in patients who did not experience an acute event. In this type of pericarditis, extensive fibrous thickening, adhesions, chronic constriction, and chronic pericardial effusion can be observed in up to 20% of patients within 2 years following irradiation [10,11].
3. *Chemotherapeutic pericarditis* (e.g., tyrosine-kinase inhibitors, interferon-α) can be detected as a pericardial effusion, often associated with varying degrees of hemodynamic impairment [7]. In patients exposed to anthracyclines, cyclophosphamide, and cytarabine, the development of pericarditis may be associated also with myocarditis. Retinoic acid pericarditis occurs in approximately 26% of patients treated with this drug and is characterized by fever, arterial hypotension, acute renal failure, and both pleural and pericardial effusions. The occurrence of pericardial and endomyocardial fibrosis years after administration of busulfan has also been described. Also, methotrexate, arsenic trioxide and, less frequently, 5-fluorouracil and docetaxel can induce pericarditis [12].

DIAGNOSIS OF PERICARDIAL DISEASE IN ONCOLOGIC PATIENTS

The first approach to the pericardial syndrome is transthoracic 2D echocardiography. In the presence of pericardial effusion, it is useful not only for diagnosis but, when needed, also as guidance of pericardiocentesis [1,2].

In patients with pericarditis, the echocardiographic findings can be entirely normal or show only a pericardial thickening, corresponding to an increased pericardial echogenicity and/or as multiple parallel reflections posterior to the left ventricle by either 2D or M-mode imaging [13]. In uncomplicated pericarditis with small or no effusion, the echocardiographic evaluation is useful to confirm the diagnosis but also to drive differential

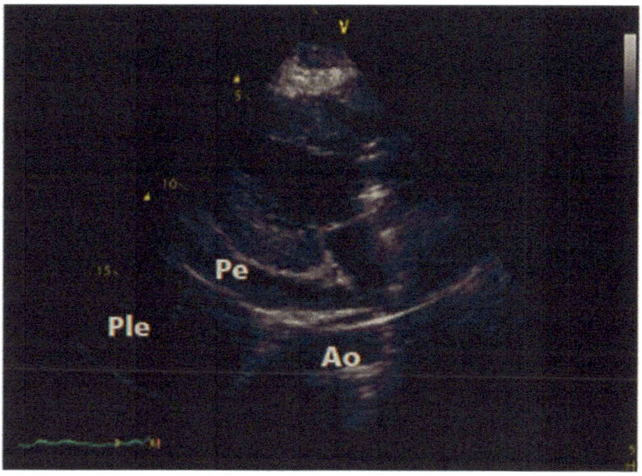

FIGURE 20.3 Parasternal long-axis view showing a moderate posterior pericardial effusion in a woman with breast cancer. *Ao*, aorta; *PE*, pericardial effusion; *PLE*, pleural effusion.

diagnosis with acute coronary syndrome, aortic dissection, and pulmonary embolism. No other imaging modalities are usually required in this setting.

In patients who have concomitant myocarditis, echocardiography also allows to evaluate localized or diffuse alterations of left ventricular (LV) function. In this clinical context CMR may add valuable information, in particular in patients with suboptimal cardiac images, highlighting "patchy" myocardial regions of late gadolinium enhancement corresponding to inflammation areas.

In the presence of moderate or large *pericardial effusion*, 2D echocardiography provides the best way to estimate the amount of pericardial effusion and assess its hemodynamic significance (Fig. 20.3). The amount of effusion can be assessed quantitatively by the end-diastolic distance of the echo-free space between the epicardium and parietal pericardium: (1) minimal pericardial effusion when seen only in systole; (2) <1 cm, corresponding to about 300 mL; (3) 1–2 cm, corresponding to 500 mL; (4) >2 cm, typically in excess of 700 mL (Fig. 20.4). The "swinging heart" (Fig. 20.5) is a very large pericardial effusion with cardiac tamponade (ECG electrical alternation of QRS complex). By using 2D echocardiography apical and subcostal views are all-important in order to determine the extent of effusion and, if there is clinical evidence of tamponade, to identify the optimal location for pericardiocentesis [2]. According to the ESC Guidelines for diagnosis and management of pericardial disease, echocardiography is the best imaging technique to evaluate size, location, and degree of hemodynamic impact of cardiac tamponade [1]. Echo signs include respiratory variation in chamber dimensions (i.e., inspiratory increase of right ventricular (RV) size with concomitant decrease in LV size), diastolic collapse of the right ventricle, late diastolic collapse of the right atrial free wall (better seen in apical four-chamber view), abnormal ventricular

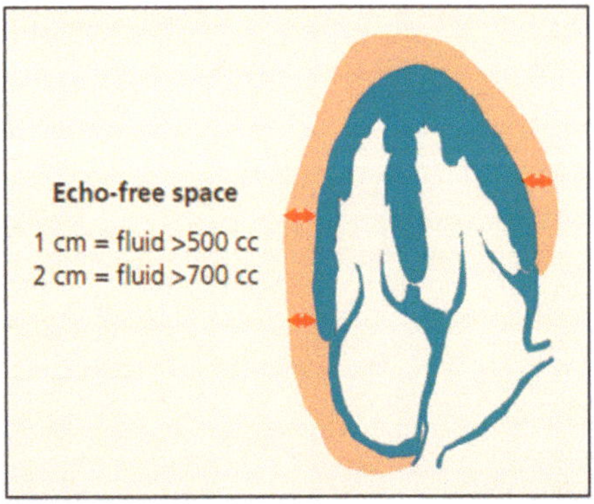

FIGURE 20.4 Schema for quantification of pericardial effusion by 2D echocardiography.

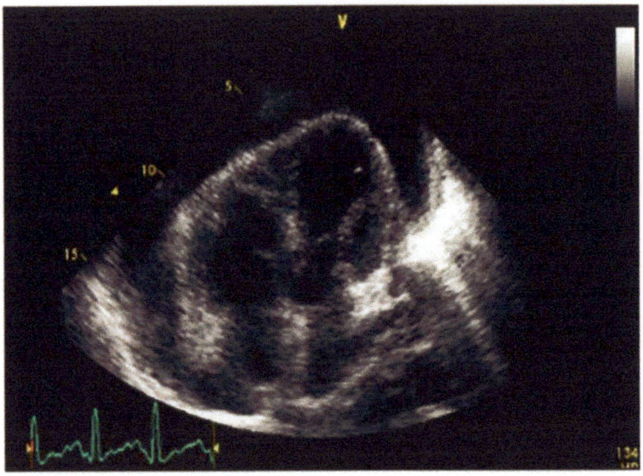

FIGURE 20.5 Severe pericardial effusion with diastolic right atrium collapse (apical four-chamber view) suggestive of pericardial tamponade in a patients with nonHodgkin lymphoma.

septal motion that shifts to the left during diastole, exaggerated respiratory variability (>25%) in mitral and tricuspid inflow velocities corresponding to "paradoxical pulsus," inspiratory decrease and expiratory increase in pulmonary vein diastolic forward flow. Transesophageal echocardiography [2] or CMR—able to detect even localized cardiac tamponade [14]—could provide valuable information but are rarely performed because of the emergency condition and the hemodynamic status of patients with cardiac tamponade [2].

Echocardiography is also used to guide percutaneous pericardiocentesis, even in unstable patients. The addition of contrast agent can improve the safety of the procedure by reducing the risk of heart puncture. The most common approach used is the subxiphoid. Under echo assistance, the

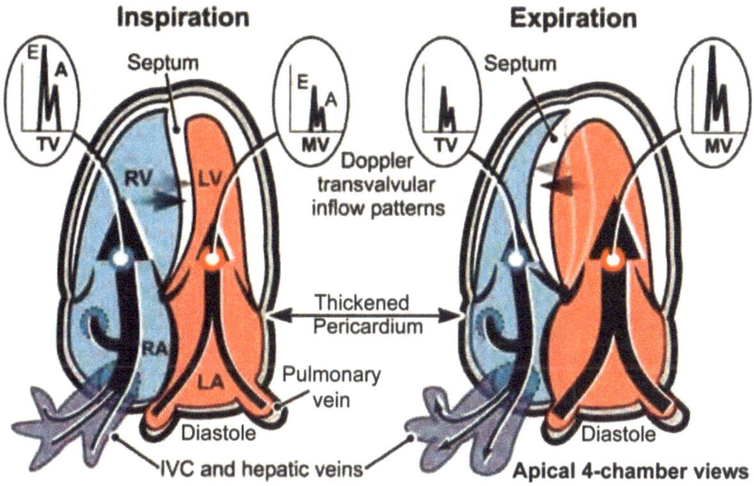

FIGURE 20.6 In constrictive pericarditis, during inspiration (left side) the mitral inflow is reduced almost immediately while there is an increase in tricuspid E-wave. Opposite and reciprocal changes during expiration (right side). *From Fauci AS, et al.* Harrison's Principles of Internal Medicine, *17th edition. McGraw-Hill Professional; New York, NY.*

operator attempts to aspirate fluid and inject immediately after agitated saline, thus confirming that the needle is entered into the pericardial sac. After the correct introduction of the needle the introduction of a catheter into the pericardial sac allows the effusion drainage [15–18].

Constrictive pericarditis in oncologic patients is mainly related to mediastinal radiation [5,10], but can be due also to high-dose chemotherapy [19]. It can be suspected if clinical signs of RV failure and of low cardiac output are evident in the presence of normal LV dimension and function. Besides pericardium thickened, other characteristic echocardiographic findings are prominent respiratory phasic diastolic bounce of interventricular septum (ventricular interdependence), restrictive diastolic filling pattern (transmitral E/A ratio >2 and E velocity deceleration time <140 ms) due to elevated LV filling pressures, diastolic flattening of LV posterior wall, inferior vena cava plethora, and expiratory diastolic flow reversal in the hepatic veins. Therefore, significant inspiratory variation of mitral E velocity ($>25\%$), associated with opposite and reciprocal changes in the right side inflow ($>40\%$ inspiratory increase in tricuspid E-velocity) and outflow, represent diagnostic criteria [20,21] (Fig. 20.6). Pulsed tissue Doppler interrogation of septal mitral annulus can be particularly useful, revealing normal or increased e′ velocity (≥ 7 cm/s), which is also higher than e′ of the lateral annulus. Conversely, in restrictive cardiomyopathy myocardial relaxation is impaired, leading to reduction of both s′ and e′ velocities [22]. CCT and CRM are indicated by ESC guidelines as second-level imaging techniques to

TABLE 20.2 Constrictive Pericarditis

Recommended	TTE to confirm clinical diagnosis
	TOE if poor TT quality of imaging (thickness of pericardium)
	CMR for planning pericardiotomy (degree of myocardial fibrosis and atrophy, lung damage, etc.)
	TTE for follow-up
Reasonable	CT/CMR to confirm clinical diagnosis if echocardiography inconclusive
	CT for planning a pericardiotomy (calcification, coronary arteries, lung damage, previous CT surgery, etc.)
	CMR for follow-up

TTE, transthoracic echocardiography; TOE, transesophageal echocardiography; CT, computed tomography; CMR, cardiovascular magnetic resonance.
Source: Modified from EACVI Recommendations for the diagnosis of constrictive pericarditis (*Eur Heart J Cardiovasc Imaging* 2015).

evaluate pericardial constriction (Table 20.2) [1,2]. CCT can detect thickened pericardium but cannot assess its hemodynamic relevance nor prove a suspected constriction. Similarly, a normal pericardial thickness cannot rule out constriction [23]. CCT imaging can clearly delineate the presence and the exact extent of pericardial calcification, that are usually associated with constrictive PD. CMR can demonstrate the thickening (Fig. 20.7) and, although less reliably than CCT, also pericardial calcification. In addition, the simple real-time cine CMR demonstrates ventricular interdependence. CMR findings are used to plan invasive treatment, such as pericardiectomy, complementing findings derived from echocardiography and/or CCT [2].

The differential diagnosis of constrictive pericarditis from restrictive cardiomyopathy by echocardiography can be challenging and the two conditions can also overlap [24]. Currently, in constrictive pericarditis E/A ratio is reduced during inspiration and increased during expiration, without any change of e′ velocity during the respiration phases (Fig. 20.8). Restrictive cardiomyopathy is characterized by a small left ventricle with an increased left atrial size. This causes an early rapid rise in LV pressure during LV filling. Typical diastolic filling pattern consists of a short mitral E velocity deceleration duration and a low A velocity resulting in a high E/A ratio. Pulsed tissue Doppler derived e′ velocity is usually reduced ($<$8 cm/s) [22]. Moreover, significant respiratory variation of mitral inflow is absent, differently from the constrictive pericarditis. Mitral inflow propagation velocity (PFV) measured by color M-mode can also be helpful in distinguishing restriction (PFV $<$45 cm/s) from constriction (PFV $>$45 cm/s) [1,25]. Actually, CCT and CMR have poor value for the diagnosis of restrictive cardiomyopathy.

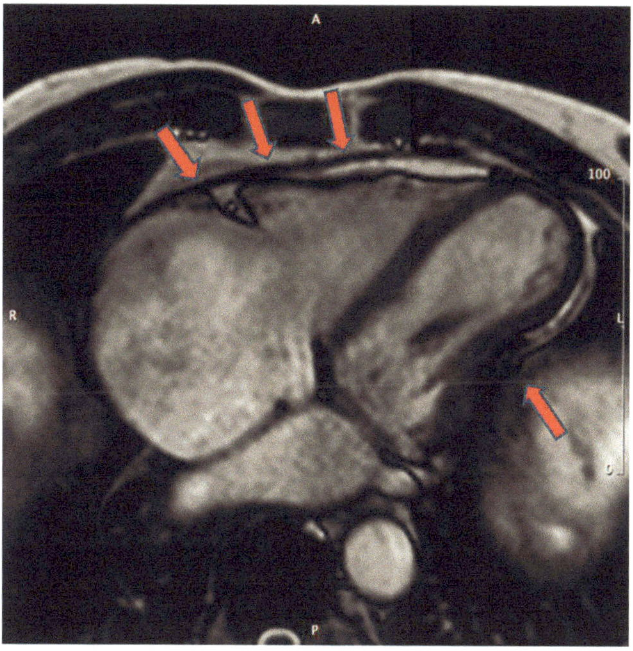

FIGURE 20.7 CMR showing areas of pericardial thickening (up to 5 mm) hampering the diastolic expansion of LV free wall in patients with pericardial constriction. *Courtesy of Dr. Santo Dellegrottaglie, Acerra (Italy).*

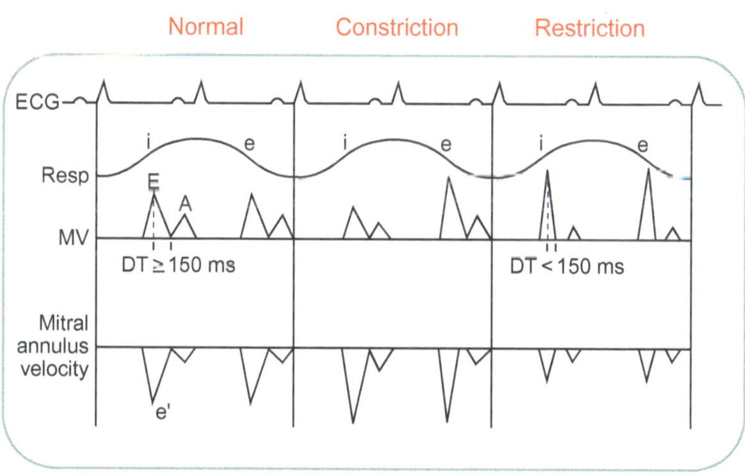

FIGURE 20.8 Respiratory variation of LV diastolic filling pattern (MV) and mitral annular velocity in normal condition (left panel), pericardial constriction (central panel) and in restrictive cardiomyopathy (right panel). *A*, transmitral A velocity; *DT*, deceleration time of E velocity; *E*, E velocity; *e′*, pulsed tissue Doppler derived e′ velocity of septal mitral annulus; *i*, inspiratory phase; *e*, expiratory phase.

REFERENCES

[1] Adler Y, Charron P, Imazio M, Badano L, Barón-Esquivias G, Bogaert J, et al. 2015 ESC Guidelines for the diagnosis and management of pericardial diseases: The Task Force for the Diagnosis and Management of Pericardial Diseases of the European Society of Cardiology (ESC) endorsed by: The European Association for Cardio-Thoracic Surgery (EACTS). Eur Heart J 2015;36:2921–64.

[2] Cosyns B, Plein S, Nihoyanopoulos P, Smiseth O, Andreade MJ, Pepi M, et al. European Association of Cardiovascular Imaging (EACVI) position paper: multimodality imaging in pericardial disease. Eur Heart J Cardiovasc Imaging 2015;16:12–31.

[3] Maisch B, Ristic A, Pankuweit E. Evaluation and management of pericardial effusion in patients with neoplastic disease. Prog Cardiovasc Dis 2010;53:157–63.

[4] Morton DL, Glancy DL, Joseph WL, Adkins PC. Management of patients with radiation-induced pericarditis with effusion: a note on the development of aortic regurgitation in two of them. Chest 1973;64:291–7.

[5] Gaya AM, Ashford RF. Cardiac complications of radiation therapy. Clin Oncol 2005;17:153–9.

[6] Krupicka J, Markova J, Pohlreich D, Kozak T, Linkova H, Diehl V, et al. Echocardiographic evaluation of acute cardiotoxicity in the treatment of Hodgkin disease according to the German Hodgkin's Lymphoma Study Group. Leuk Lymphoma 2002;43:325–2329.

[7] Perrino C, Schiattarella GC, Magliulo F, Ilardi F, Carotenuto C, Gargiulo G, et al. Cardiac side effects of chemotherapy: state of art and strategies for a correct management. Curr Vasc Pharmacol 2014;12:106–16.

[8] Halfdanarson TR, Hogan WJ, Moynihan TJ. Oncologic emergencies: diagnosis and treatment. Mayo Clin Proc 2006;81:835–48.

[9] Gornik HL, Gerhard-Herman M, Beckman JA. Abnormal cytology predicts poor prognosis in cancer patients with pericardial effusion. J Clin Oncol 2005;23:5211–16.

[10] Lancellotti P, Nkomo VT, Badano LP, Bergler J, Bogaert J, Davin L, et al. Expert consensus for multi-modality imaging evaluation of cardiovascular complications of radiotherapy in adults: a report from the European Association of Cardiovascular Imaging and the American Society of Echocardiography. Eur Heart J Cardiovasc Imaging 2013;14:721–40.

[11] Jaworski C, Mariani JA, Wheeler G, Kaye DM. Cardiac complications of thoracic irradiation. J Am Coll Cardiol 2013;61:2319–28.

[12] Plana JC, Galderisi M, Barac A, Ewer MS, Ky B, Scherrer-Crosbie M, et al. Expert consensus for multimodality imaging evaluation of adult patients during and after cancer therapy: a report from the American Society of Echocardiography and the European Association of Cardiovascular Imaging. Eur Heart J Cardiovasc Imaging 2014;15:1063–93.

[13] Galiuto L, Badano L, Fox K, Sicari R, Zamorano JL. The EAE textbook of echocardiography. Oxford: Oxford University Publishing; 2011.

[14] Francone M, Dymarkowski S, Kalantzi M, Bogaert J. Real-time cine MRI of ventricular septal motion: a novel approach to assess ventricular coupling. J Magn Reson Imaging 2005;21:305–9.

[15] Callahan JA, Seward JB, Tajik AJ. Cardiac tamponade: pericardiocentesis directed by two-dimensional echocardiography. Mayo Clin Proc 1985;60:344–7.

[16] Dubourg O, Ferrier A, Gueret P, Farcot JC, Terdjman M, Rocha P, et al. Two dimensional contrast echocardiography during the drainage of hemopericardium with tamponade. Presse Med 1983;12:2225–8.

[17] Chandraratna PA, Reid CL, Nimalasuriya A, Kawanishi D, Rahimtoola SH. Application of 2-dimensional contrast studies during pericardiocentesis. Am J Cardiol 1983;52:1120–2.

[18] Callahan JA, Seward JB, Tajik AJ, Holmes Jr DR, Smith HC, Reeder GS, et al. Pericardiocentesis assisted by two-dimensional echocardiography. J Thorac Cardiovasc Surg 1983;85:877–9.

[19] Tulleken JE, Kooiman CG, van der Werf TS, Zijlstra JG, de Vries EG. Constrictive pericarditis after high-dose chemotherapy. Lancet 1997;350:1601.

[20] Oh JK, Hatle LK, Seward JB, Danielson GK, Schaff HV, Reeder GS, et al. Diagnostic role of Doppler echocardiography in constrictive pericarditis. J Am Coll Cardiol 1994;23:154–62.

[21] Fauci AS, Kasper DL, Longo DL, Braunwald E, Hauser SL, Jameson JL, et al. Harrison's Principles of Internal Medicine, 17th edition. McGraw-Hill Professional; New York, NY.

[22] Nagueh SF, Appleton CP, Gillebert TC, Marino PN, Oh JK, Smiseth OA, et al. Recommendations for the evaluation of left ventricular diastolic function by echocardiography. J Am Soc Echocardiogr 2009;22:107–33.

[23] Talreja DR, Edwards WD, Danielson GK, Schaff HV, Tajik AJ, Tazelaar HD, et al. Constrictive pericarditis in 26 patients with histological normal pericardial thickness. Circulation 2003;108:1852–7.

[24] Klein AL, Abbara S, Agler DA, Appleton CP, Asher CR, Hoit B, et al. American Society of Echocardiography clinical recommendations for multimodality cardiovascular imaging of patients with pericardial disease: endorsed by the society for cardiovascular magnetic resonance and society of cardiovascular computed tomography. J Am Soc Echocardiogr 2013;26:965–1012.

[25] Palka P, Lange A, Donnelly JE, Nihoyannopoulos P. Differentiation between restrictive cardiomyopathy and constrictive pericarditis by early diastolic Doppler myocardial velocity gradient at the posterior wall. Circulation 2000;102:655–62.

Chapter 20.3

The Role of Contrast Echocardiography

M.J. Monaghan

Many patients undergoing cancer therapy which has involved chest irradiation, mastectomy, or breast reconstruction have very limited echocardiography windows, leading to poor endocardial definition. This can make accurate determination of left ventricular volumes (using biplane Simpson's methods) difficult.

The use of commercial ultrasound contrast agents has been demonstrated to improve the accuracy and reproducibility of 2D echo assessment of the left ventricle in patients with suboptimal echo windows. Both the European Society of Cardiovascular Imaging and the American Society of Echocardiography have created recommendations for the use of these products which state that they should be used when two or more contiguous LV segments cannot be adequately visualized in any apical views [1,2]. Although there have been limited publications on the use of contrast agents to enhance LV evaluation in patients specifically undergoing cancer therapy, one can imply from the extensive literature in the general echo population that it has a role in cancer patients with suboptimal 2D echo windows [3]. In a large prospective study of more than 600 patients with technically difficult echo studies, Kurt et al. [4] demonstrated that the addition of contrast to a 2D echo study had a significant effect upon the assessment of LVEF% in that the EF value was changed by >10% in 16.7% of patients.

In Fig. 20.9 an apical four-chamber view in a patient who is undergoing trastuzumab treatment for breast cancer and with suboptimal echo windows is shown pre (left) and postcontrast administration. The improvement in endocardial definition is readily appreciated together with the ability to perform a biplane Simpson's analysis of left ventricular volumes.

Three-dimensional echocardiography is generally accepted as a more accurate, and more importantly, a more repeatable method for measuring left ventricular volumes and ejection fraction. It does not rely on any geometric assumptions and does not suffer from fore-shortening. As detailed elsewhere in this chapter, 3D echo is a more preferable method for LV volume assessment than 2D and should be used wherever possible. However, 3D echo can suffer as much, if not more, from poor endocardial definition than 2D echo. Since most echo machine vendors have incorporated contrast-specific imaging into their 3D imaging modes, it would seem to make sense to use contrast in suboptimal imaging studies as well. In Fig. 20.10 an example of contrast-enhanced 3D analysis of LVEF% in the same patient as shown in Fig. 20.9 is illustrated.

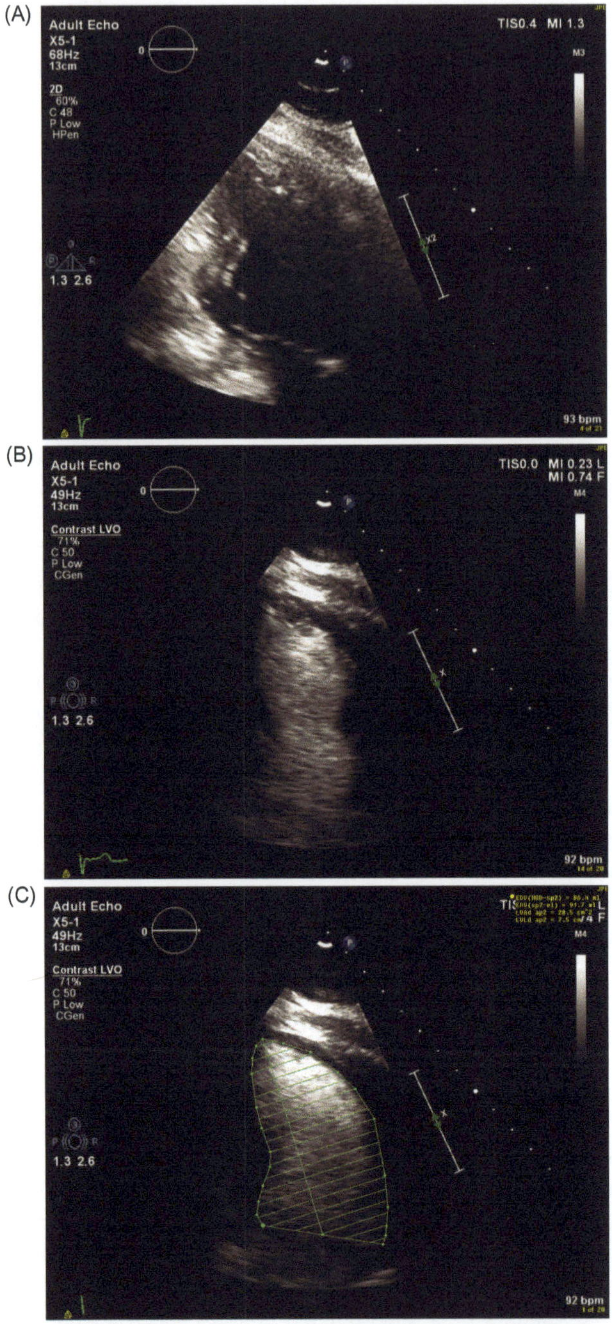

FIGURE 20.9 (A) A noncontrast apical two-chamber view in a patient undergoing trastuzumab therapy where the image quality is very poor and LV endocardial definition inadequate for analysis. (B) The same image following contrast administration. Endocardial definition is significantly improved. (C) Simpson's evaluation of LV volumes from the image shown in (B).

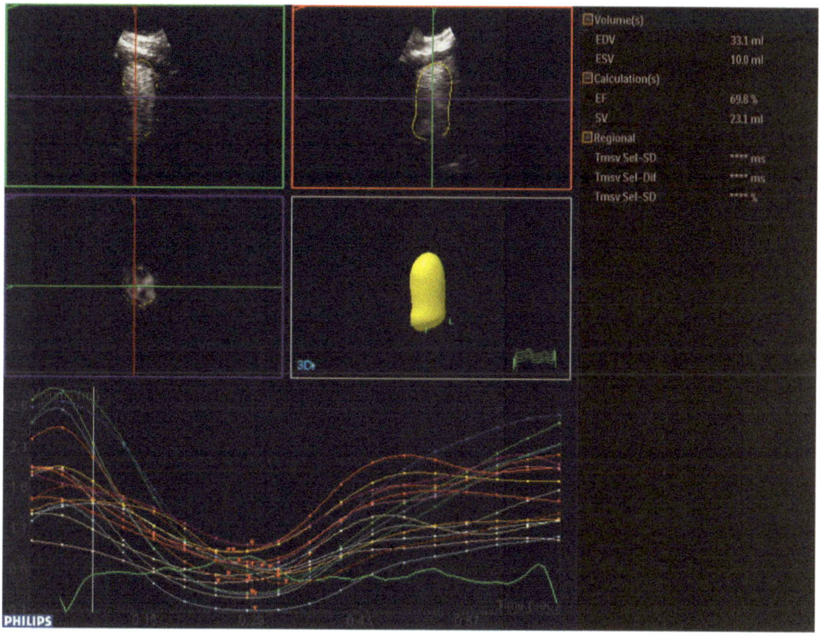

FIGURE 20.10 A contrast-enhanced 3D dataset undergoing LV volume analysis using proprietary 3D software. This is from the same patient as illustrated in Fig. 20.9 and the 3D LV ejection fraction = 69%.

However, not all studies have demonstrated any advantage when using contrast-enhanced 3D echo in patients undergoing treatment with potentially cardiotoxic drugs [5]. However, there are some technical issues including contrast-specific 3D analysis software and the fact that most patients had adequate baseline echo images anyway, that could explain the lack of benefit of 3D contrast seen in this particular study. At present, there are insufficient data to recommend the use of contrast 3D echo for the follow-up of patients undergoing therapy with cardiotoxic drugs.

The expert consensus document on the use of multimodality imaging in patients during and after cancer therapy produced by the American Society of Echocardiography and the European Association of Cardiovascular Imaging [6] clearly recommends the use of contrast to enhance 2D echo images of the left ventricle when endocardial dropout occurs. Specifically, contrast should be used when two or more contiguous left ventricular segments are not well visualized on noncontrast apical images. These recommendations are consistent with those for any 2D echo assessment of the left ventricle where imaging is suboptimal and an accurate assessment of function and volume cannot be performed.

REFERENCES

[1] Mulvagh SL, Rakowski H, Vannan MA, Abdelmoneim SS, Becher H, Bierig SM, et al. American Society of Echocardiography consensus statement on the clinical applications of ultrasonic contrast agents in echocardiography. J Am Soc Echocardiogr 2008;21:1179–201.

[2] Senior R, Becher H, Monaghan M, Agati L, Zamorano J, Vanoverschelde JL, et al. Contrast echocardiography: evidence-based recommendations by European Association of Echocardiography. Eur J Echocardiogr 2009;10:194–212.

[3] Yu EH, Sloggett CE, Iwanochko RM, Rakowski H, Siu SC. Feasibility and accuracy of left ventricular volumes and ejection fraction determination by fundamental, tissue harmonic, and intravenous contrast imaging in difficult-to-image patients. J Am Soc Echocardiogr 2000;13:216–24.

[4] Kurt M, Shaikh K, Peterson L, Kurrelmeyer K, Shah G, Nagueh S, et al. Impact of contrast echocardiography on evaluation of ventricular function and clinical management in a large prospective cohort. J Am Coll Cardiol 2009;53(11):0735–1097.

[5] Thavendiranathan P, Grant AD, Negishi T, Plana JC, Popovic ZB, Marwick TH. Reproducibility of echocardiographic techniques for sequential assessment of left ventricular ejection fraction and volumes: application to patients undergoing cancer chemotherapy. J Am Coll Cardiol 2013;61:77–84.

[6] Plana JC, Galderisi M, Barac A, Ewer MS, Ky B, et al. Expert consensus for multimodality imaging evaluation of adult patients during and after cancer therapy: a report from the American Society of Echocardiography and the European Association of Cardiovascular Imaging. J Am Soc Echocardiogr 2014;27:911–39.

Chapter 20.4

Stress Echocardiography

R. Sicari

Stress echocardiography is the combination of 2D echocardiography with a physical, pharmacologic, or electrical stress. The diagnostic endpoint for the detection of myocardial ischemia is the induction of a transient change in LV regional function during stress. The stress echo sign indicative of myocardial ischemia is a stress-induced worsening in LV regional function, i.e., worsening of LV myocardial wall thickening in a region contracting normally at baseline. The stress echo sign of myocardial viability is a stress-induced improvement of LV regional function during low levels of stress in an abnormally contracting myocardial region at rest [1,2]. Stress echocardiography is an established technique for detection and prognostication of stable coronary artery disease as recommended by guidelines. It is a second-line noninvasive imaging technique that may be useful in the evaluation of patients with intermediate probability for coronary artery disease (ECG uninterpretable or unable to exercise) [2]. The use of this technique in patients undergoing cancer treatment remains unsettled since there are no clear indications due to the lack of large clinical trials. The potential clinical use of stress echocardiography in this setting can be summarized in three large areas:

1. Patients who are undergoing regimens that may be associated with ischemia (fluorouracil, bevacizumab, sorafenib, and sunitinib) [3];
2. Evaluation of subclinical LV dysfunction;
3. Evaluation of contractile reserve in patients with cancer therapeutics-related cardiac dysfunction.

Both exercise [4] and dobutamine stress-echo [4–13] have been applied to cancer patients for the identification of anthracycline-induced cancer therapeutics-related cardiac dysfunction, however the results of these studies appear to be inconclusive and contradictory. There are several reasons for these inconsistencies: small sample sizes, inhomogeneity of the sample under investigation (patients with known coronary artery disease versus those without); different staging of disease with unbalanced follow-up. In 23 young adult acute lymphoblastic leukemia, survivors receiving doxorubicin before the onset of puberty ejection fraction at 1 month after therapy had a sensitivity of 53% and a specificity of 75% for detecting patients at risk for developing cancer therapeutics-related cardiac dysfunction. When exercise echocardiography was performed, sensitivity raised to 89% but with a significant loss of specificity which fell to 41%. [6]. Exercise may not be the perfect tool to assess these patients who may be deconditioned for the comorbidity and on-going treatment. Pharmacologic stress echocardiography seems more suitable, being able to achieve conventional diagnostic endpoints independent of physical fitness. In a study [4] from the Thoraxcenter, 31 patients were studied before chemotherapy (anthracycline), with follow-ups during, at the end, and 6 months after chemotherapy. Left ventricular function was assessed by 2D echocardiographic wall motion score index and by Doppler echocardiography of mitral valve inflow at rest and during dobutamine stress echocardiography. Radionuclide ventriculography was used as an independent reference for ejection fraction. The authors concluded that wall motion score index measured by 2D echocardiography parallels radionuclide ejection fraction at follow-up. However, assessment of contractile reserve over time did not show any incremental value for the early detection of cardiotoxicity. Consistent with these results Lanzarini et al. [10] did not report any incremental value of dobutamine stress echocardiography in young adults at 7 years from chemotherapy [10]. Other studies have tried to assess whether dobutamine stress echocardiography could potentially allow earlier identification of disease by recognizing a compromise in cardiac reserve. One of these studies prospectively assessed LV contractile reserve by low-dose dobutamine stress-echo in 49 women with breast cancer prior to each chemotherapy cycle and 1, 4, and 7 months after stopping the treatment. A reduction in left ventricular contractile reserve with dobutamine >5% appeared to be a threshold discriminating patients destined to develop a subsequent LVEF decrease [13]. Several studies demonstrated that the presence of contractile reserve is related to a lower incidence rate of events during the follow-up [1,2].

The EACVI/ASE expert consensus [14] provides two main recommendations which summarize the potential use of stress echocardiography with this particular group of patients and here reported:

- Stress echocardiography may be helpful in the evaluation of patients with intermediate or high pretest probability for coronary artery disease (CAD) (ECG uninterpretable or unable to exercise) who will receive regimens that may cause ischemia (fluorouracil, bevacizumab, sorafenib, and sunitinib).
- Stress echocardiography may be of help in the determination of contractile reserve of patients with evidence of post-therapy cardiomyopathy.

The evidence on the use of stress echocardiography in this subset of patients is scant. There are no available data on the use of speckle tracking during stress echocardiography and its potential ability to detect subtle forms of left ventricular dysfunction in a more sensitive way than wall motion analysis. The detection of microvascular dysfunction with Doppler-derived assessment of coronary flow reserve (CFR) during vasodilator stress echo, which may be related to the onset of left ventricular dysfunction may be a suitable tool to assess the early phases of the disease [2], but again no data are available.

REFERENCES

[1] Pellikka PA, Nagueh SF, Elhendy AA, Kuehl CA, Sawada SG, American Society of Echocardiography. American Society of Echocardiography recommendations for performance, interpretation, and application of stress echocardiography. J Am Soc Echocardiogr 2007;20:1021–41.

[2] Sicari R, Nihoyannopoulos P, Evangelista A, Kasprzak J, Lancellotti P, Poldermans D, et al. European Association of Echocardiography. Stress echocardiography expert consensus statement: European Association of Echocardiography (EAE) (a registered branch of the ESC). Eur J Echocardiogr 2008;9:415–37.

[3] Yeh ETH, Bickford CL. Cardiovascular complications of cancer therapy: incidence, pathogenesis, diagnosis, and management. J Am Coll Cardiol 2009;53:2231–47.

[4] Bountioukos M, Doorduijn JK, Roelandt JR, et al. Repetitive dobutamine stress echocardiography for the prediction of anthracycline cardiotoxicity. Eur J Echocardiogr 2003;4:300–5.

[5] Klewer SE, Goldberg SJ, Donnerstein RL, Berg RA, Hutter Jr. JJ. Dobutamine stress echocardiography: a sensitive indicator of diminished myocardial function in asymptomatic doxorubicin-treated long-term survivors of childhood cancer. J Am Coll Cardiol 1992;19:394–401.

[6] Jarfelt M, Kujacic V, Holmgren D, Bjarnason R, Lannering B. Exercise echocardiography reveals subclinical cardiac dysfunction in young adult survivors of childhood acute lymphoblastic leukemia. Pediatr Blood Cancer 2007;49:835–40.

[7] De Wolf D, Suys B, Maurus R, Benoit Y, Verhaaren H, Matthijs D, et al. Dobutamine stress echocardiography in the evaluation of late anthracycline cardiotoxicity in childhood cancer survivors. Pediatr Res 1996;39:504–12.

[8] De Wolf D, Suys B, Verhaaren H, Matthys D, Taeymans Y. Low-dose dobutamine stress echocardiography in children and young adults. Am J Cardiol 1998;81:895–901.

[9] Cottin Y, L'huillier I, Casasnovas O, Geoffroy C, Caillot D, Zeller M, et al. Dobutamine stress echocardiography identifies anthracycline cardiotoxicity. Eur J Echocardiogr 2000;1:180–3.

[10] Lanzarini L, Bossi G, Laudisa ML, Klersy C, Arico M. Lack of clinically significant cardiac dysfunction during intermediate dobutamine doses in long-term childhood cancer survivors exposed to anthracyclines. Am Heart J 2000;140:315–23.

[11] Elbl L, Hrstkova H, Chaloupka V, Novotny J, Michalek J. The evaluation of left ventricular function in childhood cancer survivors by pharmacological stress echocardiography. Neoplasma 2003;50:191–7.

[12] Hamada H, Ohkubo T, Maeda M, Ogawa S. Evaluation of cardiac reserved function by high-dose dobutamine-stress echocardiography in asymptomatic anthracycline-treated survivors of childhood cancer. Pediatr Int 2006;48:313–20.

[13] Civelli M, Cardinale D, Martinoni A, Lamantia G, Colombo N, Colombo A, et al. Early reduction in left ventricular contractile reserve detected by dobutamine stress echo predicts high-dose chemotherapy-induced cardiac toxicity. Int J Cardiol 2006;111:120–6.

[14] Plana JC, Galderisi M, Barac A, Ewer MS, Ky B, Scherrer-Crosbie M, et al. Expert consensus for multimodality imaging evaluation of adult patients during and after cancer therapy: a report from the American Society of Echocardiography and the European Association of Cardiovascular Imaging. Eur Heart J Cardiovasc Imaging 2014;15:1063–93.

Chapter 20.5

Advanced Echocardiography: Speckle Tracking Echocardiography and 3D Echocardiography

T. Edvardsen

THREE-DIMENSIONAL (3D) ECHOCARDIOGRAPHY

Three-dimensional echocardiography (3DE) has demonstrated superiority and better accuracy than two-dimensional echocardiography (2DE) for the measurement of left ventricular (LV) volume in several studies [1,2]. The most important reasons for this superiority is that 3DE eliminates geometric assumptions, incorrect orientation of 2D apical views, and errors caused by foreshortened views. This advantage has also been demonstrated in survivors after cancer treatment [3]. It is well known that the variability in repeated assessments of ejection fraction (EF) from 2D is high. Another advantage of 3DE is therefore lower variability in the measurements in sequentially acquired echo studies undergoing cancer chemotherapy [4]. This will make findings of a decreased LV function more reliable. The baseline and follow-up studies of patients during cancer treatment should preferably be performed by 3DE. It is, however, important to accept the limitations by this technique: 3DE requires high-quality images and operator expertise. The technique is not available in all echocardiographic laboratories due to higher cost. An EF obtained from the 2D biplane Simpson should always be stated in the echocardiographic report.

The recommendations from the European Association of Cardiovascular Imaging (EACVI) and the American Society of Echocardiography (ASE) are listed in Table 20.3.

SPECKLE TRACKING ECHOCARDIOGRAPHY

EF is a volume-based method for assessment of left ventricular (LV) function. It is the most widely used functional measurement, but initial signs of heart failure may be lost due to its inherited weaknesses even when using 3DE. It can be of major importance to discover very early changes of LV function during and after chemotherapy, and a decrease of EF can be revealed too late to receive successful treatment [5,6]. An ideal diagnostic tool is volume- and load-independent—but such a noninvasive diagnostic tool does not exist. However, one very sensitive diagnostic tool for detection

TABLE 20.3 Three-dimensional Echocardiography—Recommendations From EACVI and ASE

3DE should be the preferred echo technique for monitoring LV function and detection of cardiotoxicity in cancer patients
Advantages include better accuracy in detecting LVEF below the lower limit of normal, better reproducibility, and lower temporal variability, as compared with 2DE in cancer patients treated with chemotherapy
Costs, availability, high reliance on image quality, and need of training for operators currently limit wide application of 3DE in the oncological setting

Source: Modified from Plana JC, et al. Expert consensus for multimodality imaging evaluation of adult patients during and after cancer therapy: a report from the American Society of Echocardiography and the European Association of Cardiovascular Imaging. *Eur Heart J Cardiovasc Imaging* 2014;15(10):1063–93.

of early and subtle LV changes is speckle tracking echocardiography (STE) [7,8]. The principle is that dedicated software can follow ultrasonic speckles in the B-mode image and calculate the strain between these speckles. Numerous studies have shown the advantages of this technique in several cardiac diseases [9]. A very robust method appears to be assessment of global longitudinal strain (GLS). GLS is obtained from the average peak systolic strain of the 16 LV segments from all three apical views. In the similar way from the three levels of the LV short-axis views, one can obtain global radial strain (GRS) and global circumferential strain (GCS).

These techniques have successfully been used in several recent studies in the detection of subclinical LV dysfunction in patients treated for cancer before a drop in EF can be discovered [10,11]. The decrease in myocardial deformation by GLS will almost always precede a decrease in EF and other measurements of myocardial function. Most studies showing the superiority of the STE technique have recommended assessment of the longitudinal function, i.e., from the apical views [12–15]. Assessment of circumferential and radial function might also be useful, but these have generally lower reproducibility than measures from the longitudinal function [10,16]. A growing body of literature supports the use of myocardial strain in detection of early cardiotoxicity in patients undergoing cancer therapy [10].

GLS by STE is the most reported method and should be assessed before the start of cancer treatment in order to have a baseline measurement of LV function. GLS should be repeated during treatment with anthracyclines alone or combined with other regimens like trastuzumab and similar. A reduction of GLS between 9% and 19%, even without an evident drop in EF, is reported to be common during anthracycline therapy [17–19]. The prognostic value of discovering early changes in ventricular function is evaluated in

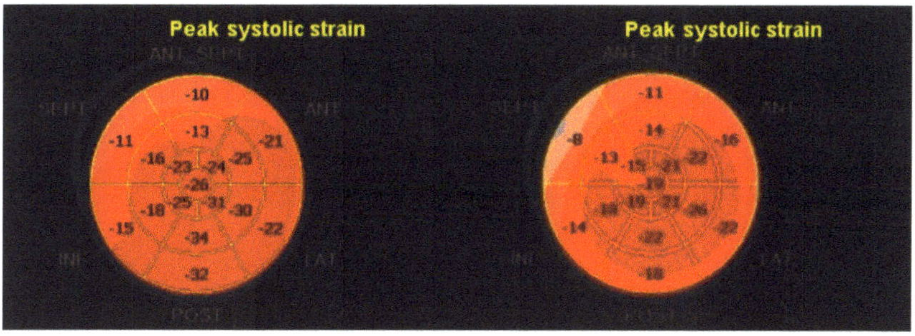

FIGURE 20.11 The left panel shows a bull's-eye plot of GLS before start of cancer treatment in a 40-year-old women with lymphoma. The average GLS was −22.2%. The right panel shows GLS 2 months later after treatment with anthracycline. The average GLS was now −17.2%.

TABLE 20.4 Deformation Imaging—Recommendations From EACVI and ASE

Myocardial strain can be measured using Doppler tissue imaging (DTI) or 2D STE. 2D STE is preferred due to lack of angle dependency
Global longitudinal strain (GLS) is the optimal parameter for the early detection of subclinical LV dysfunction
Measurements during chemotherapy should be compared with the baseline value
A relative percentage reduction of GLS of 15% from baseline is very likely to be abnormal
When applying STE for the longitudinal follow-up of cancer patients, the same vendor-specific ultrasound machine should be used

Source: Modified from Plana JC, et al. Expert consensus for multimodality imaging evaluation of adult patients during and after cancer therapy: a report from the American Society of Echocardiography and the European Association of Cardiovascular Imaging. *Eur Heart J Cardiovasc Imaging* 2014;15(10):1063–93.

several studies and a reduction of GLS of 10−15% seems to predict cardiotoxicity [13,16,20,21] (Fig. 20.11).

The same equipment should be used in all studies of one patient, due to differences in vendor software [22,23]. It is also important to acknowledge that expertise imaging proficiencies are needed before decisions on cancer treatment are concluded from a drop in GLS. The recommendations from EACVI and ASE are listed in Table 20.4 [6].

REFERENCES

[1] Badano LP, Boccalini F, Muraru D, Bianco LD, Peluso D, Bellu R, et al. Current clinical applications of transthoracic three-dimensional echocardiography. J Cardiovasc Ultrasound 2012;20:1–22.

[2] Shimada YJ, Shiota T. Meta-analysis of accuracy of left ventricular mass measurement by three-dimensional echocardiography. Am J Cardiol 2012;110:445–52.

[3] Armstrong GT, Plana JC, Zhang N, Srivastava D, Green DM, Ness KK, et al. Screening adult survivors of childhood cancer for cardiomyopathy: comparison of echocardiography and cardiac magnetic resonance imaging. J Clin Oncol 2012;30:2876–84.

[4] Thavendiranathan P, Grant AD, Negishi T, Plana JC, Popović ZB, Marwick TH. Reproducibility of echocardiographic techniques for sequential assessment of left ventricular ejection fraction and volumes: application to patients undergoing cancer chemotherapy. J Am Coll Cardiol 2013;61:77–84.

[5] Cardinale D, Colombo A, Lamantia G, Colombo N, Civelli M, Giacomi G, et al. Anthracycline-induced cardiomyopathy: clinical relevance and response to pharmacologic therapy. J Am Coll Cardiol 2010;55:213–20.

[6] Plana JC, Galderisi M, Barac A, Ewer MS, Ky B, Scherrer-Crosbie M, et al. Expert consensus for multimodality imaging evaluation of adult patients during and after cancer therapy: a report from the American Society of Echocardiography and the European Association of Cardiovascular Imaging. Eur Heart J Cardiovasc Imaging 2014;15:1063–93.

[7] Edvardsen T, Gerber BL, Garot J, Bluemke DA, Lima JAC, Smiseth OA. Quantitative assessment of intrinsic regional myocardial deformation by Doppler strain rate echocardiography in humans: validation against three-dimensional tagged magnetic resonance imaging. Circulation 2002;106:50–6.

[8] Gjesdal O, Helle-Valle T, Hopp E, Lunde K, Vartdal T, Aakhus S, et al. Noninvasive separation of large, medium, and small myocardial infarcts in survivors of reperfused ST-elevation myocardial infarction: a comprehensive tissue Doppler and speckle-tracking echocardiography study. Circ Cardiovasc Imaging 2008;1:189–96.

[9] Edvardsen T, Haugaa KH. Imaging assessment of ventricular mechanics. Heart Br Card Soc 2011;97:1349–56.

[10] Thavendiranathan P, Poulin F, Lim K-D, Plana JC, Woo A, Marwick TH. Use of myocardial strain imaging by echocardiography for the early detection of cardiotoxicity in patients during and after cancer chemotherapy: a systematic review. J Am Coll Cardiol 2014;63:2751–68.

[11] Tsai H-R, Gjesdal O, Wethal T, Haugaa KH, Fosså A, Fosså SD, et al. Left ventricular function assessed by two-dimensional speckle tracking echocardiography in long-term survivors of Hodgkin's lymphoma treated by mediastinal radiotherapy with or without anthracycline therapy. Am J Cardiol 2011;107:472–7.

[12] Ganame J, Claus P, Uyttebroeck A, Renard M, D'hooge J, Bijnens B, et al. Myocardial dysfunction late after low-dose anthracycline treatment in asymptomatic pediatric patients. J Am Soc Echocardiogr 2007;20:1351–8.

[13] Negishi K, Negishi T, Hare JL, Haluska BA, Plana JC, Marwick TH. Independent and incremental value of deformation indices for prediction of trastuzumab-induced cardiotoxicity. J Am Soc Echocardiogr 2013;26:493–8.

[14] Negishi K, Negishi T, Haluska BA, Hare JL, Plana JC, Marwick TH. Use of speckle strain to assess left ventricular responses to cardiotoxic chemotherapy and cardioprotection. Eur Heart J Cardiovasc Imaging 2014;15:324–31.

[15] Stoodley PW, Richards DAB, Boyd A, Hui R, Harnett PR, Meikle SR, et al. Altered left ventricular longitudinal diastolic function correlates with reduced systolic function immediately after anthracycline chemotherapy. Eur Heart J Cardiovasc Imaging 2013;14:228–34.

[16] Sawaya H, Sebag IA, Plana JC, Januzzi JL, Ky B, Tan TC, et al. Assessment of echocardiography and biomarkers for the extended prediction of cardiotoxicity in patients treated with anthracyclines, taxanes, and trastuzumab. Circ Cardiovasc Imaging 2012;5:596–603.

[17] Stoodley PW, Richards DAB, Boyd A, Hui R, Harnett PR, Meikle SR, et al. Left ventricular systolic function in HER2/neu negative breast cancer patients treated with anthracycline chemotherapy: a comparative analysis of left ventricular ejection fraction and myocardial strain imaging over 12 months. Eur J Cancer Oxf Engl 1990 2013;49:3396–403.

[18] Zhang H, Shen W, Gao C, Deng L, Shen D. Protective effects of salidroside on epirubicin-induced early left ventricular regional systolic dysfunction in patients with breast cancer. Drugs RD 2012;12:101–6.

[19] Motoki H, Koyama J, Nakazawa H, Aizawa K, Kasai H, Izawa A, et al. Torsion analysis in the early detection of anthracycline-mediated cardiomyopathy. Eur Heart J Cardiovasc Imaging 2012;13:95–103.

[20] Mornoş C, Petrescu L. Early detection of anthracycline-mediated cardiotoxicity: the value of considering both global longitudinal left ventricular strain and twist. Can J Physiol Pharmacol 2013;91:601–7.

[21] Fallah-Rad N, Walker JR, Wassef A, Lytwyn M, Bohonis S, Fang T, et al. The utility of cardiac biomarkers, tissue velocity and strain imaging, and cardiac magnetic resonance imaging in predicting early left ventricular dysfunction in patients with human epidermal growth factor receptor II-positive breast cancer treated with adjuvant trastuzumab therapy. J Am Coll Cardiol 2011;57:2263–70.

[22] Edvardsen T. Can modern echocardiographic techniques predict drug-induced cardiotoxicity?. J Am Coll Cardiol 2011;57:2271–2.

[23] Voigt J-U, Pedrizzetti G, Lysyansky P, Marwick TH, Houle H, Baumann R, et al. Definitions for a common standard for 2D speckle tracking echocardiography: consensus document of the EACVI/ASE/Industry Task Force to standardize deformation imaging. Eur Heart J Cardiovasc Imaging 2015;16:1–11.

Chapter 21

The Role of Cardiovascular Magnetic Resonance (CMR)

C. Bucciarelli-Ducci

Chapter Outline

INTRODUCTION

Cardiovascular magnetic resonance (CMR) is a noninvasive tomographic imaging technique. Its intrinsic advantages are the ability to acquire images in multiple planes without limitation of the acoustic window and patients' body habitus, lack of radiation exposure, high contrast-to-noise ratios, and true 3D volumetric coverage with no geometric assumptions. However, the unique opportunity that CMR offers is noninvasive myocardial tissue characterization.

CMR is contraindicated in patients with ferromagnetic implants, including non-MR conditional cardiac devices. In particular, in patients with breast cancer caution should be used in evaluating breast tissue expanders which might contain some ferromagnetic components. Additional limitations of CMR include limited (but increasing) availability and expertise, cost, and potential patient claustrophobia. In patients with renal dysfunction and eGFR <30 mL/min/1.73 m^2 administration of gadolinium-chelate contrast should be considered with caution due to the potential, albeit minimal, risk of nephrogenic systemic sclerosis [1].

STANDARD ANALYSIS OF CARDIAC STRUCTURE AND FUNCTION

Cine images are typically acquired in the long- and short-axis views using a standard steady-state free precession pulse sequence. Complete left and right

Anticancer Treatments and Cardiotoxicity. DOI: http://dx.doi.org/10.1016/B978-0-12-802509-3.00021-2

ventricular (RV) coverage is achieved by obtaining contiguous short-axis slices from the atrioventricular plane to the apex. Endocardial and epicardial contours are then drawn in the end-diastolic and end-systolic frames of each short-axis slice and normally performed with semiautomated software, in accordance with the Society for Cardiovascular Magnetic Resonance (SCMR) guidelines on standardized image interpretation and postprocessing of CMR images [2]. Myocardial deformation and in particular circumferential and longitudinal strain can be assessed by CMR using a spatial modulation of magnetization sequence, myocardial tagging, or a feature tracking postprocessing algorithm applied to cine images.

CMR is highly accurate and reproducible with excellent interstudy reproducibility and superior to 2D echocardiography in measuring left ventricular (LV) volumes and LV mass in normal, dilated, and hypertrophic hearts. This allows to considerably lower the sample sizes to detect clinically significant changes in end-diastolic volume, end-systolic volume, ejection fraction, and LV mass when using CMR [3]. For example, showing a 3% absolute change in ejection fraction in patients with heart failure would require 14 patients with CMR versus 115 patients with echocardiography (power of 90%, α-error of 0.05) with a reduction in sample size of 88% [4]. CMR is therefore considered the reference standard for measuring LV/RV volumes and function [4], making it well suited for assessing potential cardiotoxic effects of chemotherapy.

In most studies there is a good correlation between CMR and echocardiographic measurement [5], particularly with 3D echocardiography [6]. In a cohort of long-term survivors of childhood cancer, 3D was superior to 2D echocardiography, but both techniques were suboptimal in reproducibly identifying patients with left ventricular ejection fraction (LVEF) $< 50\%$ compared to CMR [7]. It is also important to recognize that different imaging techniques use different normal reference values and therefore are not interchangeable [8].

The joint ASE/EACVI expert consensus document for multimodality imaging evaluation of adult patients during and after cancer therapy recommends echocardiography (preferably 3D) as the method of choice for the evaluation of patients before, during, and after cancer therapy [5]. However, it is recognized that CMR is the reference standard in the evaluation of LV/RV volumes and LVEF, and that it may be particularly useful for accurate LV assessment when discontinuation of chemotherapy is being considered, or when echocardiographic assessment is suboptimal [4]. The high accuracy and precision of CMR may allow to detect subtle abnormalities that might not meet the criteria for cardiotoxicity, albeit representing early markers of cardiac injury.

A recent systematic review comprehensively illustrates the role of CMR in the detection of cardiac toxicity from cancer chemotherapy [9]. A number of studies have adopted CMR to assess LV/RV volumes, ejection fraction, LV mass, and strain in adult or pediatric patients receiving anthracycline, trastuzumab, or doxorubicin chemotherapy [10].

A significant deterioration of CMR LVEF and LV end-systolic volume (LVESV) was observed in patients with breast cancer, lymphoma, and leukemia following anthracycline chemotherapy treatment [10–12].

Anthracycline cardiomyopathy can also be characterized by a reduction in CMR LV mass, which was the strongest predictor of major cardiovascular events [13].

Early development of subclinical abnormalities, such as deterioration of LVESV and ventricular strain, were demonstrated using CMR in both breast and hematological cancer [14] and in patients with nonHodgkin lymphoma [15].

There are limited data on the cardiotoxic effect of chemotherapy in the RV. A reduction of right ventricular ejection fraction (RVEF) after anthracycline was documented by CMR in the absence of heart failure symptoms [11]. This tends to be a later marker of disease and occult cardiotoxicity can occur in asymptomatic patients despite a normal LVEF and RVEF [16].

CMR was used for serial assessments in patients with HER2 positive breast cancer trastuzumab in whom cardiomyopathy developed within 3 months of treatment, with a progressive decline in LVEF up to 9 months stabilizing at $38 \pm 6\%$ [17]. However, the majority of patients were asymptomatic (86%).

In long-term survivors of childhood cancer (mean age 14.6 years, mean follow-up 7.8 years) treated with anthracycline, CMR demonstrated a significant prevalence of impaired left and right EF and increased volumes [18].

Vascular Function

During a single CMR exam both the heart and the vasculature can be simultaneously assessed. Mitochondrial dysfunction after anthracycline treatment can be experienced both at the level of the cardiomyocytes and of the arterial endothelial cells. Aortic stiffness is a known independent predictor of adverse cardiovascular events. Early onset (within 4 months) of aortic stiffness has been described after anthracycline chemotherapy compared to age-matched controls, even after adjusting for covariates [12]. This correlated with higher cumulative dose of anthracycline. These findings were confirmed in a larger cohort of patients receiving anthracycline [14] and trastuzumab [19] and these changes partially reverse a year after therapy discontinuation, with the more severe effects observed with anthracycline [19].

TISSUE CHARACTERIZATION BY LGE CMR AND T1 MAPPING

CMR offers the unique opportunity to perform noninvasively myocardial tissue characterization by exploiting the magnetic properties of hydrogen nuclei protons within a determined magnetic field. Myocardial tissue characterization can be achieved in health and disease by imaging the native magnetic properties of the heart (T1 longitudinal relaxation time and T2 transverse relaxation time) with several pulse sequences and by using a gadolinium-chelate contrast agent. CMR can identify the presence and extent of myocardial edema/inflammation, as well as focal, replacement, and interstitial myocardial fibrosis.

Myocardial replacement fibrosis is imaged using a T1-weighted inversion-recovery gradient echo sequence after the administration of a gadolinium-chelate contrast agent. These are extracellular contrast media which accumulate in the increased myocardial extracellular space due to a pathological process. This leads to increased signal intensity compared to the normal myocardium (late gadolinium enhancement (LGE)). This is a very well-established technique to image focal myocardial fibrosis in both ischemic and nonischemic cardiomyopathies [20].

The first report of abnormal contrast-enhanced images in patients treated with anthracycline was in 2001 by Wassmuth. Higher myocardial signal intensity was noted at day 3, predicting a future drop in LVEF. However, whether this demonstrates increased myocardial extracellular distribution volume (fibrosis) or enhanced water exchange (edema) between the compartments remains undetermined given the use of a (now antiquate) spin-echo sequence, a precursor of the inversion-recovery gradient echo sequence now considered the gold standard technique for LGE.

Overall, the incidence of LGE is low ($\sim 5\%$) and the pattern of LGE described in anthracycline-treated patients can be epicardial, mid-wall, and focal fibrosis of the insertion points of the RV into the LV [9].

In trastuzumab, cardiomyopathy CMR identified epicardial linear LGE of the lateral wall [17,21]. This is a pattern suggesting trastuzumab induced myocarditis. Mid-wall LGE of the basal inferolateral wall can present in the absence of systolic or diastolic dysfunction and with no symptoms of heart failure during or after treatment with trastuzumab [22]. Mid-wall LGE was also observed in 30% of patients with nonHodgkin lymphoma 3 months after treatment, including in the presence of preserved LVEF [15]. Conversely, no LGE was identified in long-term survivors of childhood cancer treated with anthracycline [16,18]. Similarly, in an adult population receiving low to moderate doses of anthracycline, no LGE was identified despite a significant drop in LVEF at sixth month [14]. Currently, there are limited data on the prognostic significance of LGE in patients receiving cancer treatment. Only one study demonstrates that LGE in patients with anthracycline cardiomyopathy was not an independent predictor of cardiovascular outcome at 27-month follow-up [13].

A novel myocardial relaxometry technique called T1 mapping offers the opportunity to detect and quantify diffuse myocardial processes, adding a new dimension in the assessment of cardiac injury with and without the need of a contrast agent. The native (noncontrast) T1 relaxation time in the heart is prolonged with fibrosis, edema, and amyloid and reduced in lipid accumulation (Anderson–Fabry disease), cardiac siderosis, and hemorrhage in acute infarction [23]. However, alteration in native T1 may result from processes affecting the myocardium, the interstitium, or both.

ECV (extracellular volume fraction) is another novel biomarker that specifically quantifies expansion of the interstitial space. The latter technique requires the acquisition of the T1 mapping images pre- and postcontrast [22]. Measurement of ECV correlates with collagen volume fraction [23,24].

Myocardial ECV was found to be elevated in 42 patients treated with anthracycline (mean age 55 ± 17 years, median 84 months after treatment) compared to control, and associated with indexes of diastolic dysfunction and increased atrial volumes [25].

ECV was also increased in asymptomatic long-term childhood cancer survivors studied by CMR 2.5–26.9 years after treatment [16]. This abnormal myocardial characteristic was present despite normal LVEF but associated with abnormal global circumferential and longitudinal CMR strain.

Increased diffuse myocardial fibrosis measured by native T1 and ECV was observed in children ($n = 30$, 15 ± 3 years) at least 2 years after anthracycline chemotherapy despite normal LVEF. This was related to cumulative dose, exercise capacity, and myocardial wall thinning, suggesting that it could represent an early marker of disease [26].

Finally, both T1- and T2-weighted CMR signal changes measured at baseline and 3 months after initiation of treatment occur diffusely and they are commensurate with small to significant changes in LVEF 3 months after potential cardiotoxic chemotherapies confirming that tissue characterization could serve as an early marker of subclinical cardiotoxicity [27].

REFERENCES

[1] Nandwana SB, Moreno CC, Osipow MT, Sekhar A, Cox KL. Gadobenate dimeglumine administration and nephrogenic systemic fibrosis: is there a real risk in patients with impaired renal function? Radiology 2015;276:741–7.

[2] Schulz-Menger J, Bluemke DA, Bremerich J, Flamm SD, Fogel MA, Friedrich MG, et al. Standardized image interpretation and post processing in cardiovascular magnetic resonance: Society for Cardiovascular Magnetic Resonance (SCMR) board of trustees task force on standardized post processing. J Cardiovasc Magn Reson 2013;15:3.

[3] Grothues F, Smith GC, Moon JC, Bellenger NG, Collins P, Klein HU, et al. Comparison of interstudy reproducibility of cardiovascular magnetic resonance with two-dimensional echocardiography in normal subjects and in patients with heart failure or left ventricular hypertrophy. Am J Cardiol 2002;90:29–34.

[4] Pennell DJ, Sechtem UP, Higgins CB, Manning WJ, Pohost GM, Rademakers FE, Society for Cardiovascular Magnetic Resonance; Working Group on Cardiovascular Magnetic Resonance of the European Society of Cardiology. Clinical indications for cardiovascular magnetic resonance (CMR): Consensus Panel report. Eur Heart J 2004;25:1940–65.

[5] Plana JC, Galderisi M, Barac A, Ewer MS, Ky B, Scherrer-Crosbie M, et al. Expert consensus for multimodality imaging evaluation of adult patients during and after cancer therapy: a report from the American Society of Echocardiography and the European Association of Cardiovascular Imaging. Eur Heart J Cardiovasc Imaging 2014;15:1063–93.

[6] Ylänen K, Eerola A, Vettenranta K, Poutanen T. Three-dimensional echocardiography and cardiac magnetic resonance imaging in the screening of long-term survivors of childhood cancer after cardiotoxic therapy. Am J Cardiol 2014;113:1886–92.

[7] Armstrong GT, Plana JC, Zhang N, Srivastava D, Green DM, Ness KK, et al. Screening adult survivors of childhood cancer for cardiomyopathy: comparison of echocardiography and cardiac magnetic resonance imaging. J Clin Oncol 2012;30:2876–84.

[8] Bellenger NG, Davies LC, Francis JM, Coats AJ, Pennell DJ. Reduction in sample size for studies of remodeling in heart failure by the use of cardiovascular magnetic resonance. J Cardiovasc Magn Reson 2000;2(4):271–8.

[9] Thavendiranathan P, Wintersperger BJ, Flamm SD, Marwick TH. Cardiac MRI in the assessment of cardiac injury and toxicity from cancer chemotherapy: a systematic review. Circ Cardiovasc Imaging 2013;6:1080–91.

[10] Wassmuth R, Lentzsch S, Erdbruegger U, Schulz-Menger J, Doerken B, Dietz R, et al. Subclinical cardiotoxic effects of anthracyclines as assessed by magnetic resonance imaging-a pilot study. Am Heart J 2001;141:1007–13.

[11] Oberholzer K, Kunz RP, Dittrich M, Thelen M. Anthracycline-induced cardiotoxicity: cardiac MRI after treatment for childhood cancer. Rofo 2004;176:1245–50.

[12] Chaosuwannakit N, D'Agostino Jr R, Hamilton CA, Lane KS, Ntim WO, Lawrence J, et al. Aortic stiffness increases upon receipt of anthracycline chemotherapy. J Clin Oncol 2010;28:166–72.

[13] Neilan TG, Coelho-Filho OR, Pena-Herrera D, Shah RV, Jerosch-Herold M, Francis SA, et al. Left ventricular mass in patients with a cardiomyopathy after treatment with anthracyclines. Am J Cardiol 2012;110:1679–86.

[14] Drafts BC, Twomley KM, D'Agostino Jr R, Lawrence J, Avis N, Ellis LR, et al. Low to moderate dose anthracycline-based chemotherapy is associated with early noninvasive imaging evidence of subclinical cardiovascular disease. J Am Coll Cardiol Cardiovasc Imaging 2013;6:877–85.

[15] Lunning MA, Kutty S, Rome ET, Li L, Padiyath A, Loberiza F, et al. Cardiac magnetic resonance imaging for the assessment of the myocardium after doxorubicin-based chemotherapy. Am J Clin Oncol 2015;38:377–81.

[16] Toro-Salazar OH, Gillan E, O'Loughlin MT, Burke GS, Ferranti J, Stainsby J, et al. Occult cardiotoxicity in childhood cancer survivors exposed to anthracycline therapy. Circ Cardiovasc Imaging 2013;6:873–80.

[17] Wadhwa D, Fallah-Rad N, Grenier D, Krahn M, Fang T, Ahmadie R, et al. Trastuzumab mediated cardiotoxicity in the setting of adjuvant chemotherapy for breast cancer: a retrospective study. Breast Cancer Res Treat 2009;117:357–64.

[18] Ylänen K, Poutanen T, Savikurki-Heikkilä P, Rinta-Kiikka I, Eerola A, Vettenranta K. Cardiac magnetic resonance imaging in the evaluation of the late effects of anthracyclines among long-term survivors of childhood cancer. J Am Coll Cardiol 2013;61:1539–47.

[19] Grover S, Lou PW, Bradbrook C, Cheong K, Kotasek D, Leong DP, et al. Early and late changes in markers of aortic stiffness with breast cancer therapy. Ann Intern Med 2015; 45:140–7.

[20] Jiji RS, Kramer CM. Cardiovascular magnetic resonance: applications in daily practice. Cardiol Rev 2011;19:246–54.

[21] Fallah-Rad N, Lytwyn M, Fang T, Kirkpatrick I, Jassal DS. Delayed contrast enhancement cardiac magnetic resonance imaging in trastuzumab induced cardiomyopathy. J Cardiovasc Magn Reson 2008;22(10):5.

[22] Lawley C, Wainwright C, Segelov E, Lynch J, Beith J, McCrohon J. Pilot study evaluating the role of cardiac magnetic resonance imaging in monitoring adjuvant trastuzumab therapy for breast cancer. Asia Pac J Clin Oncol 2012;8:95–100.

[23] Bulluck H, Maestrini V, Rosmini S, Abdel-Gadir A, Treibel TA, Castelletti S, et al. Myocardial T1 mapping. Circ J 2015;79:487–94.

[24] Miller CA, Naish JH, Bishop P, Coutts G, Clark D, Zhao S, et al. Comprehensive validation of cardiovascular magnetic resonance techniques for the assessment of myocardial extracellular volume. Circ Cardiovasc Imaging 2013;6:373–83.

[25] Neilan TG, Coelho-Filho OR, Shah RV, Feng JH, Pena-Herrera D, Mandry D, et al. Myocardial extracellular volume by cardiac magnetic resonance imaging in patients treated with anthracycline-based chemotherapy. Am J Cardiol 2013;111:717–22.

[26] Tham EB, Haykowsky MJ, Chow K, Spavor M, Kaneko S, Khoo NS, et al. Diffuse myocardial fibrosis by T1-mapping in children with subclinical anthracycline cardiotoxicity: relationship to exercise capacity, cumulative dose and remodelling. J Cardiovasc Magn Reson 2013;15:48.

[27] Jordan JH, D'Agostino Jr RB, Hamilton CA, Vasu S, Hall ME, Kitzman DW, et al. Longitudinal assessment of concurrent changes in left ventricular ejection fraction and left ventricular myocardial tissue characteristics after administration of cardiotoxic chemotherapies using T1-weighted and T2-weighted cardiovascular magnetic resonance. Circ Cardiovasc Imaging 2014;7:872–9.

Chapter 22

Nuclear Medicine Imaging and Cardiotoxicity

P.A. Erba, R. Boni and M. Sollini

Chapter Outline

INTRODUCTION

Cardiotoxicity represents a frequent complication secondary to the intake of some classes of chemotherapeutic agents, with significant consequences on patients' outcome [1]. The majority of studies on cardiotoxicity focus on patients treated with anthracyclines and trastuzumab, but cardiotoxic effect has been described for classes of drugs such as inhibitors of tyrosine kinases, inhibitors of vascular endothelial growth factor (VEGF) or multikinase inhibitors (imatinib, dasatinib, nilotinib, sunitinib, sorafenib, and bevacizumab), antimetabolites (5-fluorouracil), alkylating agents (cisplatin, cyclophosphamide), and taxanes (docetaxel and paclitaxel) [2]. Radiotherapy (RT), that is often associated with standard chemotherapy treatment, is also associated with cardiotoxicity appearing as (acute) myocardial infarction, pericardial disease, valvular heart disease, and heart failure (HF). The incidence of late irradiation-induced cardiac disease depends on the irradiated volume, total irradiation dose, dose per fraction, and on the presence or absence of preexisting cardiovascular risk factors. Irradiation of the mediastinum with a cumulative dose >30 Gy and a daily fractioning >2 Gy appeared to be related to a high risk of developing cardiac dysfunction [3].

Anticancer Treatments and Cardiotoxicity. DOI: http://dx.doi.org/10.1016/B978-0-12-802509-3.00022-4

Two groups of patients, i.e., those suffering from Hodgkin's disease and breast cancer, are particularly at risk of developing late myocardial damage, since RT treatment techniques for both patient groups may include (large) parts of the heart, and adjuvant systemic therapy, in particular anthracycline-containing chemotherapy, is frequently administered to these patient.

Over the last few decades, several clinical guidelines have emphasized the need for monitoring cardiotoxicity [4–10]. Timely detection of cardiotoxicity allows initiation of cardioprotective medication. Several clinical parameters have been identified that can be used for periodic evaluation of various aspects of cardiac performance prior to, during, and after therapy. Myocardial biopsy is still considered the most accurate and specific method in identifying the myocardial damage induced by chemotherapy, detecting the ultrastructural alteration of cardiomyocytes [11]. Nevertheless, its invasiveness limited its use in clinical practice. The most validated definition of cardiotoxicity has been established by the cardiac review and evaluation committee based either on the onset of HF symptoms and signs or by an asymptomatic decrease of left ventricular ejection fraction (LVEF) [12]. Therefore, assessment of LVEF is the most widely utilized parameter in monitoring the cardiac function in clinical practice.

Imaging techniques, such as echocardiography (ECHO), multigated equilibrium radionuclide venticulography (MUGA), and cardiovascular magnetic resonance (CMR) nowadays allow accurate and reproducible evaluation of volumes and of alteration of LVEF. However, the drop of LVEF represents a late phenomenon in the physiopathology of the chemotherapy-induced cardiotoxicity and has low sensitivity in the presence of subclinical myocardial dysfunction. This evidence has led researchers to look to other imaging methods that evaluate cardiac function independently of cardiac volume changes to detect the earliest manifestation of cardiotoxicity. Some of these methods, such as speckle tracking imaging, have been already introduced in clinical practice whereas others are under investigation in experimental settings.

Nuclear imaging techniques, besides providing sensitive and accurate estimation of LVEF, represent an emerging tool for noninvasive detection of myocardial damage induced by antineoplastic drugs [13]. In fact, nuclear imaging techniques by the use of radioactive tracers (chemical compounds linked to short-lived isotopes) provide quantitative detection of the molecule and molecule-based events related to the pathological process, in vivo in living subjects with the potential to speed laboratory discovery and to personalize the care of an individual patient with a certain disease. The peculiarity of these techniques, that makes the fundamental difference between nuclear medicine imaging and other imaging techniques, is represented by the radiopharmaceutical, the key molecule of the whole process. In fact, for a certain biologic-physiologic process one (or more than one) specific radiopharmaceutical has been designed. Indeed, the radiopharmaceutical is a function of its chemical nature (Table 22.1), it produces a physical signal

TABLE 22.1 Examples of Radiotracers Used to Evaluate Cardiotoxicity and Their Own "Target" Biologic-Physiologic Process

Technique	Tracer	Mechanism/Action
Scintigraphy	^{99m}Tc-erythrocyte	Contractile function
	^{201}Thallium	Myocradial perfusion (reflecting viable myocytes)
	^{99m}Tc-tetrofosmin	Myocradial perfusion (reflecting viable myocytes)
	^{99m}Tc-sestamibi	Myocradial perfusion (reflecting viable myocytes)
	^{111}In-antimyosin	Necrosis/cell death
	^{123}I-MIBG	Neuronal imaging (false neurotransmitters)
	^{111}In-trastuzumab	Therapeutic target imaging (HER2 mAb)
	^{99m}Tc-annexin V	Apoptosis
	^{123}I-BMIPP	Fatty acid use
PET	[^{18}F]FDG	Glucose metabolism
	^{13}N-ammonia	Myocradial perfusion
	^{82}Rb	Myocradial perfusion
	^{11}C-HED	Neuronal imaging (false neurotransmitters)
	^{11}C-CGP-12177	Neuronal imaging (adrenoceptor antagosists)
	[^{11}C]-rolipram	Intracellular signaling (second messenger)
	[^{18}F]-CP18	Apoptosis
	^{11}C-acetoacetate	Fatty acid use

Source: Modified from D'Amore C, et al. Nuclear imaging in detection and monitoring of cardiotoxicity. *World J Radiol* 2014;6:486–92.

(emission of γ-rays and/or $\beta+$ particles) that medical equipment can detect (gamma camera or positron emission tomography (PET) nowadays, often combined with computed X-ray tomography (CT) scans to give coregistration of the two images, SPECT/CT and PET/CT).

In this chapter, we will review nuclear imaging techniques used to image cardiotoxicity.

Radionuclide Blood-Pool Imaging

First-pass (FP) and equilibrium radionuclide venticulography (RVG, also known as multigated acquisition, MUGA) has long been considered the gold standard for chemotherapy-related cardiotoxicity screening.

The key principle of ventriculography is to image the blood-pool over time. Afterwards the radiopharmaceutical injection electrocardiograph (ECG)-gated cardiac scintigraphy is obtained. Indeed, concomitant registration of ECG signal allows to assign counts into specific intervals within the cardiac cycle.

For FP radionuclide ventriculography (FPRNV) study a short sequence of cardiac cycles acquired during the transit of a bolus through the heart is acquired, whereas for equilibrium RVG data are collected from several hundred cardiac cycles to generate an image set of the beating heart that is presented as a single, composite cardiac cycle (Fig. 22.1).

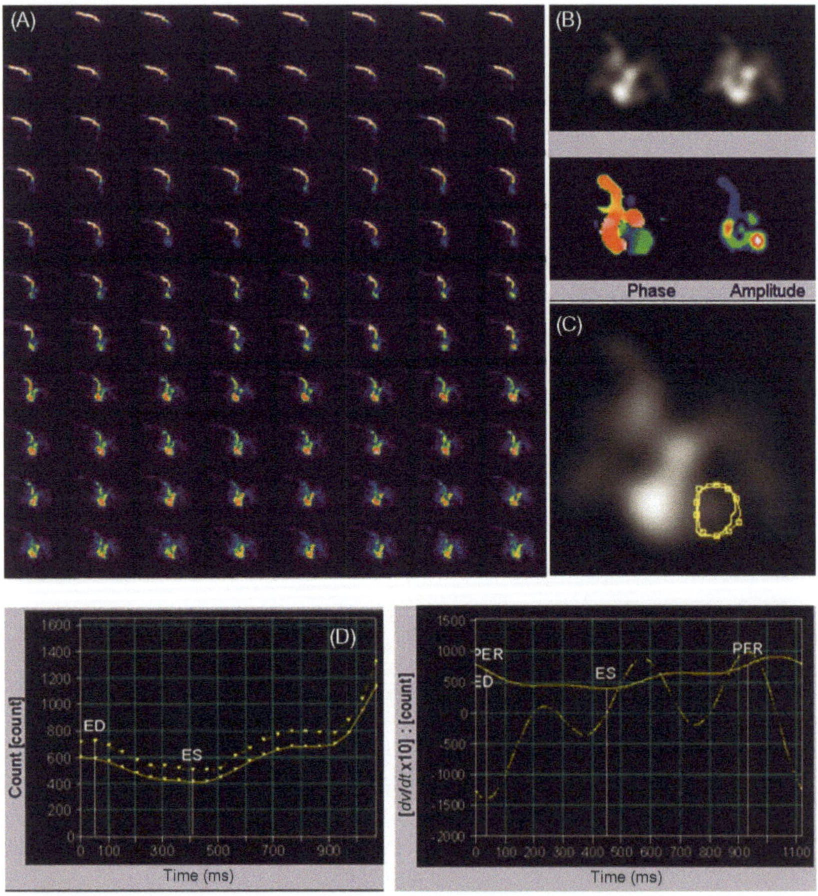

FIGURE 22.1 Baseline rest first-pass radionuclide angiography in a 72-year-old female with pulmunary hypertension and breast cancer (A–D). Visualization of the end-diastolic (ED), end-systolic (ES), phase and amplitude images (B) generated by software after region of interest (ROI) positioning (C). (D) The volumes curves and the peak ejection rate (PER). Ejection fraction = 51%.

FPRNV provides high target-to-background ratio with temporal separation of the right ventricular (RV) and left ventricular (LV), but imaging is possible in only one projection. The quality of FPRNV may be affected by many factors, regarding data acquisition, as well as processing parameters. Like other modalities addressing ventricular function, FPRNV requires that the cardiac rhythm remains stable during acquisition. FPRNV is achievable with many compounds that do not undergo substantial FP pulmonary uptake. Otherwise, only the RV can be assessed. If a series of studies is required (e.g., stress/rest), the tracer must be rapidly cleared from the blood pool (^{99m}Tc-DTPA or ^{99m}Tc-sulfur colloid). FPRNV can be performed just before equilibrium radionuclide venticulography (RNV); acquisition is then performed during tracer injection (^{99m}Tc-pertechnetate, labeled red cells, or ^{99m}Tc-HSA). FPRNV is also achievable with myocardial perfusion tracers such as ^{99m}Tc-sestamibi or ^{99m}Tc-tetrofosmin.

FPRNV requires a rapid injection of the radiopharmaceutical bolus using a large-gauge cannula in a proximal vein (usually antecubital), preferring a medial vein in the right arm because venous return has the shortest and least tortuous course to the right atrium, and the arm may be abducted to straighten the veins [14]. Injection into a central venous catheter should be avoided for right ventricular ejection fraction (RVEF) determination, as the bolus passage through the RV will then often include less than four heartbeats. For LV evaluation, a central venous catheter is well suited for tracer administration. FPRNV requires a minimum activity amount of 700 MBq, and the bolus must be highly concentrated (<1 mL) and rapidly flushed by at least 10 mL saline.

FPRNV study requires a high-count rate. Some prefer a high-sensitivity, parallel-hole collimator for FPRNV studies, especially for LV studies [15], whereas others prefer, especially for RV studies, a general-purpose or even a high-resolution, parallel-hole collimator to more accurately define the cardiac chambers and the valve planes, moving during the cardiac cycle [16]. During imaging postprocessing, background subtraction is necessary to remove scatter (spillover), approximately 20–30% during the LV phase [17]. Background can be identified with an region of interest (ROI) defined immediately outside the apical perimeter of the LV. Time–activity curves (TAC) from cardiac cycles containing the maximum activity are summed in phase as for the RV ejection fractions measurement. For equilibrium RVG two radiopharmaceuticals are used: ^{99m}Tc-labeled erythrocyte (^{99m}Tc-RBCs) or human serum albumin (^{99m}Tc-HSA). Three methods are available to label red blood cells (RBCs): in vitro, modified in vivo, and in vivo. The basic mechanism of the labeling in all approaches is the same. The RBCs are "pretinned" by stannous (Sn^{2+}) ions, which may be present in different compounds, followed by addition of ^{99m}Tc-pertechnetate after 10–30 min. The amount of Sn^{2+} required for optimal labeling is in the range of 0.03–0.15 mg/mL of blood or 10–20 mg/kg body weight. Deviation from that range may reduce labeling efficiency by up to 20% [14]. The in vitro method using a commercially available kit yields the highest labeling efficiency (>95%) [18,19]. A further advantage of the in vitro method is that a sample can be evaluated for radiolabeling efficiency with a centrifuge method as described in the manufacturer's package insert. Additionally, if radiolabeling is substandard because of a drug interaction (iodinated contrast, chemotherapy, digoxin, calcium channel blockers, cyclosporin, metronidazole, ranitidine, propanolol, quinidine, dipyridamole, heparin, low hematocrit level, sickle-cell disease or thalassemia, circulating antibodies from prior transfusion or transplantation or other factor such as excessive ^{99m}Tc-sodium pertechnetate volume, excessive generator in-growth time, excessively aged generator eluates, anticoagulant sequestration of stannous ions), or because of a procedural deviation, a salvage technique may be attempted [20]. This procedure involves transferring the in vitro ^{99m}Tc-RBCs into a sterile 15 mL polypropylene centrifuge tube and centrifuging at 400 g for 5 min. The supernatant is then removed with a sterile pipette, and the ^{99m}Tc-RBCs are resuspended in 2 mL of 0.9% sodium chloride. If the radiochemical purity of the ^{99m}Tc-RBCs is then more than 95% and adequate radioactivity remains, the salvage is deemed successful. The modified in vivo label (90% labeling efficiency) can serve as an alternative when the in vitro method is not available [21–23]. In vitro labeling should be performed under strictly aseptic conditions in a laminar airflow unit dedicated to cell labeling. In vitro labeling gives by far the highest labeling efficiency and, over time, the most stable labeling. Measurement of erythrocyte volume by in vitro labeled RBCs with ^{99m}Tc gives values similar to labeling with the gold standard ^{51}Cr; this is not the case with the in vivo or in vivo/in vitro method nor with ^{99m}Tc-labeled HSA, calculated from total blood volume and hematocrit. Therefore, determination of absolute LV volumes with RNV must be performed using in vitro labeled RBCs.

In the vivo/in vitro labeling of RBCs consist of intravenous (iv) administration of a stannous agent followed 15–30 min later by withdrawal of an aliquot (3–10 mL) of pretinned blood through a cannula into a shielded syringe containing an anticoagulant (ACD or heparin) and the required amount of ^{99m}Tc-pertechnetate. The blood is mixed with the ^{99m}Tc-pertechnetate and allowed to incubate for 10–20 min at room temperature with occasional mixing. The unbound activity may be washed away by centrifugation before reinjection via the same cannula. Alternatively, the radiolabeled RBCs can be reinjected without the washing step.

The in vivo method may be used in patients who will not accept injection of blood. The recommended administered activity of ^{99m}Tc-RBCs is 555–1110 MBq (15–30 mCi) in adults [14]. In children under 18 years old, the recommended administered activity is based on the EANM Pediatric Dosage Card, which uses a baseline activity of 56 MBq (1.51 mCi) multiplied by a weight-based multiple [23,24]. The resulting minimum administered activity is 80 MBq (2.16 mCi) for a 3-kg patient and the maximum administered activity is 784 MBq (21.19 mCi) for a 68-kg patient.

^{99m}Tc-HSA may be used as an alternative to radiolabeled RBCs [14]. ^{99m}Tc-HSA is prepared from radiopharmaceutical kits containing stannous ion as the reducing agent for ^{99m}Tc [25,26]. However, albumin escapes from the intravascular space, and the ^{99m}Tc-binding is not very stable; therefore, ^{99m}Tc-HSA is inferior to ^{99m}Tc-labeled RBCs as a blood-pool imaging agent and should not be used for volume determination or LVEF monitoring over hours. The usual administered activity is 800 MBq (range of 370–925 MBq) for an adult patient [27]. The activity for children may be adjusted according to body weight, with a minimum activity of 80 MBq to obtain images of sufficient quality [24].

Equilibrium RVG assess (1) regional and global wall motion; (2) cardiac chamber size and morphology; and (3) ventricular systolic and diastolic function, including left and RV ejection fractions (LVEF and RVEF, respectively). Typical acquisitions for RVG last for 10–15 min and include supine imaging in the LAO view at 30–45° ("best septal" for RV–LV separation). Other views may be relevant for assessing regional LV function: anterior view (0° or 45° less than "best septal" view), a lateral view (left cross-table lateral or 45° greater than "best septal"). For an accurate measurement of EF, a minimum of 16 frames/R–R interval are required, with R–R interval tolerance window set to 10–20%. A higher framing rate (32–64 frames/R–R) is preferred for the measurement of diastolic functional parameters [28]. Fig. 22.2 shows an example of RVG in a patients after doxorubicin chemotherapy.

RNV might also be obtained after exercise (supine ergometer exercise, the most convenient form of stress; upright ergometer exercise or pharmacological stress with a vasodilator or inotropic drug) allowing LVEF measurement for comparison with the rest [29]. The radioactive amount injected is similar to the amount used in a resting RNV study, although a larger activity amount may be given to shorten acquisition times during exercise.

Imaging processing consists of drowing ventricular and background ROIs either manually by the operator, with support of the cine loop and phase image for an accurate definition of valvular planes, or automatically by the computer. Automatic programs, provided the acquisition data are appropriate (projection separating RV from LV, counting statistics, etc.), only require a master ROI drawn by the operator over the LV, which includes the whole ventricle. Then, end-diastolic (ED) and end-systolic (ES) ROIs, as well as a background ROI, are defined for calculation of the LVEF and for a TAC showing emptying and filling of the LV. The efficiency of automatic methods is influenced by count statistics, target/background ratio, wall motion (WM), and pixel size. Parametric images, such as phase and amplitude images, may be useful for identification of the valve plane. From the first derivative of the TAC, additional indices of systolic function may be calculated: peak ejection rate, the minimum value of the first derivative in the systolic interval, the corresponding time and the time-to-peak ejection rate can

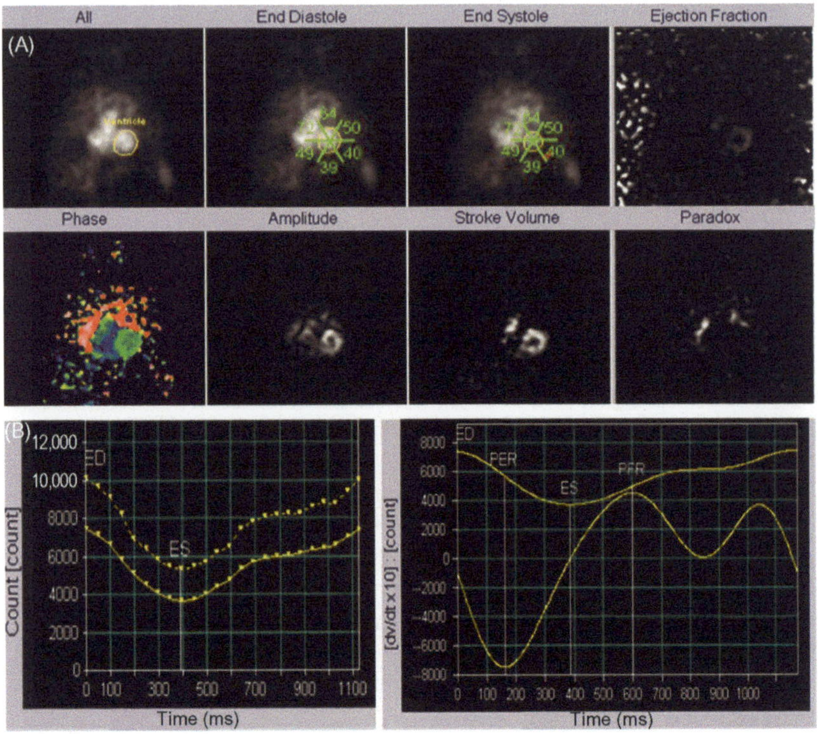

FIGURE 22.2 (A) Baseline rest equilibrium angiography in a 72-year-old female with pulmonary hypertension and breast cancer with the visualization of the end-diastolic (ED), end-systolic (ES) and ejection fraction, phase, amplitude, stroke volume and paradox images generated by software after region of interest (ROI) positioning. (B) The volume curves and the peak ejection rate (PER). Ejection fraction = 50%.

be also calculated. In addition, the pattern of contraction of all LV segments might be assessed using the cinematic display of each view and described using a standard scoring system (normal, mild–moderate–severe hypokinesia, akinesia, and dyskinesia).

Normal values for the LVEF based on RNV range from 55% to 75%; a LVEF <50% indicating a lower cardiac function. A decline below 50% or a drop in LVEF >10% compared to baseline indicates worsening of cardiac function. However, it should be remembered that physiologic variability may affect sequential assessment of LVEF.

The single largest study monitoring cardiotoxicity with RVG (or SPECT) in 1487 patients receiving doxorubicin shows that 19% of patients will be at high risk for developing cardiotoxicity. Among those at high risk for developing cardiotoxicity, patients developing clinical HF had the greater absolute drop in LVEF compared to those who did not (mean drop in LVEF 23% ± 14% vs 12% ± 10%) [30]. RVG screening in patients receiving doxorubicin led to early discontinuation of treatment in 13% of patients due to criteria for cardiotoxicity, the majority of whom were asymptomatic [31]. These data highlight the importance of routine screening, as many patients will demonstrate signs of cardiotoxicity by a drop in LVEF in the absence of HF symptoms.

However, whether the LVEF is the most appropriate measure for the early detection of LV dysfunction is controversial. A decline in systolic function, and hence LVEF, is considered a late sign of cardiotoxicity, revealing in the case of type I toxicity that irreversible damage to the myocardium has already occurred. Many patients present with histological evidence of anthracycline-related changes with normal resting LV function [32]. The addition of exercise stress RVG may identify a reduced contractily reserve in asymptomatic patients with normal resting LVEF [33]. Adding exercise stress RVG in patients with endomyocardial biopsy-proven cardiotoxicity increased sensitivity from 58% to 100% at the cost of a drop in specificity [34]. No large-scale studies in this population have yet demonstrated whether the routine addition of exercise RVG to screening would be cost-effective or alter dose recommendations of chemotherapeutic regimens.

In addition to changes in systolic function, RVG can provide information regarding diastolic function [35]. Theoretically, diastolic abnormalities occur prior to a drop in LV systolic function. Several factors may contribute, such as alterations of intracellular calcium handling [36] or increased coronary resistance resulting in acute elevations in LV end-diastolic pressure as in the case of exposure to anthracyclines [37]. Among the diastolic parameters, a significant decrease in the peak filling rate (PFR) has been described after 1 month of anthracycline treatment [38]. In this study, despite the PFR value still being within the normal range (PFR > 2.5), this correlates with a simultaneous decrease in LVEF (remaining within the normal range), suggesting that the same underlying process impairs both systolic and diastolic functions. More recently, Lapinńska et al. [39] confirmed the usefulness of RNV to evaluate cardiotoxicity in breast cancer patients undergoing chemotherapy (adriamycin plus cyclophosphamide or adriamycin plus docetaxel) associated with RT. Reductions in LVEF and PFR and an increase in the end-systolic and end-diastolic volumes were observed with all parameters significantly worsened in patients undergoing adriamycin plus cyclophosphamide where cumulative anthracycline dose is higher as compared to the adriamycin plus docetaxel regimen. RT did not significantly lower the value of EF as compared to the group of patients who underwent chemotherapy alone.

Nousiainen et al. [40] documented good diagnostic performances (sensitivity = 90% and specificity = 72%) of RNV in the prediction of chronic HF development in 28 patients treated with increasing cumulative doses of doxorubicin for nonHodgkin lymphoma. However, results of this little prospective study were not confirmed by a large retrospective study [41]. In fact, Swain et al. [41] observed that 66% of patients experiencing doxorubicin-related chronic HF showed no clinically relevant decline in LVEF value assessed by RNV scan from baseline levels (ranging from 0% to 30% of the absolute value), suggesting that it is not accurate in HF prediction. More recently, Fatima et al. [42] performed RNV and echo in 42 patients with different cancers during chemotherapy with adriamycin (65 ± 10 mg/m^2), determining the percentage of LVEF (%LVEF) at baseline and after each cycle (six in total). A significant decline ($P < 0.001$) in %LVEF was noted at the end of adriamycin therapy, using both RNV (12.17 ± 5.01) and echo (9.26 ± 4.82); however, RNV identified many more patients who developed protocol-defined cardiotoxicity than echo (31% vs 14%). Subclinical adriamycin cardiotoxicity was detectable from the third cycle and if not detected earlier continued therapy may progress to severe and irreversible cardiotoxicity. Skovgaard et al. [43] compared RNV to brain natriuretic peptide (BNP) as predictors of developing congestive heart failure (CHF) or death in a population of anthracycline-treated cancer patients. They found that in cancer patients treated with cardiotoxic chemotherapy both BNP and LVEF can significantly predict subsequent hospitalization with CHF but only BNP (and not LVEF) had a prognostic value in detecting overall death.

In the pediatric population, echo is the preferred method of surveillance as it does not deliver radiation and RNV is reserved for confirmation of LVEF decline in high-risk patients. However, when compared to echocardiography to assess LV function in children with Hodgkin disease (HD) receiving doxorubicin, before RT both early (≤ 2 cycles) and late (≥ 6 cycles) during treatment, RVG was more sensitive than echo in detecting early impairment of LV function at low cumulative doses of doxorubicin [44].

Table 22.2 reports the main results of literature searching on the use of radionuclide blood-pool imaging to image cardiotoxicity.

^{99m}Tc Gated Blood-Pool Single-Photon Emission Tomography (SPECT, GBPS)

The use of ECG-gated blood pool SPECT has recently gained some popularity. Tomographic acquisition should overcome the difficulties of planar RNV in the separation of cardiac chambers, allowing the simultaneous evaluation of RV and LV function and LV volumes without any geometrical assumptions. Currently used acquisition protocols are largely identical or strongly inspired by protocols used for myocardial perfusion SPECT (MPI). Tomographic RNV is most commonly acquired with a two-headed gamma camera, collimator, energy window, orbit, matrix size, and zoom similar to MPI. Sixteen frames/cycle are preferred to eight frames, which may lead to overestimation of end-systolic counts and, hence, underestimation of the EF values and the gating and R–R interval tolerance window should be set to 10–20%, similar to planar RNV.

TABLE 22.2 Summary of the Main Publications on Cardiotoxicity Imaged By Radionuclide Blood-pool Imaging

References	Patients (*n*)	Treatment	Test(s)	Parameter(s) Evaluated	Main Findings
Aapro et al. 1983 [45]	10	Mitoxantrone	MUGA, endomyocardial biopsy	LVEF, wall motion, cardiac status	None of pts showed evidence of clinically significant myocardial damage. Endomyocardial biopsy showed grade 2.5 anthracyclin-type cardiotoxicity in 1 case suggesting the indication of serial endomyocardial biopsy in pts on long-term drug therapy to determine the incidence, dose-relationship, and severity of potential mitoxantrone-associated endomyocardial damage
Abu-Khalaf et al. 2007 [46]	85	Doxorubicin + paclitaxel + cyclophosphamide	ERNA	LVEF	Clinical HF in one patient. LVEF< 50% at the end of therapy in 8% of pts. At a median follow-up of 7 years, the median absolute change in LVEF from baseline was −5.5% (LVEF < 50% in 12% of cases)
Agarwala et al. 2000 [47]	55[a]	Adriamycin	MUGA	LVEF	Cardiotoxicity in 13 pts (3/13 clinical evidence of CHF). In 10 pts, timely discontinuation of adriamycin, based on the MUGA report, probably has helped avoid the development of CHF
Alcan et al. 1985 [48]	33	Anthracycline	RNV stress/rest	LVEF, Fourier image analysis	The exercise RNV performed better than rest RNV alone in the early detection of anthracycline-related cardiotoxicity. The single most sensitive indicator of cardiotoxicity was the Fourier image analysis. Sequential rest/stress RNV studies with Fourier amplitude and phase analysis were the most sensitive to evaluate pts who receive potentially cardiotoxic agents

(Continued)

TABLE 22.2 (Continued)

References	Patients (*n*)	Treatment	Test(s)	Parameter(s) Evaluated	Main Findings
Alexander et al. 1979 [49]	55	Doxorubicin	RNV	LVEF	Severe cardiotoxicity (CHF) in 9% of pts. Moderate toxicity in 11% of pts in whom doxorubicin was discontinued (no subsequent HF or a further decline in EF during the follow-up period)
Appel et al. 1990 [50]	980	Cyclophosphamide + epirubicin + 5-fluorouracil vs cyclophosphamide + methotrexate + 5-fluorouracil	RNV, TDI, echo, blood test	LVEF, NT-proBNP	Epirubicin-containing regimen showed no cardiac impairment when compared to methotrexate-based ones
Barendswaard et al. 1991 [51]	52	Doxorubicin	RNV	Wall motion	Increased number of wall motion abnormalities in the RV (20%) compared with the LV (4.5%), particularly in the RV septum
Basar et al. 2014 [52]	56[a]	Anthracycline	MUGA, ECG, Holter, echo, MRI	n.r.	Subclinical cardiac dysfunction detected in 20 pts by at least one of echo, MRI, or MUGA
Carrió et al. 1993 [53]	30	Doxorubicin	MUGA, ^{111}In-antimyosin scintigraphy	LVEF, HLR	Intense antimyosin uptake at intermediate cumulative doses identified pts at risk of cardiotoxicity before EF deteriorates
Carrió et al. 1995 [54]	36	Doxorubicin	RNV, ^{111}In-antimyosin scintigraphy, ^{123}I-MIBG scintigraphy	LVEF, H/M, HLR	Cell damage and impaired adrenergic neuron activity was found in pts with maintained or slightly decreased EF

Cassidy et al. 1988 [55]	14	Vincristine + mitozantrone + prednisolone	RNV stress/rest	LVEF	Abnormalities of LVEF in 46% of pts. Clinical signs of HF in 1 case
Choi et al. 1983 [56]	337	Doxorubicin	FPRNV	LVEF	Abnormal baseline LV performance in 13% of pts (antecedent cardiovascular disease ± previous thoracic RT). Small but significant fall in LVEF in the 12 pts who received a cumulative dose ≥350 mg/m^2. Only 1 pt had CHF
Cochet et al. 2011 [57]	118	Tratuzumab	RNV	LVEF, PFR, PER, TPFR	During follow-up trastuzumab-mediated cardiotoxicity in 15% of pts. Impaired LV diastolic function before treatment resulted in an independent predictor of trastuzumab-mediated cardiotoxicity. The evaluation of diastolic function could allow optimal risk stratification before the introduction of trastuzumab
Coleman et al. 1984 [58]	34	Mitoxantrone	RNV stress/rest	LVEF	Deterioration in EF in 29% of pts (CHF in 2/10)
Constine et al. 1997 [59]	50	RT (mantle)	ERNA, MPI (^{201}Tl or ^{99m}Tc-MIBI), ECG	LVEF, PFR perfusion defect(s), wave alteration(s)	Generally normal measures of LVEF and myocardial perfusion
Cottin et al. 1998 [60]	99	Epirubicin vs doxorubicin	RNV	LVEF, PER, PFR	Advantage of epirubicin over doxorubicin in terms of cardiotoxicity
de Bree et al. 2007 [61]	13	Cytoreductive surgery + intraoperative hyperthermic intrathoracic doxorubicin + cisplatin	RNV, ECG, echo, blood test	LVEF, wave alteration(s), troponin	The degree of LVEF reduction was statistically related to maximal intrathoracic doxorubicin concentration and total cisplatin dose
de Leonardis et al. 1991 [62]	16	Mitoxantrone	RNV	LVEF	Pts treated with mitoxantrone may develop late cardiotoxicity

(*Continued*)

TABLE 22.2 (Continued)

References	Patients (*n*)	Treatment	Test(s)	Parameter(s) Evaluated	Main Findings
Dresdale et al. 1983 [63]	101	Doxorubicin	RNV	LVEF	Clinical CHF doxorubicin-related in 14% of pts. Incidence of cardiomyopathy in the asymptomatic group (detected by RNV) of 52%. Overall incidence of cardiomyopathy detected either clinically or by RNA of 46%
Druck et al. 1984 [64]	38	Doxorubicin	MUGA stress/rest, ECG, endomyocardial biopsy	LVEF, wave alteration(s), cardiac status	All abnormal MUGA were associated with abnormal biopsies (no false-positive scans). Stress MUGA uncovered 6 abnormal cases which could have been missed with a rest scan alone
Duan et al. 2003 [65]	23	Anthracycline	RNV, MPI (^{99m}Tc-MIBI), ECG, blood test	LVEF, myocardial relative quantity (MRQ), myocardial enzyme (CK-MB)	MPI was useful to monitor cardiotoxicity and its changes occurred earlier than LVEFs
Eising et al. 1997 [66]	43	Cyclosporin A + doxorubicin or epirubicin	RNV stress/rest	LVEF	Cyclosporin A did not cause any significant increase in cardiotoxicity
Estabragh et al. 2011 [67]	59	Imatinib	MUGA, echo, ECG	LVEF, wave alteration(s)	No evidence of myocardial deterioration, either at baseline or over 12 months of imatinib treatment
Ettinghausen et al. 1986 [68]	118	Doxorubicin	RNV stress/rest	LVEF	High-dose doxorubicin regimen resulted in significantly greater declines in EF than the low-dose protocol, the use of the low-dose regimen decreases the magnitude of the cardiomyopathic changes
Fatima et al. 2011 [42]	42	Adriamycin	MUGA, echo	LVEF, %LVEF	Subclinical cardiotoxicity was detectable from the 3rd cycle. Protocol-defined cardiotoxicity in 31% and 14% of pts using MUGA and echo, respectively

Feola et al. 2011 [69]	53	Anthracyclines	RNV, blood test	LVEF, troponin I, BNP	LVEF ≥10% reduction at 2 years in 32% of pts (higher baseline plasma BNP compared to normal group). LVEF and BNP modified early after anthracycline chemotherapy
Geidel et al. 1991 [70]	785	Adriamycin	RNV, echo	Fractional shortening rate, EF at rest	Sub/clinical heart damage (frequency/severity) increased with cumulative adriamycin and time since cessation of therapy
Gill et al. 2013 [71]	141	Pegylated liposomal doxorubicin	MUGA	LVEF	Pegylated liposomal doxorubicin did not carry a significant risk of cardiotoxicity, as evidenced by the stability of LVEF even after treatment with large cumulative doses
Goffette et al. 2005 [72]	52	Mitoxantrone	RNV	LVEF	No cardiotoxicity during the course of the treatment. CHF 24–80 months after the last dose of mitoxantrone in 6% of pts
Haas et al. 2015 [73]	1943	Sunitinib or sorafenib	MUGA	LVEF	Within 6 months, about 1% of pts experienced a cardiac event (LVEF decline from baseline >15% and below the institutional lower limit of normal). With dose interruption or adjustment, 16/21 cases recovered their LVEF to >50%
Harris et al. 2002 [74]	224	Liposome-encapsulated doxorubicin vs conventional doxorubicin	MUGA	LVEF	Liposome-encapsulated doxorubicin produced less cardiotoxicity than conventional doxorubicin (13% vs 19%)
Hofheinz et al. 2005 [75]	27	Anthracycline	MUGA	LVEF	Neither relevant LVEF decreases nor hints of cardiac toxicity were observed
Jain et al. 1985 [76]	54	Epirubicin or doxorubicin	MUGA stress/rest	LVEF	Symptomatic CHF in 17% of pts (at a cumulative dose of 1134 mg/m^2 of epirubicin compared with 492 mg/m^2 of doxorubicin)
Jensen et al. 2010 [77]	106	Fluorouracil + oxaliplatin	RNV, ECG, blood test	LVEF, wave alteration(s), NT-proBNP, lactic acid	Fluorouracil induced myocardial neuroendocrine changes with increasing plasma NT-proBNP and lactic acid but without long-term dysfunction of LV

(Continued)

TABLE 22.2 (Continued)

References	Patients (*n*)	Treatment	Test(s)	Parameter(s) Evaluated	Main Findings
Kingwell et al. 2010 [78]	163	Mitoxantrone	MUGA; blood test	LVEF, blood cell counts, liver function	Cardiotoxicity evident after doses (14% of pts) well below current maximum recommended levels
Knesewitsch et al. 1987 [79]	348	Adriamycin	ERNV rest	EF, EDV, ESV, SV, PFR, PER	Subnormal EF in 14% of pts at beginning of treatment, increased up to 86% (doses >500 mg/m^2)
Knesewitsch et al. 1987 [80]	348	Adriamycin	ERNV stress vs rest	EF, EDV, ESV, SV, PFR, PER	Pathologic results at rest were detected earlier than subnormal changes of exercise values
Lahtinen et al. 1991 [81]	24	Epirubicin or doxorubicin	RNV rest	LVEF	LVEF decreased significantly more in the doxorubicin than in the epirubicin group (at cumulative doses of 400–500 mg/m^2). During epirubicin therapy LVEF decrease >10% in 33% of pts without clinically significant cardiotoxicity. During doxorubicin therapy LVEF decrease >10% in 58% of pts (1 case of CHF at 200 mg/m^2)
Landys et al. 1985 [82]	42	Mitoxantrone	RNV, echo	LVEF	Decreased LVEF in 7% of pts without signs of overt LV failure during the treatment period
Lapińska et al. 2012 [39]	71	Adriamycin + cyclophosphamide ± RT vs adriamycin + docetaxel ± RT	RNV	EF, EDV, ESV, PFR	All parameters evaluated resulted in early indicators of myocardial damage. Adriamycin + cyclophosphamide caused more cardiotoxic effects than adriamycin + docetaxel chemotherapy. Additional RT did not significantly increase cardiotoxicity

Lee et al. 1987 [83]	12	Doxorubicin	RNV	LVEF, rapid-filling velocity, slow-filling velocity, filling volume ratio, total diastolic time, diastolic time ratio	Average rapid-filling velocity and slow-filling velocity were both significantly reduced after doxorubicin treatment. No significant changes in filling volume ratio, total diastolic time or diastolic time ratio
Lekakis et al. 1996 [84]	37	Doxorubicin	RNV, ^{123}I-MIBG scintigraphy	LVEF, H/M	In pts receiving doxorubicin H/M was significantly lower and correlated with cumulative dose compared to pts not treated with doxorubicin
Lopez et al. 1998 [85]	129	Epirubicin ± dexrazoxane	MUGA, ^{111}In-antimyosin scintigraphy	LVEF, HLR	All methods of cardiac evaluation clearly documented the cardioprotective effect of dexrazoxane
Lu et al. 2012 [86]	3779	Trastuzumab	MUGA, echo	LVEF	The introduction of mandatory cardiac testing for early-stage disease spilled over to the metastatic setting. While deviation from guidelines may be warranted in some cases, this study suggested underutilization of cardiac testing among pts treated with trastuzumab in the metastatic setting
Luk et al. 2014 [87]	30	n.r.	MUGA, MRI	LVEF	A semiautomated technique in MRI resulted time saving and comparable with the MUGA for an accurate LVEF determination
Maini et al. 1997 [88]	36	Epirubicin	RNV, ^{111}In-antimyosin scintigraphy	LVEF, HLR	LVEF appeared more useful at high cumulative dosages and during follow-up to monitor late pump dysfunction, HLR may be effective during the early phase of the therapy in determining which pts are at risk for development of late cardiac dysfunction

(*Continued*)

TABLE 22.2 (Continued)

References	Patients (*n*)	Treatment	Test(s)	Parameter(s) Evaluated	Main Findings
McKillop et al. 1983 [34]	37	Adriamycin	RNV rest/stress, echo, endomyocardial biopsy	LVEF, %FS, cardiac status	An abnormal LVEF at rest (≤45%) had a sensitivity of 53% and a specificity of 75% for detecting pts at moderate or high risk of developing CHF. The addition of exercise LVEF increased the sensitivity of detection of moderate or high-risk patients to 89% (specificity of 41%). Echo yielded lower sensitivities than RNV. As a single test, exercise LVEF possesses the sensitivity for use as a screening method, but the lack of specificity prevents its use as a definitive test; rest LVEF determinations, although more specific, do not possess the sensitivity for its use as screening or definitive tests
Mitani et al. 2003 [31]	265	Doxorubicin	ERNA	LVEF	Incipient fall in LVEF provided an appropriate and cost-effective approach for predicting and preventing impending CHF
Morgan et al. 1981 [89]	292	Doxorubicin	FPRNV	EF	Prior to the first dose of doxorubicin, all patients should have a baseline EF and risk factor assessment assessment (e.g., cardiovascular disease, mediastinal RT within 6 months of starting treatment, total doxorubicin dose >550 mg/m^2). The evaluation of EF may be performed before each subsequent dose in pts with risk factors or with initial EF <45%, while in the remaining cases, serial studies are not required (until a cumulative dose of 450 mg/m^2)
Morgan et al. 1985 [90]	25	RT (mantle)	ERNV stress/rest, MPI (^{201}Tl)	LVEF, perfusion defect(s), wall motion	Abnormalities of myocardial function in 24% of pts. MPI normal in all pts

Neri et al. 1989 [91]	22	Epirubicin	RNV	LVEF	Epirubicin, at a dose of 120 mg/m^2, not increased hematological or cardiac toxicity
Neri et al. 1991 [92]	26	Anthracycline	RNV, blood test	LVEF, atrial natriuretic factor	Atrial natriuretic factor provided a simple noninvasive method of assessing ventricular dysfunction related to cardiac toxicity
Nony et al. 2000 [93]	6	Doxorubicin	RNV, PET (^{11}C-acetate)	LVEF, oxidative metabolism, blood flow	Using PET to evaluate both acute and chronic toxicity, no significant effect was observed either on the flux through the tricarboxylic acid cycle or on myocardial blood flow. Systolic LV function showed a significant impairment after 300 mg/m^2 of doxorubicin
Nousiainen et al. 2002 [40]	30	Doxorubicin	RNV	LVEF	Clinical HF in 7% of pts (dose of 500 mg/m^2). LVEF decreased >10% absolute ejection fraction units to a LVFF ≤50% in 36% of pts. Significant impairment of LV function during doxorubicin therapy may be predicted early, already at low cumulative doxorubicin doses (200 mg/m^2)
Nousiainen et al. 2001 [94]	27	Doxorubicin	RNV, blood test	LVEF, plasma norepinephrine, natriuretic peptide	Doxorubicin-induced LV dysfunction was associated with an early change in sympathovagal balance towards sympathetic predominance
Parmentier et al. 1988 [95]	30	Anthracycline	RNV	EF, PFR, TPFR, filling fraction	Diastolic dysfunction uncommon in anthracycline-treated pts prior to systolic dysfunction
Pauwels et al. 1983 [96]	23	Doxorubicin	ERNA stress/rest	RVEF, LVEF	The effect of an incremental dose was not a function of the cumulative dose. No significant changes were detected in RVEF. LVEF at standardized exercise levels did not correlate with cumulative doses or change as a function of interval dosage

(*Continued*)

TABLE 22.2 (Continued)

References	Patients (*n*)	Treatment	Test(s)	Parameter(s) Evaluated	Main Findings
Pichon et al. 2005 [97]	70	Anthracycline or trastuzumab	RNV, blood test	LVEF, cardiac output, BNP	Anthracycline-induced HF in 6% of pts. BNP concentrations were found to be positively correlated to anthracycline cumulative dose and negatively to LVEF values. Patients who developed HF showed a continuous BNP increase and concentrations >100 ng/mL
Pihkala et al. 1996 [98]	91[a]	Anthracyclines vs anthracyclines + RT vs RT	RNV, echo	LVEF	RNV identified less cases of LVEF dysfunction compared to echo
Piver et al. 1985 [99]	73	Adriamycin	RNV	EF	All patients should have an initial RNV before adriamycin therapy. Pts with low normal initial EF or significant difference between the initial EF and minimum EF, or who develop below normal EF should have RNV studies performed at more frequent intervals
Rabinovitch et al. 1989 [100]	26	Doxorubicin	MUGA	LVEF	Multivariate model was useful in timing discontinuation of doxorubicin prior to the development of a clinically significant deterioration in LVEF
Reuvekamp et al. 2015 [101]	77	Trastuzumab	MUGA	LVEF, PFR, TPFR	Systolic and diastolic dysfunction during treatment in 47% and 58% of pts, respectively. 67% of pts with systolic dysfunction also developed diastolic dysfunction

Ritchie et al. 1980 [102]	36	Anthracycline	RNV	EF	Depression of EF in 22% of pts at 3 weeks following drug administration ($\geq$280 mg/m^2). Definite clinical syndromes of congestive cardiomyopathy developed only in pts showing EF depression (in some cases it developed without signs of CHF). Serial EF determinations prior to anthracycline administration is a potentially useful predictor of cardiac toxicity. EF depression and/or preservation of a normal EF should be weighed in the decision for administering high-dose anthracycline
Robinson et al. 1983 [103]	56	Adriamycin	MUGA	LVEF	Serial cardiac scan enabled irreversible HF due to adriamycin toxicity to be averted, by allowing cessation of drug administration in 5% of pts who had not yet reached the predicted limit of adriamycin
Rohde et al. 2005 [104]	51	Adriamycin	RNV, blood test	LVEF, enzymatic (SOD) and nonenzymatic (TRAP-U) antioxidants	Significant LV systolic dysfunction in 12% of pts. SOD activity increased after treatment and high baseline levels predicts adriamycin-induced cardiotoxicity
Rohde et al. 2007 [105]	55	Adriamycin	RNV, echo	LVEF, Tei index	After treatment of systolic dysfunction (final LVEF <50%) in 14% of pts. Tei index did not appear useful to detect early adriamycin cardiotoxicity
Safra et al. 2000 [106]	42	Doxil	MUGA, endomyocardial biopsies	LVEF, cardiac status	Cumulative doses in excess of 500 mg/m^2 of doxil appear to carry a considerably lesser risk of cardiomyopathy than is generally associated with free doxorubicin

(*Continued*)

TABLE 22.2 (Continued)

References	Patients (*n*)	Treatment	Test(s)	Parameter(s) Evaluated	Main Findings
Saito et al. 2003 [107]	25	Taxan	RNV, MPI (^{99m}Tc-MIBI), ^{123}I- BMIPP scintigraphy	LVEF, perfusion defect(s), TAC	Taxan impairs myocardial fatty acid metabolism. Mean LVEF showed a significant decrease after chemotherapy
Sartori et al. 1995 [108]	11	Interferon	RNV	LVEF	LVEF decreased after 1 month of therapy (reduction >10% in 45% of pts). Three months after therapy was stopped and 82% of pts showed an LVEF close to the pretreatment level
Savage et al. 1990 [109]	16	RT	RNV, MPI (^{201}Tl)	LVEF, PFR, perfusion defect(s)	Pts who received RT to the entire cardiac volume had a lower mean LVEF and PFR than those who had some portion of the heart shielded throughout treatment. No perfusion defects were evident in either group
Scopinaro et al. 1993 [110]	25	Blood transfusion + intensive iron removal therapy	ERNA stress/rest, echo	LVEF, PFR	PRF did not show diagnostic value in the early detection of iron cardiotoxicity
Shpall et al. 1988 [111]	27	Mitoxantrone	RNV	LVEF	Cardiotoxicity in 37% of pts
Skovgaard et al. 2014 [43]	333	Anthracycline	MUGA, blood test	LVEF, BNP	Higher BNP and lower LVEF in pts who developed congestive HF
Sobić-Saranović et al. 1997 [112]	32	Anthracycline	RNV	EF, PFR, TFR, R–R intervals	Diastolic LV parameters and R–R intervals significantly differed before and after chemotherapy

Steinherz et al. 1995 [113]	15	Anthracycline ± RT	RNV, ECG, continuous taped ECG, echo, cardiac catheterization, endomyocardial biopsy	Fractional shortening, LVEF, wave alteration(s), cardiac status	Pts with early cardiac symptoms improved transiently but decompensated later. Pts with no early symptoms developed cardiac symptoms > 10 years after therapy
Strashun et al. 1986 [114]	101	Doxorubicin	MUGA, nonimaging scintillation probe	EF	Clinical cardiotoxicity in 13% of pts. Eight asymptomatic patients presenting decline in absolute EF had therapy terminated before the development of clinical cardiotoxicity. The majority of patients (83%) did not have a decline ≥15% from baseline into the abnormal range at 450 mg/m^2 cumulative dose levels
Suzuki et al. 1999 [115]	37	Anthracycline	RNV, ECG, Echo	LVEF, PFR, end-diastolic count, filling fraction, wave alteration(s)	None of the patients developed clinical CHF. No significant changes of LVEF detected by RNV and echo/ECG parameters after drug administration.
					The RNV indices of early diastolic function showed a significant decrease suggesting usefulness for detecting silent myocardial damage induced by anthracyclines
Tantawy et al. 2011 [44]	39[a]	Anthracycline	RNV, echo, endomyocardial biopsy	LVEF, cardiac status	Cardiotoxicity occurred early and at low cumulative doses of doxorubicin. RNV was more sensitive than echo in detecting early impairment of LV function

(Continued)

TABLE 22.2 (Continued)

References	Patients (*n*)	Treatment	Test(s)	Parameter(s) Evaluated	Main Findings
Trappolini et al. 1988 [116]	13	Daunorubicin	RNV	EF, PFR	Early reduction of PFR in pts who underwent daunorubicin induction therapy also in case of normal EF
Valdés Olmos et al. 1992 [117]	13	Doxorubicin	RNV, ^{123}I-MIBG scintigraphy	LVEF, washout rate	In spite of a localized loss of LV function, doxorubicin-related cardiotoxicity appeared to be based on a global process of myocardial adrenergic derangement
Vici et al. 1998 [118]	95	Epirubicin ± dexrazoxane	MUGA, ^{111}In-antimyosin scintigraphy	LVEF, HLR	Dexrazoxane significantly protects against the development of high-dose epirubicin cardiotoxicity apparently without evidence of an adverse impact on antitumor activity and noncardiac toxicity
Vorobiof et al. 1983 [119]	6	Amsacrine	RNA	LVEF	Significant decrease in LVEF in pts (33%) who received doses ≥580 mg/m^2 while no significant change in cardiac function in pts who received total doses of 325–510 mg/m^2
Vorobiof et al. 1985 [120]	50	Epidoxorubicin or mitoxantrone	RNA	LVEF	Decrease of LVEF ≥10% in 30% of pts treated with epidoxorubicin at doses of 143–1200 mg/m^2 and in 30% of pts treated with mitoxantrone at a dose of 26–98 mg/m^2. Clinical signs of cardiotoxicity in 7% of pts treated with epidoxorubicin at doses >1000 mg/m^2

Wachters et al. 2004 [121]	69	Gemcitabine + cisplatin vs epirubicin + gemcitabine	MUGA	LVEF	Difference in decline in LVEF from baseline in 2% in the gemcitabine + cisplatin arm vs 6% in the epirubicin +gemcitabine arm. No clinical evidence of HF during 12 months follow-up
Walker et al. 2010 [122]	50	Doxorubicin and trastuzumab	MUGA, echo (2D and 3D), MRI	LVEF	MUGA and 3D-echo resulted in alternate imaging modality for the serial monitoring of LVEF
Wheeler et al. 1982 [123]	27	Doxorubicin	MUGA	LVEF	Clinical evaluation did not suggest an increased risk of cardiotoxicity at 120 mg/m^2
Yabuta 1990 [124]	15	Cytoxan, adriamycin, cisplatin	MUGA	LVEF	LVEF during treatment was significantly lower than the pretreatment values

BNP, brain natriuretic peptide; ECG, electrocardiogram; echo, echocardiography; ERNA, equilibrium radionuclide angiocardiography, FPRNV, first-pass radionuclide ventriculography, HLR, heart-to-lung ratio; H/M, heart-to-mediastinum ratio; LVEF, left ventricle ejection fraction; MPI, myocardial perfusion scintigraphy; MRI, magnetic resonance imaging; MUGA, multigated equilibrium radionuclide venticulography; PFR, peak filling rate; PER, peak ejection rate; pts, patients; RT, radiotherapy; TAC, time–activity curve; TDI, tissue-Doppler imaging; TFR, time to filling rate; RNV, radionuclide venticulography.

[a]*Pediatric patients.*

The reconstruction and processing can be done using commercially available software programs that allow sophisticated wall motion analysis, which seems valuable in monitoring and tailoring the treatment of congestive HF patients [41].

The performance of GBPS for LVEF has been analyzed in several studies. Comparison of the commercially available software packages revealed acceptable agreement both among the methods and with planar RNV [125–127]. However, GBPS tends to underestimate LVEF values compared to other imaging modalities such as RNV, FPRNV, and echo [128]. In addition it is less reliable in patients with normal small cavities. Luk et al. [87] found comparable value of LVEF between MUGA and cardiac MRI using a semiautomatic or a manual drawing technique while a significant difference was observed in the case of in-line tracking. LVEF measurements may be more easily and as reproducibly obtained using other methods, including planar RNV and the advantage of tomographic ERNV for LVEF lies mainly in the concomitantly acquired RV function.

In addition, in GBPS the RVEF should be interpreted with caution [128] and the method for its calculation needs to be improved before routine clinical application [129,130].

Myocardial Perfusion Imaging

Cardiac perfusion can be evaluated by both SPECT- and PET-based radiopharmaceuticals. SPECT is still the predominant technique in this clinical setting.

Although MPI has been available in routine clinical settings since the 1970s, the development of gated SPECT over the past two decades has made possible a combined assessment of myocardial perfusion and LV function.

Thallium-201 thallous chloride, a potassium analogue, was the first radionuclide used widely for myocardial perfusion studies, but due to its several limitations it is nowadays substituted by ^{99m}Tc-labeled perfusion tracers: ^{99m}Tc-2-methoxyisobutylisonitrile (sestamibi) and ^{99m}Tc-1,2-bis[bis(2-ethoxyethyl) phosphino] ethane (tetrofosmin). They both are cationic complexes that diffuse passively through the capillary and cell membrane, resulting in relatively slower immediate extraction. Myocardial uptake of the ^{99m}Tc-labeled tracers increases almost proportionately with an increase in perfusion, reaching a plateau in myocardial uptake at a myocardial perfusion around twice resting levels. Within the cell it is retained in intact mitochondria, reflecting viable myocytes.

The general protocol for an MPI with ^{99m}Tc-labeled perfusion tracers includes separate injections at stress and rest, if a rest study is deemed necessary. Resting injections should ideally be given after the administration of sublingual nitrate, in particular in patients with a suspicion of severe myocardial or old infarction. This is important because without the administration of sublingual nitrate myocardial viability may be underestimated in areas with reduced resting perfusion [131]. For stress imaging, in patients with suspected or known coronary artery disease (CAD), dynamic exercise is the first test of choice. Alternatively vasodilator stress testing with adenosine, regadenoson, dipyridamole, or catecholamine agonist dobutamine are used. The administered activity is dependent on the type of equipment (single-head or a multiple-head scintillation camera, or a camera based on a CZT detector), patient characteristics (body weight), acquisition protocol (1-day or 2-day protocols, imaging time, pixel size, gated acquisition), and the radiopharmaceutical (^{99m}Tc-compounds or ^{201}Tl-chloride). The reconstruction method may also be of importance, i.e., filtered back-projection versus iterative reconstruction. There is limited evidence in the literature demonstrating activity amounts to be injected for optimal images in the different settings of patients and instrumentation. For a classical SPECT acquisition, according to the "as low as reasonably achievable" (ALARA) principle, for a normal weight adult patient (i.e., BMI <25) for a gated study on a multiple-head scintillation camera, using filtered back-projection, an acquisition duration of 15 min and a pixel size of around 6 mm EANM guideline recommend the following activities: for ^{99m}Tc-coumpound for 2-day protocol, 350–700 MBq/study and for 1-day protocol about 250–400 MBq for the first injection, three times more for the second injection [132]. Camera systems based on new technology (e.g., CZT cameras) have improved count sensitivity that can be used to either reduce the amount of activity accordingly or decrease image acquisition duration [133–135].

Myocardial perfusion studies acquired in a gated mode using an ECG-trigger "gated" mode (gated MPI), have the clear advantage of evaluating LVEF, volumes, and evaluation of LV regional wall motion and thickening, diastolic function as well as perform phase analysis for assessment of LV dyssynchrony. The gating of a SPECT acquisition is easily implemented using the QRS complex of the ECG signal, since the *R*-wave corresponds to end diastole [14]. Using ECG gated SPECT the heartbeat is usually divided into eight or 16 temporal frames or gates. The *R*-wave of the QRS complex serves as the signal and starting point (triggering point) of the cardiac cycle. The cardiac cycle is divided into frames representing different phases of the cardiac cycle. After a gated SPECT acquisition with eight gates and 64 projections, eight raw data files each with 64 projection images are recorded. While eight-frame gating is still prevalent in gated perfusion SPECT imaging, it is obvious that the cardiac cycle can be more accurately described with more frequent temporal sampling. Sixteen-frame gating offers the opportunity to assess diastolic LV function. Eight-frame gating seems to be a reasonable compromise between the count statistics that should provide accurate edge definitions of the ventricular walls and the temporal resolution that is required to record the short end-systolic period [136].

Information on ventricular function has proven to be useful for both the diagnosis and prognosis of CAD. Using gated studies, the quantification of poststress wall motion abnormalities or LVEF increases the sensitivity of stress-rest MPI SPECT, especially in patients with three-vessel CAD, in whom a diffuse decrease in subendocardial blood flow may cause an impairment of ventricular function without focal perfusion defects [137,138]. Moreover, the ability to observe myocardial contraction in segments with apparent fixed perfusion defects permits the nuclear test reader to discern attenuation artifacts from true perfusion abnormalities, thus leading to better specificity of gated MPI SPECT [139]. Finally, poststress LVEF and end-systolic volumes measured by gated MPI SPECT are independent predictors of cardiovascular events and have incremental prognostic values over myocardial perfusion and clinical data in predicting cardiac death [140].

MPI SPECT may be combined with a CT scan for attenuation, calcium scoring (CACS), or coronary CT angiography. For the latter, an intravenous injection of iodine-based contrast agent is needed. Coronary CT in combination with ECG-gating and a contrast agent allowed the visualization of the coronary artery lumen and detection of coronary artery stenosis [141]. For coronary imaging in general, a contrast agent with a high concentration of iodine is used (300–400 mg/mL) to ensure adequate opacification of the small coronary arteries [132], about 60–90 mL injected at an injection speed of 4–6 mL/s. Often, the bolus is split between a first bolus of pure contrast and then a bolus with a mix of contrast and saline, to reduce streak artefacts from contrast enhancement of the vena cava and the right side of the heart. Otherwise, the contrast bolus is followed by a saline flush of 40–70 mL. With the newest generation of CT scanners, a smaller contrast bolus with lower iodine concentration is likely sufficient to obtain good contrast enhancement of the coronary arteries [142].

The combined diagnostic information from myocardial perfusion SPECT imaging and CCTA is complementary: CCTA presents a very high negative predictive value to exclude CAD [143], whereas it is associated with a general overestimation of the severity of CAD stenosis and difficulties to differentiate between slight differences in stenosis severity. SPECT provides the true hemodynamic significance of coronary artery lesions detected by CCTA, also the in presence of strong calcifications or artefacts. On the other hand, CCTA offers the complementary information to SPECT through documentation of multivessel disease (i.e., presence of balanced ischemia not detectable by semiquantitative SPECT analysis) and subclinical atherosclerosis.

Beside being extensively used for preoperative cardiac risk assessment in candidate oncological patients to surgery, MPI have been evaluated as a screening tool to prevent cardiac side effects in cancer patients undergoing RT.

In long-term survivors with HD treated with mediastinal RT (combined in some cases with chemotherapy), several pilot studies using MPI suggested that RT produced no significant functional sequelae at long-term follow-up. Normal ^{201}Tl MPI was found in asymptomatic HD patients 5–16 years after RT associated with MOPP (mechlorethamine, vincristine, procarbazine, and prednisone) chemotherapy [90] or without any chemotherapy [109]. In this latter study although LVEF and PFR were within the normal range, patients irradiated to large cardiac volumes had lower LVEF and PFR compared with patients who had some part of the heart volume shielded. Similar results were found when ^{99m}Tc-sestamibi was used with myocardial ischemia documented in up to 5% of patients in two different studies. The first was in a group of 112 (out of 352) treated with mediastinal RT at intermediate total doses (30–45 Gy) with partial inclusion of the heart eventually associated with chemotherapy (including doxorubicin) [144]. The second was in 50 asymptomatic and youthful patients treated by mantle RT with modern techniques of whom 17 also received chemotherapy where the use of combined MPI and RNV showed only mild myocardial ischemia [59].

In contrast to the studies mentioned above, Gustavsson et al. [145] reported that only nine out of 23 HD patients treated with RT to the mediastine had normal ^{201}thallium MPI, whereas they presented disturbed LV function based on echo findings. In two different studies by Maunoury et al. [146] and Pierga et al. [147], evaluating clinically asymptomatic patients after mantle field RT (in some cases combined with doxorubicin-containing chemotherapy) abnormalities on both visual and quantitative analysis of ^{201}Tl MPI were found in about 84% and 85% of patients, respectively. More recently, in a follow-up study, a high rate of MPI defects post-RT was reported. However, in this study 66% of patients had received doxorubicin-containing chemotherapy before RT [148].

In patients with left-sided breast cancer the very first study with ^{201}Tl MPI was normal in about 90% of patients after RT (and no adjuvant chemotherapy) [149], whereas using ^{99m}Tc-sestamibi, a variable degree of perfusion defects was described. In a prospective study in patients before and after adjuvant RT (and in some cases doxorubicin-containing chemotherapy) 50% new fixed LV perfusion defects were found in about three-quarters of patients [150]. The localization of the defects corresponded well with the irradiated volume of the LV. Interestingly, neither ECG changes nor LV segmental wall motion abnormalities could be detected by echo [151]. Later studies including patients with either left- or right-side breast cancer treated with or without adjuvant RT $\pm$ cyclophosphamide, showed at MPI with a ^{99m}Tc-based lower degree of reversible, fixed, or mixed perfusion defects [152], mostly affecting the apex in left-breast patients [153]. In both studies, LVEF was normal in all patients, few signs of diastolic and no valvular dysfunction of clinical significance were observed by echo. In addition, no cardiac deaths among the total of patients included in these studies were recorded, despite the fact that in some patients older radiation techniques had been applied [154].

More recent data indicate that cardiac injury after irradiation of the thorax is detectable using MPI as moderately reduced perfusion or hypoperfusion of the anterior wall segments [155]. Volume-dependent perfusion defects in approximately 40% of patients within 2 years of RT were observed. These perfusion defects were associated with corresponding wall-motion abnormalities [156]. In a selected study population of relapse-free breast cancer patients treated with RT at least 5 years previously and without history of ischemic heart disease prior to RT to the left breast was associated with a significantly greater number of myocardial perfusion abnormalities than RT to the right breast. These abnormalities were both reversible and irreversible, suggesting that RT can lead to both myocardial damage and to epicardial coronary disease. However, LVEF was normal in all patients in whom it was measured, and with a minimum of 5 years follow-up since treatment, no abnormalities were considered to be clinically significant [153]. RT-induced perfusion defects may persist or initially appear at gated-SPECT 3–6 years post-RT in a high percentage of patients (52% and 57%, respectively). However, these defects were not associated with changes in regional wall motion or EF, therefore, their clinical relevance is still unclear [157]. No significant difference in ^{99m}Tc-sestamibi MPI defects was found in clinically asymptomatic patients treated after surgery for left-sided breast cancer treated either with RT plus systemic hormonal treatment (35%) or CMF (cyclophosphamide, methotrexate, and 5-fluorouracil) chemotherapy (65%) or without RT [158]. In the same population after RT (total dose of 46–50 Gy by tangent beams) with and without doxorubicin, MPI demonstrated a dose-dependent perfusion defect at 6 months with minimal defects appreciated at 0–10 Gy, and a 20% decrease in regional perfusion at 41–50 Gy. A decrease in LVEF >10% at 6 months was present only in one case while two patients had developed transient pericarditis [159].

The use of more advanced techniques, such as ^{99m}Tc-Sestamibi gated-SPECT, in patients with breast cancer treated with RT and doxorubicin-based chemotherapy demonstrated that cardiac function, as assessed by LVEF, was not altered by the combined treatment of RT and chemotherapy, except in patients with known cardiovascular risk factors. On the other hand, the appearance of new perfusion defects was observed in all patients treated with the combination of doxorubicin and RT when portions of the LV received >50% of the RT dose. In this study, the perfusion defects did not seem to correlate with clinical events, but follow-up was short and thus clinical significance was still not determined [159]. However, the gated-derived data of ventricular systolic performance after a stress test can give information on the coronary reserve and the contractile reserve, allowing an early appropriate treatment of patients [160]. ^{99m}Tc-tetrofosmin-gated SPECT/CT was also use in combination with CACS in patients with left-sided breast cancer with cardiac risk factor candidate to postsurgical RT after a doxorubicin-based chemotherapy, resulting in a reliable screening method to prevent cardiac damage in cancer patients [161].

These data are warrant of a critical reading and require some considerations. The first is about the outdated RT treatment regimens the oldest studies refer to, which are no longer used. Such older RT techniques employed higher radiation doses and lacked appropriate cardiac shielding that have undoubtedly influenced the development of cardiac damage. Nowadays, orthovoltage RT, as well as the use of tangential fields, which seem to spare the heart from harmful irradiation, is recommended, whenever this option is available, whereas high fraction doses should be avoided to minimize late tissue damage to the heart [162]. The second point is related to the nuclear medicine procedure used for MPI. The high rates of myocardial perfusion defects in patients treated with RT ± chemotherapy found in the oldest studies refer to the use of ^{201}Tl MPI, often planar images that might suffer from false-positive findings as well as of temporary reversible abnormalities detected after sustained exercise. Indeed, when scintigraphy with ^{99m}Tc-labeled radiopharmaceuticals was used, studies indicated an incidence of ~5% for myocardial perfusion defects. Recent SPECT studies with ^{99m}Tc-labeled radiopharmaceuticals, using more strict inclusion criteria, seem to confirm a low rate of late perfusion deficits following external RT ± chemotherapy, and an increased risk for ischemic cardiac disease only for patients with known cardiovascular risk factors [144,152,158,159]. Finally, the low number of patients included in some studies may have reduced the statistical power of these studies, and observed differences between patients treated with and without RT could simply arise by chance [158,159].

The prevalence of myocardial perfusion abnormalities detected using gated MPI has also been evaluated in patients with esophageal cancer after RT. RT resulted in an association with a high prevalence of inferior LV ischemia in patients with distal esophageal cancer. Most perfusion defects were encompassed within an isodose line ≥45 Gy in the RT plan [163].

In patients with lung cancer, chemoradiation (CRT) or RT to centrally located lung tumors tends to cause anterior/septal MPI defects. Abnormal MPI segments in the CRT/RT group have received significantly higher radiation than normal segments [164].

Cardiac symptoms occur more frequently in patients with perfusion abnormalities by SPECT after RT than in patients with normal SPECT scans, suggesting that such perfusion defects may be clinically significant. One confounding factor is that women who know they have RT-induced perfusion defects may be more likely to report episodes of chest pain. Long-term follow-up will be necessary to better assess the clinical significance of RT-induced perfusion defects [164].

Despite its success in research applications, the limited availability of PET technology, its increased cost, and the limited data supporting its use and reimbursement have all contributed to the relatively limited clinical acceptance of this imaging technology for MPI studies. However, the emergence of hybrid PET/CT equipment holds great promise for cardiac imaging as it provides a potential opportunity to increase the application of PET/CT technologies in cardiology. Several PET radiopharmaceuticals have been used for evaluating myocardial perfusion with PET, the most widely used in clinical practice are ^{13}N-ammonia and ^{82}Rb. Myocardial retention of ^{13}N-ammonia is heterogeneous, with retention in the lateral LV wall being about 10% lower than that of other segments. Retention of ^{13}N-ammonia by the myocardium has a nonlinear and inverse relationship with blood flow, with the net tissue extraction (the product of the retained fraction during FP and myocardial blood flow) decreasing as myocardial blood flow increases. For ^{13}N-ammonia, the relation between net tissue extraction and blood flow is linear for values of blood flow up to 2.5 mL/min/g. At high flow rates, "metabolic trapping" of ^{13}N-ammonia becomes the rate-limiting factor affecting tracer retention. This leads to underestimation of blood flow at high flow rates [165]. Therefore, to quantify myocardial blood flow using ^{13}N-ammonia, it becomes necessary to correct for flow-dependent changes in net tissue extraction. ^{13}N-ammonia allows the acquisition of ungated and gated images of good quality. Gated ^{13}N-ammonia imaging can provide accurate assessments of both regional and global cardiac function [166]. However, this imaging agent is not well suited for peak stress gated imaging because of the 3–4-min time interval between radiotracer injection and the start of imaging and the relatively long (20 min) acquisition time. For an ^{13}N-ammonia study lower activity is used for the rest images (0.37 GBq, 10 mCi) and a higher activity (1.11 GBq, 30 mCi) for the stress images.

^{82}Rb is a potassium analogue with kinetic properties similar to those of ^{201}Tl [167]. Myocardial uptake of ^{82}Rb requires active transport via the sodium/potassium adenosine triphosphate transporter, which is dependent on coronary blood flow [168]. The single-capillary transit extraction fraction of ^{82}Rb exceeds 50%. However, its net extraction fraction decreases in a nonlinear fashion with increasing myocardial blood flow [169]. For ^{82}Rb, approximately the same activity (1.48–2.22 GBq, 40–60 mCi) is injected for the rest and the stress myocardial perfusion studies.

The general protocol for a complete PET/CT MPI consists of a CT scout image or topogram followed by a low-dose CT scan covering the heart region. Emission images can be acquired as ECG-gated imaging (most typically used) or dynamic acquisition. Imaging begins 90–120 s after ^{82}Rb injection, or 3–5 min after ^{13}N-ammonia injection and the scan duration is approximately 5 or 20 min, respectively. The number of gated frames is usually set to 8 or 16, with rejection of ectopic beats outside the acceptance window. When dynamic images are recorded they start with the bolus of ^{82}Rb or ^{13}N-ammonia and continue for 7–8 min or 20 min, respectively [167]. The advantage of this approach is that it allows quantification of myocardial blood flow (in mL/min/g), by fitting regional tissue and blood TAC to a suitable kinetic model. However, its main disadvantage is that one needs to perform a separate radionuclide injection to obtain ECG-gated images from which to assess cardiac function, especially when using ^{82}Rb. Using

^{13}N-ammonia, one can acquire a short multiframe or dynamic scan (4 min) that can be followed with a separate 15-min ECG-gated scan to assess myocardial perfusion and LVEF, without the need for an additional radionuclide injection because of its longer physical half-life. Stress testing can be performed by pharmacologic means (e.g., adenosine, dipyridamole, or dobutamine) or with exercise [170]. The latter is easier with ^{13}N-ammonia than with ^{82}Rb because of its longer half-life (9.96 min vs 76 s). In selected patients, it is also possible to obtain a CTA immediately after the MPI.

PET radiopharmaceuticals for blood flow and metabolism have been extensively studied for evaluation of myocardial viability. The most commonly used PET protocol involves evaluation of myocardial glucose metabolism with [^{18}F]FDG in conjunction with PET or SPECT examination of MBF with ^{13}N-ammonia or ^{99m}Tc-sestamibi, respectively. This approach appears to have slightly better overall accuracy for predicting recovery of regional function after revascularization than do single-photon techniques [171]. In patients with HF with LV dysfunction, the magnitude of symptom improvement after revascularization correlates with the preoperative extent of [^{18}F]FDG "mismatch" pattern [172].

The role of PET in the early detection of cardiotoxicity is still debated. Nony et al. [93] showed a significant decrease in LVEF assessed by RNV after treatment with doxorubicin impairment after the administration of 300 mg/m^2, without significant alteration in myocardial blood flow evaluated with ^{11}C-acetate PET in female cancer patients without heart disease. Borde et al. [173] analyzed changes in myocardial glucose metabolism using [^{18}F]FDG PET and suggested increased glucose utilization was evidence of cellular alteration preceding the cardiotoxicity cascade in patients treated with adriamycin. Similar promising observations has been reported by Basu et al. [173,174] in patients with lymphoma.

Several studies have found that focal increased [^{18}F]FDG uptake in the irradiation field is sometimes seen in patients with thoracic tumors after RT [175–177]. Abnormal [^{18}F]FDG uptake might be related to radiation-induced cardiotoxicity. However, the value of [^{18}F]FDG PET for the diagnosis of radiation-induced cardiotoxicity has not been fully explored since these studies are retrospective in nature, and lack a pre-RT scan. Therefore it is not possible to exclude the presence of increased [^{18}F]FDG uptake before RT. In addition, almost all of the cancer patients in these studies were treated with concurrent chemotherapy, and some patients were at high risk for cardiovascular disease or diabetes mellitus. These multiple confounding factors may have an unclear effect of RT on changes in myocardial metabolism. In addition, the high variability of physiological myocardial FDG might be an important confounding factor of these studies. In fact, variable focus of diffuse physiological [^{18}F]FDG uptake is often observed in the normal myocardium of fasting nondiabetic patients (6–12 h to overnight) with normal glucose levels [178]. Accumulation of [^{18}F]FDG is most notable in the

LV myocardium, which has a greater muscle mass than other cardiac chambers. Uptake in the wall of the right ventricle is typically equal to or less intense than that in the LV myocardium; uptake in the wall of the right and left atria is usually not detected. Factors possibly influencing myocardial uptake of [^{18}F]FDG include patients' age, fasting time, blood glucose levels, and a low-carbohydrate diet. In particular, age and fasting time do not affect physiological [^{18}F]FDG uptake in the myocardium, whereas blood glucose levels may have a nonlinear effect on myocardial uptake [179]. Low-carbohydrate diet [180] and a very high-fat, low-carbohydrate, protein-permitted meal followed by fasting for 3–6 h [181] before [^{18}F]FDG injection might be adopted to decrease myocardial uptake. Alternatively, unfractionated heparin (50 IU/kg iv) could be administered before [^{18}F]FDG injection [182]. Heparin acts by activating lipoprotein lipase and hepatic lipase, enhances plasma lipolytic activity, and elevates plasma levels of FFA [183].

Another potential confounding factor for [^{18}F]FDG-PET/CT is represented by increased metabolic activity along the posterior aspect of the heart, where lipomatous hypertrophy of the interatrial septum may appear as a fat-containing mass with increased [^{18}F]FDG uptake [184]. In addition, a number of pathologic conditions can mimic the pattern of focally increased [^{18}F]FDG uptake [185]. Therefore, whether focal increased [^{18}F] FDG uptake is related to radiation-induced cardiac damage is unclear. A recent study in an animal model investigated cardiac [^{18}F]FDG uptake after heart irradiation (a single dose of 20 Gy for radiation), as well as the pathology of those changes [186]. Focal increased [^{18}F]FDG uptake was observed in the anterior myocardium corresponding to the irradiated field. In addition, the ratio of the irradiated field to the nonirradiated field SUV was significantly higher 3 months after irradiation than before irradiation (animals were prepared with a LCHF diet). At histology, the irradiated myocardium showed obvious perivascular fibrosis and mild myocardial degeneration without inflammatory cell infiltration. However, no cardiac dysfunction was found at irradiation by echo.

Table 22.3 summarizes the main results of a literature search on the use of MPI to image cardiotoxicity.

Sympathetic Nervous Innervation Imaging

Sympathetic nervous innervation imaging of the heart with SPECT and PET radiopharmaceuticals is a promising technique for detection of early anthracycline injury and for identification of patients at high risk of developing cardiotoxicity [13].

The sympathetic nervous system uses norepinephrine (NE). NE exerts its effect through binding and activation of adrenergic receptors on target cells (α- and β-receptors) [192]. In human heart, β1-adrenoceptors are predominant (β1–β2 ratio = 3:1) and are distributed in all cardiac regions.

TABLE 22.3 Summary of the Main Publications on Cardiotoxicity Imaged by Myocardial Perfusion Imaging

Reference	Patients (*n*)	Treatment	Test(s)	Parameter(s) Evaluated	Main Findings
Borde et al. 2012 [173]	18	Adriamycin	PET ([^{18}F]FDG)	Glucose metabolism (SUV)	Significant change in SUV_{mean} values in the myocardium (≥20%) in 67% of pts
Constine et al. 1997 [59]	50	RT (mantle)	MPI (^{201}Tl or ^{99m}Tc-MIBI), ERNA, ECG	Perfusion defect(s), LVEF, PFR, wave alteration(s)	Generally normal measures of LVEF and myocardial perfusion
Duan et al. 2003 [65]	23	Anthracycline	MPI (^{99m}Tc-MIBI), RNV, ECG, blood test	Myocardial relative quantity, LVEF, myocardial enzyme (CK-MB)	MPI was useful to monitor cardiotoxicity and its changes occurred earlier than LVEFs
Gallucci et al. 2010 [160]	30	Anthracycline-containing chemotherapy + RT (left side)	MPI	Perfusion defect(s)	Myocardial perfusion defect in 26% of pts (fixed = 3%; reversible = 23%). Normal perfusion scan but depressed rest and stress LVEF in 3% of cases
Gardner et al. 1993 [187]	12	Cyclophosphamide	PET (^{13}N-ammonia, [^{18}F]FDG), ECG	Perfusion defects, glucose metabolism, wave alteration(s)	Substantial increase in ^{13}N-ammonia perfusion in the inferior region simultaneously with electrocardiographic T wave inversions in the inferior leads in a single pt
Gayed et al. 2006 [163]	51	RT	MPI	Perfusion defect(s)	RT was associated with a high prevalence (54%) of inferior LV ischemia
Gayed et al. 2009 [188]	44	Chemoradiation or RT	MPI	Perfusion defect(s)	RT (±chemotherapy) to centrally located lung tumors tends to cause anterior/septal MPI defects

(*Continued*)

TABLE 22.3 (Continued)

Reference	Patients (*n*)	Treatment	Test(s)	Parameter(s) Evaluated	Main Findings
Glanzmann et al. 1998 [144]	112	RT ± chemotherapy	MPI, rest/stress ECG, echo	Perfusion defect(s), wave alteration, wall motion, EF	In pts without hypertension and coronary artery disease, findings of MPI and echo evaluation of systolic and diastolic function were normal. Treatment with chemotherapy was not a significant risk factor for cardiac events
Hardenbergh et al. 2001 [159]	20	RT (left side) ± doxorubicin	MPI	Perfusion defect(s), LVEF	Cardiac perfusion defects 6 months post-RT in 60% of pts
Marks et al. 2005 [156]	111	RT	MPI (^{99m}Tc-MIBI or ^{99m}Tc-tetrofosmin)	Perfusion defect(s), wall motion, EF	RT caused volume-dependent perfusion defects associated with corresponding wall-motion abnormalities in about 40% of pts within 2 years of RT
Morgan et al. 1985 [90]	25	RT (mantle)	MPI (^{201}Tl), ERNV stress/rest	Perfusion defect(s), wall motion, LVEF	MPI normal in all pts. Abnormalities of myocardial function in 24% of pts
Pach et al. 1998 [189]	7	Carbon monoxide	MPI (^{99m}Tc-MIBI), blood test, blood gas analysis, ECG	Perfusion defect(s), COHb, blood lactate level, enzymes activity (ALT, AST, CPK), wave alteration(s)	Considering the results of ECG and enzyme activity only, no objectives were found to diagnose the cardiac dysfunction. MPI indicated regions of myocardium that have decreased blood flow in all pts
Pach et al. 2001 [190]	29	Carbon monoxide	MPI (^{99m}Tc-MIBI), blood test, blood gas analysis, ECG	Perfusion defect(s), COHb, blood lactate level, enzymes activity (ALT, AST, CPK), wave alteration(s)	All pts had abnormal MPI scan (differently intensified pathological changes: degree I of pathological changes in 5 pts, degree II in 7 pts, degree III in 16 pts, and degree IV in 1 pt). MPI results were more sensitive than ECG and enzymes activity for the evaluation of CO cardiotoxicity in acute poisoning, enabling the evaluation of localization and disease extent

Pistevou-Gompaki et al. 2003 [154]	22	RT (left side)	MPI (^{99m}Tc-tetrofosmin), ECG, echo	Perfusion defect(s), LVEF, wave alteration(s)	No signs of ischemic heart disease in any pts with methods used. Some type of abnormal nonischemic echo findings 6 months after RT in 32% of pts
Prosnitz et al. 2007 [157]	44	RT	MPI	Perfusion defect(s), wall motion, EF	RT-induced perfusion defects may persist or initially appear 3–6 years post-RT in a high percentage of pts (up to 71%). These defects were not associated with changes in regional wall motion or EF
Saito et al. 2003 [107]	25	Taxan	MPI (^{99m}Tc-MIBI), RNV, ^{123}I- BMIPP scintigraphy	Perfusion defect(s), LVEF, TAC	Taxan impairs myocardial fatty acid metabolism. Mean LVEF showed a significant decrease after chemotherapy
Savage et al. 1990 [109]	16	RT	MPI (^{201}Tl), RNV	Perfusion defect(s), LVEF, PFR	Pts who received RT to the entire cardiac volume had a lower mean LVEF and PFR than those who had some portion of the heart shielded throughout treatment. No perfusion defects were evident in either group
Seddon et al. 2002 [153]	24	RT	MPI	Perfusion defect(s), EF	RT to the left breast was associated with a significantly greater number of myocardial perfusion abnormalities than RT to the right breast (71% vs 17%)
Tzonevska et al. 2006 [155]	56	RT	MPI (^{99m}Tc-MIBI)	Perfusion defect(s)	Moderately reduced perfusion in 24% of pts
Tzonevska et al. 2011 [191]	24	Chemotherapy + RT	MPI, echo, ECG, blood test	Perfusion defect(s), LVEF, wave alteration(s), ProBNP	Early signs of cardiotoxicity in 42% of pts

(*Continued*)

TABLE 22.3 (Continued)

Reference	Patients (*n*)	Treatment	Test(s)	Parameter(s) Evaluated	Main Findings
Tzonevska et al. 2014 [161]	28	Doxorubicin-based chemotherapy + RT	MPI (^{99m}Tc-tetrofosmin) G-SPECT/CT	QGS/QPS quantitative analysis, calcium scores	GSPECT/CT + calcium scores provided combined cardiac assessment serving as reliable screening method to prevent cardiac damage caused by RT in left-sided breast cancer pts, who have cardiac risk factors and have been administered doxorubicin-based chemotherapy
Unal et al. 2013 [177]	28	RT	PET ([^{18}F]FDG)	Glucose metabolism (SUV)	Regional myocardial [^{18}F]FDG uptake in 74% of pts and diffuse myocardial [^{18}F]FDG uptake in 13% of pts. SUV of the pts with regional uptake revealed significantly higher values in the irradiated segments compared to nonirradiated segments
Yu et al. 2003 [164]	114	RT	MPI	Perfusion defect(s)	Cardiac symptoms occurred more frequently in pts with perfusion abnormalities after RT than in pts with normal MPI (29% vs 2%)

BNP, brain natriuretic peptide; echo, echocardiography; ERNA, equilibrium radionuclide angiocardiography; HLR, heart-to-lung ratio; H/M, heart-to-mediastinum ratio; LVEF, left ventricle ejection fraction; MPI, myocardial perfusion scintigraphy; MRI, magnetic resonance imaging; MUGA, multigated equilibrium radionuclide venticulography; PFR, peak filling rate; PER, peak ejection rate; pts, patients; RT, radiotherapy; SUV, standardized uptake values TAC, time–activity curve; TDI, tissue-Doppler imaging; TFR, time to filling rate; RNV, radionuclide venticulography.

β2-adrenoceptors are instead mainly concentrated in the ventricle and atria where they are functionally linked to inotropic response. The presence of β3-adrenoceptors in the human heart is still a matter of debate [193,194].

Terminal release of neurotransmitters occurs from localized swelling of the axons (varicosity or boutons) where NE is stored in neuronal vesicles and synthesized from tyrosine in a series of reactions (tyrosine is converted to dihydrxoyphenylalanine, than to dopamine that is converted by dopamine-β-hydroxylase to NE). Following sympathetic impulse, vesicles dock to the axonal membrane of the varicosity via scaffolding proteins and the contents of the vesicle are released into a synaptic cleft. The sympathetic signal is terminated by the active recapture of NE to the neuron via an NE reuptake transporter. Postsynaptically sympathetic signaling is conducted by neurotransmitter stimulation of G-protein-coupled adrenoceptor expressed at the target tissue surface.

Overall, the sympathetic system had an excitatory effect on most heart function, being the major target organ in the "fight-or-flight" response associated with sympathetic c activation in physical or stressful conditions (i.e., increase in heart rate, cardiac electrical activation, contractility). The sympathetic system in the heart also considerably contributes to the regulation of coronary artery tone and myocardial blood flow both in direct and indirect ways, together with biochemical and physical factors. The direct effect of sympathetic stimulation on coronary tone and myocardial blood flow depends on the balance between α- and β-adrenoceptors located in coronary vessel walls: stimulating α1-adrenoceptors results in coronary vasoconstriction, stimulating β2-adrenoceptors in vasodilatation. Since smaller coronary arteries mainly contain β2-adrenoceptors, whereas epicardial larger coronary arteries mainly have α1-adrenoceptors, the final physiologic effect of sympathetic activation is mild to moderate vasodilation and an increase in myocardial blood flow. The indirect effect is a consequence of sympathetic effect on cardiac metabolism (mainly increased oxygen consumption), which results in a local release of vasodilator substances and increased myocardial blood flow. In the presence of decreased myocardial performances a compensatory sympathetic drive is activated, which determines increases in contractility, conduction, and heart rate [195]. Chemotherapy-induced cardiomyopathy activates a compensatory response that increases adrenergic sympathetic and renin–angiotensin system activity to preserve organ perfusion [196]. In patients with chronic HF, increased release of NE with depletion of NE deposits and downregulation of human NE transporter (hNET1) have been shown [197]. These may contribute to vasoconstriction and progressive impairment of LV function [195].

Several SPECT and PET radiopharmaceuticals for imaging the cardiac autonomic nervous system have been developed, the majority based on the structure of NE and other catecholamines. This class of tracers includes labeled neurotransmitters ([^{18}F]-fluorodopamine, [^{11}C]-epinephrine), substrate analogues termed "false neurotransmitters" (^{123}I-metaiodobenzylguanidine, ([^{18}F]-LMI1195, ^{123}I-MIBG, [^{11}C]-metahydroxyephedrine, [^{11}C]-mHED, [^{11}C]-phenylephrine, [^{11}C]-phenethylguanidines) and uptake-1 inhibitors ([^{11}C]-methyreboxetine, [^{11}C]-desipramine). The most widely utilized in clinical practice are ^{123}I-MIBG and [^{11}C]-mHED. A second class of sympathetic nervous system radiotracers are labeled adrenoceptor antagonists ((S)-(3′-terbutylamino-2′-hydroxypropoxy)-benzimidazol-2-[^{11}C]-one, [^{11}C]-CGP-12177 [198], (S)-4-(3′-[^{11}C]isopropylamino-2-hydroxypropoxy)-2H-benzimidazol-2-one, [^{11}C]-CGP-12388 [199], a prazosin like drug [^{11}C]-GB-67 [200]). In addition, radiotracers of intracellular signaling have been used, such as second messenger ((R)-[^{11}C]-rolipram [201]), the protein kinase A signaling axis ([^{11}C]- and [^{18}F]-forskolin for adenylate cyclase [202,203], an analogue of sildenafil [^{11}C]-RAL-01 for phosphodiesterase-5 [204] and isoquinolinesufonamide protein kinase inhibitor analogues [205]) and protein kinase C signaling axis ([^{11}C]-diacylglycerol [206,207]).

Despite PET radiotracers more closely resembling the endogenous neurotransmitters than SPECT ones (e.g., ^{123}MIBG), and the variety of available tracers that may allow for more detailed analysis of neuronal signaling [195,208], only few PET centers are capable of producing this class of PET tracers. In fact, the complex, laborious, and demanding radiolabeling process of most of the ligands requires specific knowledge and sophisticated infrastructure. Radiochemical purity and specific activity are the two main critical factors in practical applications. Low specific activity resulting in exposure of the myocardium to unlabeled catecholamines has to be prevented so that competition with the labeled tracer does not hamper image quality and to avoid pharmacologic action due to adrenoceptor activation [195].

^{123}I-MIBG is a NE analogue, showing the same uptake, storage, and release mechanisms of NE. It is an aralkylguanidine NE analogue not metabolized by catechol-*O*-methyl transferase and monoamine oxidase [209]. ^{123}I-MIBG was first developed as an oncological radiopharmaceutical for neuroendocrine tumors; however, uptake in the myocardium in an early study prompted further exploration. ^{123}I-MIBG presents high affinity for uptake-1 with extended neuronal retention time with evidence for a significant extraneuronal uptake-2 accumulation [210–212]. After administration (about 111–370 MBq in adult patients of normal weight for a study on a multiple-head camera) ^{123}I-MIBG initial concentration apparently depends primarily on blood flow. The extravesicular concentration of ^{123}I-MIBG decreases rapidly, whereas the intravesicular concentration remains relatively constant, thus the concentration plateaus after 4 h indicating the adrenergic neuron terminal concentration [84]. Therefore, the rate of ^{123}I-MIBG washout based on early and late measurements of myocardial uptake provides an estimation of sympathetic tone [213]. Indeed, after ^{123}I-MIBG administration, early (15 min) and late (4 h) planar images of the thorax with the patient lying in the same supine position are acquired (for about 10 min), to determinate heart-to-mediastinal ratio (H/M) and washout rate (WR). To calculate an H/R ratio ROIs are drawn at the heart (H, including or not including the cavity) and the upper mediastinum (M, avoiding the thyroid gland) in the planar anterior view. The mean count density in each ROI is obtained. Myocardial WR from initial to late images is also calculated, and expressed as a percentage, as the rate of decrease in myocardial counts over time between early and late imaging (normalized to mediastinal activity). Optionally, a SPECT study after early and late planar imaging could be performed. Compared to myocardial perfusion SPECT imaging, 64 projections over 180° or 128 projections over 360° are usually recommended. The majority of data on ^{123}I-MIBG SPECT refer to images obtained 3–4 h after ^{123}I-MIBG administration (late SPECT). When regional ^{123}I-MIBG distribution is evaluated a characteristic finding of these images is that the inferior wall has a relatively lower activity as compared to the other walls, with a considerable variation in uptake [214]. Such heterogeneity might be explained as a reflection of variation in physiology [215] due to a predominant sympathetic innervation in the anterior wall [216]. However, equally, distribution to inferoposterior and anterior myocardial wall has been also reported in later studies [217]. A decrease in myocardial ^{123}I-MIBG uptake is observed with aging, especially in patients >60 years [218]. Therefore, myocardial ^{123}I-MIBG uptake has to be corrected for age.

The neurohumoral response to the presence of dysfunctional myocytes results in a compensatory sympathetic drive, which increases the contractility, conduction, and heart rate. Therefore, ^{123}I-MIBG might be used to obtain images of the efferent sympathetic innervation of the heart before significant reduction in LVEF is noted [219]. For example, patients with HF presented reduced ^{123}I-MIBG cardiac uptake and accelerated the washout rate, as a consequence of increased NE in the cardiac synaptic space and a reduction in the presynaptic space [13]. ^{123}I-MIBG H/M ratio on the delayed image and WR have been found to be significantly associated with brain natriuretic peptide serum NE concentration, and heart-type fatty acid binding protein, which is a marker for ongoing myocardial damage [220,221]. The H/M ratio has also been associated with myocardial contractile reserve [222]. ^{123}I-MIBG parameters have also been successfully used in monitoring the effect of HF treatment, representing an excellent predictor of prognosis [223,224]. In patients with HF with LVEF <45% a H/M ratio <1.2 was a strong predictor of mortality [225] and a H/M ratio <1.74 was demonstrated to be an independent predictor of cardiac death [226]. The normal reference value of H/M ratios varies widely between institutions, ranging from 1.4 to 2.8, emphasizing the need to standardize acquisition protocols and methods for quantitation to create appropriate conditions to perform large-scale clinical studies with the aim of establishing evidence for the usefulness of ^{123}I-MIBG [227].

^{123}I-MIBG has also been investigated as an early marker for cardiotoxicity after antracycline therapy. In a rat model, a clear dose-dependent reduction of ^{123}I-MIBG has been observed after 6 weeks treatment with doxorubicin, when only mild myocyte damage at histopathology examination was detected [228]. In the same model, a remarkable decrease in LVEF was evident starting 2 weeks later [229]. Studies in asymptomatic patients treated with anthracyclines revealed that ^{123}I-MIBG uptake (H/M rate) is useful to assess myocardial adrenergic derangement and to identify patients at risk of developing cardiotoxicity [54,230]. The H/M ratio result was lower both in patients treated with anthracyclines and with other chemotherapeutic agents, decreasing in a dose-dependent way and even at very low dosage of doxorubicin, when LVEF is preserved [54,229,231]. Two mechanisms have been suggested to explain decreased ^{123}I-MIBG uptake in a heart with doxorubicin cardiomyopathy. The first imputes the decrease in ^{123}I-MIBG uptake to the destruction of adrenergic nerve tissue whereas the second explains the reduction of H/M ratio as a functional alteration of adrenergic nerves, as a result of hyperexcitation of nerve endings as a compensatory mechanism for impaired cardiac pump function [232,233]. Using SPECT, a reduction in myocardial accumulation of ^{123}I-MIBG after doxorubicin was larger in the LV than in the RV myocardium [234]. In addition, a regional correspondence between ^{123}I-MIBG decrease and histopathologic finding of atrophic and fibrotic nerve fibers [234,235] was demonstrated as well as greater vulnerability of the subendocardial layer as compared to the subepicardium [232].

In a recent pilot study ^{123}I-MIBG was also used in the setting of trastuzumab (humanized monoclonal antibody against HER2) cardiotoxicity. Since this drug typically causes a transient, asymptomatic decline in LVEF, distinguishing patients that would recover LVEF from patients most likely to develop HF (about 10%) is fundamental to decide treatment discontinuation. This study included patients with an asymptomatic decrease in LVEF. An impairment in both H/M ratio (<1.6) and WR rate ($>25\%$) was a predictor of persistent LVEF impairment within the 13 months of follow-up. On the contrary, normal (or near-normal) ^{123}I-MIBG parameters were associated with LVEF recovery [236].

In only one study was ^{123}I-MIBG scintigraphy used to evaluate cardiotoxicity in cancer patients treated with chest RT and anthracyclines or chest RT alone. In these patients ^{123}I-MIBG cardiac H/M ratio was significantly decreased compared to controls. Also, the ^{123}I-MIBG WR and the LVEF showed significant differences, but with some overlap in individual cases.

Critical open issues ^{123}I-MIBG are represented by the definition of a valid cut-off for H/M ratio and WR for early recognition of cardiotoxicity, the identification of its role in monitoring the effect of therapy to prevent or treat early-stage chemotherapy-induced HF as well as on late cardiotoxicity with long-term follow-up.

PET imaging can play a key role in the evaluation of cardiac autonomic dysfunction associated with HF [192] providing some advantages over SPECT (e.g., higher spatial and temporal resolution). A series of different pre- and postsynaptic tracers has been developed [195]. However, the clinical use of receptor-target tracers for adrenergic system has been limited to a few studies and is still facing significant challenge.

[^{11}C]-mHED and [^{11}C]-CGP-12177 are the most widely used radiopharmaceuticals for PET imaging of the autonomic nervous system. The use of [^{11}C]-mHED demonstrated superior results as compared to ^{123}I-MIBG in terms of resolution, homogeneity of tracer distribution [237], better regional abnormality analysis [238], and the advantage of absolute quantification by using kinetic modeling. An important advance in the field has been reached by the organization of the PARAPET, the first large-scale PET clinical trial, which evaluated the autonomic neuronal system to predict arrhythmia in patients with ischemic cardiomyopathy eligible for ICD as primary prevention [239,240]. In patients with idiopathic dilated cardiomyopathy [241,242] and myocardial ischemia [243,244] a decrease of β-adreceptor density was shown by using [^{11}C]-CGP-12177.

However, up to now no data in humans have been published on the specific issue of cardiotoxicity. The only available data are derived from a recent animal study [245] that exploited the early alterations in sympathetic signaling associated with doxorubicin-induced cardiotoxicity at presynaptic (NA reuptake), postsynaptic (adrenergic receptors), and intracellular second messenger (PDE4) sites using [^{11}C]-HED, [^{3}H]CGP-12177, and (R)-[^{11}C]-rolipram. In this study, despite the absence of any change in the echo-measured physiological indices or relative heart size, decreased postsynaptic β-adreceptors assessed by [^{3}H]CGP-12177 as well impaired intracellular signaling response at the PDE4 level evaluated using (R)-[^{11}C]rolipram and administration of desipraminel were found. Reduced β-adrenoreceptor and downstream impairment of second messenger signaling response appeared early in this model and may precede changes in LV function, suggesting the potential for use of imaging with PET.

A novel ^{18}F based PET tracer, LMI1195, a NE transporter substrate with very similar molecular proprieties to ^{123}I-MIBG, has finished a phase I trial. Preliminary results show its favorable safety, dosimetry, biodistribution, and tolerability profile [246,247]. In the near future, this radiopharmaceutical might represent an option to apply on a larger-scale PET for the evaluation of cardiotoxicity in patients receiving anticancer treatment.

Table 22.4 summarizes the main results of a literature search on the use of sympathetic nervous innervation imaging for cardiotoxicity. Fig. 22.3 shows an example of sequential ^{123}I-MIBG scintigraphy in patients treated with doxorubicin.

^{111}In-Antimyosin Imaging

The immunoscintigraphic agent ^{111}In-antimyosin is a specific marker of myocardial cell injury and necrosis. Antimyosin antibodies bind to intracellular

TABLE 22.4 Summary of the Main Publications on Cardiotoxicity Imaged by Sympathetic Innervation Imaging

References	Patients (*n*)	Treatment	Test(s)	Parameter(s) Evaluated	Main Findings
Carrió et al. 1995 [54]	36	Doxorubicin	^{123}I-MIBG scintigraphy, RNV, ^{111}In-antimyosin scintigraphy	H/M, LVEF, HLR	Cell damage and impaired adrenergic neuron activity was found in pts with maintained or slightly decreased EF
Lekakis et al. 1996 [84]	37	Doxorubicin	^{123}I-MIBG scintigraphy, RNV	H/M, LVEF	In pts receiving doxorubicin H/M was significantly lower and correlated with cumulative dose compared to pts not treated with doxorubicin
Ono et al. 1994 [248]	19	Multiagent including adriamycin	^{123}I-MIBG scintigraphy	WR	Low uptake in the myocardium and rapid WR especially in the lateral and inferior segments, in pts with cardiotoxicity. Such cardiotoxic effect is dose-dependent
Stokkel et al. 2013 [236]	9	Trastuzumab	^{123}I-MIBG scintigraphy	H/M, WR	In pts with a persistently decreasing LVEF, ^{123}I-MIBG scintigraphy might indicate whether recovery will occur and, consequently, whether retreatment may be initiated
Takano et al. 1996 [234]	27	Doxorubicin	^{123}I-MIBG scintigraphy	H/M, WR	The H/M and the WR of the doxorobucin group were respectively lower and higher than those of the control group
Valdés Olmos et al. 1992 [117]	13	Doxorubicin	^{123}I-MIBG scintigraphy, RNV	WR, LVEF	In spite of a localized loss of LV function, doxorubicin-related cardiotoxicity appeared to be based on a global process of myocardial adrenergic derangement
Valdés Olmos et al. 1995 [219]	21	Doxorubicin or epirubicin	^{123}I-MIBG scintigraphy	WR	^{123}I-MIBG uptake tended to be significantly impaired, at higher cumulative chemotherapy dose levels, before significant LVEF changes in 62% of pts

BNP, brain natriuretic peptide; echo, echocardiography; ERNA, equilibrium radionuclide angiocardiography; HLR, heart-to-lung ratio; H/M, heart-to-mediastinum ratio; LVEF, left ventricle ejection fraction; MPI, myocardial perfusion scintigraphy; MRI, magnetic resonance imaging; MUGA, multigated equilibrium radionuclide venticulography; PFR, peak filling rate; PER, peak ejection rate; pts, patients; RT, radiotherapy; TAC, time–activity curve; TDI, tissue-Doppler imaging; TFR, time to filling rate; RNV, radionuclide venticulography.

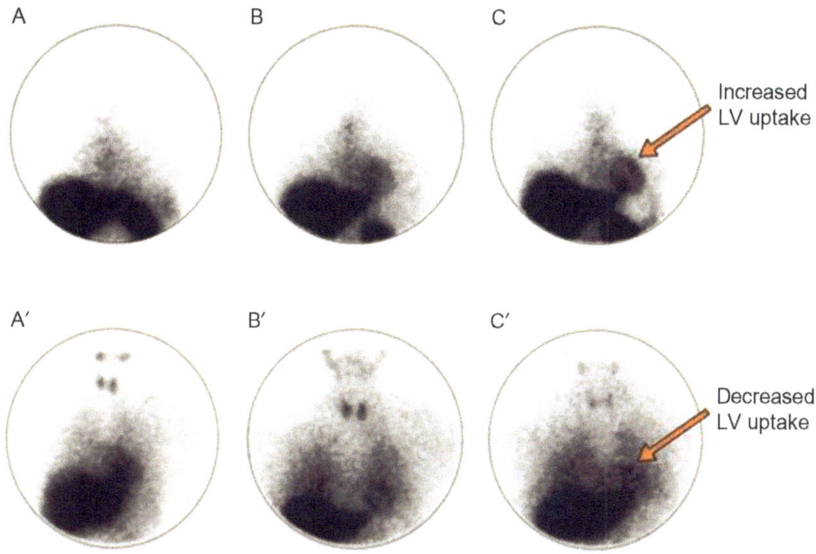

FIGURE 22.3 ^{111}In-antimyosin and ^{123}I-MIBG: sequential ^{111}In-antimyosin (A, B, and C) and ^{123}I-MIBG (A′, B′, and C′) studies in patients treated with doxorubicin at baseline (A and A′) at 240–300 mg/m^2 (B and B′) and at 420–600 mg/m^2 (C and C′) of doxorubicin. A pattern of increasing myocardial ^{111}In-antimyosin uptake with decreasing myocardial ^{123}I-MIBG uptake is present, reflecting the presence of progressive myocellular injury from anthracycline-based chemotherapy. *Adapted from Kongbundansuk S, et al. Noninvasive imaging of cardiovascular injury related to the treatment of cancer. Am Coll Cardiol Img 2014;7(8):824–38.*

myosin when sarcolemma disruption occurs and the cell is irreversibly damaged [13], as in the case of doxorubicin cardiotoxicity [195]. Therefore, ^{111}In-antimyosin can represent potential biomarkers for the assessment of patients with subclinical LV dysfunction [53,218].

Uptake of ^{111}In-antimyosin in the myocardium, quantified by calculating the heart-to-lung (HLR) ratio on the images acquired 24–48 h after tracer injection [54,88,218] was significantly correlated with cumulative epirubicin administered dose, remaining substantially unmodified up to 6 months after therapy discontinuation. A value of HLR >1.85 at intermediate epirubicin dosage level showed a sensitivity of 95% and a specificity of 57% as a predictor of late LVEF impairment [88].

Similarly, in breast cancer patients treated with or without anthracycline chemotherapy (doxorubicin or mitoxantrone) and without any cardiovascular risk factors or previous chemotherapy or mediastinal RT, increased ^{111}In-antimyosin uptake correlated with changes in LVEF [218]. More interestingly, increased uptake was also demonstrated in patients without a significant reduction in LVEF after chemotherapy. In patients with sarcoma, a HLR ≥1.90 at ^{111}In-antimyosin scan at a low cumulative dose (240–300 mg/m^2) predicted a reduction in LVEF ≥10% at a subsequent high cumulative doxorubicin dose (420–600 mg/m^2) [53]. These findings strongly suggest the potential use of this radiopharmaceutical to detect cellular damage before the onset of LV functional impairment, allowing the identification of patients at risk of developing HF, in particular when treated with an increasing dose of chemotherapeutic drugs [13]. The cardiac uptake of ^{111}In-antimyosin could also be useful to discriminate between patients with transient and persistent LV dysfunction and to guide clinical decisions about discontinuation of anthracycline therapy. In fact, patients with a persistent reduction in LVEF after chemotherapy show significantly higher HLR compared to patients with a transient reduction of LVEF [230]. However, since patients with a history of severe anthracycline-induced cardiomyopathy might present persistent myocardial cell injury up to 10 years after the development of HF, regardless of recovery of LV function [249] it is still unknown whether abnormal antimyosin uptake is temporary or permanent [195].

Abnormal ^{111}In-antimyosin uptake, associated with a greater decrease in LVEF, was also observed early with a progressive trend during treatment, in patients with advanced breast cancer and soft tissue sarcomas treated with high-dose epirubicin with or without dexrazoxane compared to the control group [85,118].

^{111}In-antimyosin scintigraphy was also assessed in a limited number of pediatric patients treated with doxorubicin (cumulative dose of 150 mg/m^2). This tracer seems to be able to detect early myocardial damage and to identify children who are at increased risk of developing cardiac sequelae [250].

In Table 22.5 the main articles published on the use of radiolabeled antimyosin imaging for cardiotoxicity are listed. Fig. 22.3 shows an example of sequential ^{111}In-antimyosin scintigraphy in patients treated with doxorubicin.

Radiolabeled Trastuzumab

In 1998, antihuman epidermal growth factor receptor 2 (HER2) trastuzumab (Herceptin, Roche) became the first humanized monoclonal antibody (mAb) approved by US Food and Drug Administration. Trastuzumab, as a single agent, is indicated for the treatment of patients with metastatic breast cancer whose tumors overexpress the HER2 protein and who have received one or more chemotherapy regimens. Trastuzumab is also approved for use in combination with paclitaxel for the treatment of patients with HER2-expressing metastatic breast cancer who have not received chemotherapy for their metastatic disease. HER2, a transmembrane receptor tyrosine kinase, is overexpressed in 25–30% of breast cancers. HER2-positivity increases the likelihood of invasion and survival of tumor cells at the site of metastasis [253]. In these patients, targeted treatment using monoclonal antibodies such as trastuzumab can be used to reduce tumor recurrence and improve survival [254]. Trastuzumab selectively binds to the extracellular domain of HER2 receptors,

TABLE 22.5 Summary of the Main Publications on Cardiotoxicity Imaged by ^{111}In-antimyosin Scan

References	Patients (*n*)	Treatment	Test(s)	Parameter(s) Evaluated	Main Findings
Carrió et al. 1993 [53]	30	Doxorubicin	^{111}In-antimyosin scintigraphy, MUGA	HLR, LVEF	Intense antimyosin uptake at intermediate cumulative doses identified pts at risk of cardiotoxicity before EF deteriorates
Carrió et al. 1995 [54]	36	Doxorubicin	^{111}In-antimyosin scintigraphy, ^{123}I-MIBG scintigraphy, RNV	HLR, H/M, LVEF	Cell damage and impaired adrenergic neuron activity were found in pts with maintained or slightly decreased EF
Erselcan et al. 2000 [251]	32	Fluorouracil + epirubicin + cyclophosphamide or fluorouracil + epirubicin + cyclophosphamide + high-dose alkylating agents or cyclophosphamide + methotrexate + fluorouracil	^{111}In-antimyosin scintigraphy	HLR	Cardiac antimyosin antibody uptake was considerably higher among pts treated with fluorouracil + epirubicin + cyclophosphamide compared to other arms. A linear association was found between the cumulative dose of epirubicin and the cardiac antimyosin uptake
Estorch et al. 1993 [218]	35	Doxorubicin or mitoxantrone	^{111}In-antimyosin scintigraphy	HLR	^{111}In-antimyosin uptake without a decrease in LVEF after treatment with mitoxantrone indicated the presence of myocyte cell damage, but not to the extent necessary to deteriorate function
Kremer et al. 1999 [250]	8[a]	Doxorubicin	^{111}In-antimyosin scintigraphy	HLR	^{111}In-antimyosin scintigraphy detected early myocardial damage after a cumulative doxorubicin dose (of 150 mg/m^2) identifying pts at increased risk of developing cardiac sequelae
Lopez et al. 1998 [85]	129	Epirubicin ± dexrazoxane	^{111}In-antimyosin scintigraphy, MUGA	HLR, LVEF	All methods of cardiac evaluation clearly documented the cardioprotective effect of dexrazoxane

(Continued)

TABLE 22.5 (Continued)

References	Patients (*n*)	Treatment	Test(s)	Parameter(s) Evaluated	Main Findings
Maini et al. 1997 [88]	36	Epirubicin	^{111}In-antimyosin scintigraphy, RNV	HLR, LVEF	LVEF appeared more useful at high cumulative dosages and during follow-up to monitor late pump dysfunction, HLR may be effective during the early phase of the therapy in determining which pts are at risk for development of late cardiac dysfunction
Valdés Olmos et al. 1994 [230]	27	Anthracycline	^{111}In-antimyosin scintigraphy	HLR	^{111}In-antimyosin scintigraphy can be used as an important confirmatory criterion for the clinical decision to discontinue anthracycline therapy since it can differentiate cardiac dysfunction caused by severe myocardial injury from temporary decreases in LVEF, without severe concomitant myocyte damage, which may occur during anthracycline therapy
Valdés Olmos et al. 2002 [252]	24	Doxorubicin or epirubicin	^{111}In-antimyosin scintigraphy	HLR, LVEF, PFR	Myocyte damage appeared to precede LV systolic and diastolic dysfunction in anthracycline treatment. Antimyosin scintigraphy was sensitive in detecting myocardial damage even after low cumulative dose
Vici et al. 1998 [118]	95	Epirubicin ± dexrazoxane	^{111}In-antimyosin scintigraphy, MUGA	HLR, LVEF	Dexrazoxane significantly protects against the development of high-dose epirubicin cardiotoxicity apparently without evidence of an adverse impact on antitumor activity and noncardiac toxicity

HLR, heart-to-lung ratio; H/M, heart-to-mediastinum ratio; LVEF, left ventricle ejection fraction; MUGA, multigated equilibrium radionuclide venticulography; PFR, peak filling rate; pts, patients.
[a]*Pediatric patients.*

where it inhibits downstream signaling pathways, resulting in a reduced proliferation of tumor cells. This is achieved by identifying tumor cells for immune destruction, and then, by initiation of antibody-dependent cellular cytotoxicity, causing apoptosis of tumor cells [255]. In addition, trastuzumab undergoes internalization (endocytosis) into the tumor cells and subsequently increases the expression of HER2 on the cellular surface. This enhances the immune effects of trastuzumab and reduces tumor expression. Therefore, patients with HER2-positive tumors may also have increased resistance to common anticancer treatments, such as chemotherapy and radiation therapy. Using immunohistochemistry, the patient's tumor HER2 expression must score a 2+ or 3+ to be eligible for therapy [256]. In monotherapy, trastuzumab results in a response in only 12–35% of the patients, whereas when this agent is combined with paclitaxel, response rates increase to 40–60% [257]. This response rate is further complicated by the fact that the majority of the patients who initially respond to trastuzumab will experience progression of their disease within 1 year of beginning therapy with the mAb [258]. Radiolabeling trastuzumab with γ- or $\beta+$-emitting radionuclides provides a means to visualize and quantitate the HER2 target with a noninvasive methodology [259–261]. Preclinical and clinical studies have demonstrated the feasibility of targeting HER2 with trastuzumab conjugated with radionuclides [257]. Trastuzumab has been labeled with ^{111}In [262] for SPECT imaging and with ^{64}Cu [263], ^{124}I [260], ^{89}Zr [264], and ^{68}Ga (F(ab′)$_2$ fragments) [265] for PET imaging.

Radiolabeled trastuzumab may be exploited as a tool in nuclear medicine to select patients for targeted therapy, monitor treatment responses of patients, determine the emergence of resistance and therefore treatment failure, provide dosimetric calculations and predictions for radioimmunotherapeutic regimens, and restage patient's disease. In addition, it might also be used to identify those patients at risk for cardiac toxicity (Table 22.6).

The potential to image HER2 expression with radiolabeled trastuzumab offers a unique opportunity to assess whether HER2 is expressed in the heart, i.e., in the case of combination therapy with anthracyclines and trastuzumab. In a small series of patients with metastatic breast cancer scheduled for trastuzumab as second-line therapy after anthracyclines, Behr et al. [266] showed myocardial uptake of ^{111}In-trastuzumab prior to treatment in seven patients. Of these, six developed clinical HF (II-IV NYHA class), whereas none of 13 patients without baseline uptake had adverse cardiac events, suggesting that pretreatment scanning with ^{111}In-trastuzumab could predict cardiotoxicity [267]. In contrast, Perik et al. [268] documented increased ^{111}In-trastuzumab uptake at the start of trastuzumab therapy in only one of 17 studied patients, who received extensive anthracycline pretreatment, and normal ^{111}In-trastuzumab uptake at baseline scintigraphy in three patients who developed trastuzumab-induced cardiomyopathy. More recently De Korte et al. [267] investigated whether myocardial HER2 expression is upregulated by anthracycline-induced cardiac stress. They performed ^{111}In-

TABLE 22.6 Summary of the Main Publications on Cardiotoxicity Imaged by ^{111}In-Trastuzumab Scintigraphy

Reference	Patients (*n*)	Treatment	Test(s)	Parameter(s) Evaluated	Main Findings
Behr et al. 2001 [266]	20	Trastuzumab	^{111}In-DTPA-trastuzumab scintigraphy	HER2 expression	HER2 overexpression in 35% of pts (NYHA II-IV cardiotoxicity subsequently developed or cardiac arrhythmia). In all pts without myocardial uptake, no adverse cardiac effects occurred
de Korte et al. 2007 [267]	10	Anthracycline	^{111}In-DTPA-trastuzumab scintigraphy	HER2 expression	Shortly after completion of anthracycline treatment, myocardial HER2 overexpression was detectable in 50% of the pts. ^{111}In-DTPA-trastuzumab scintigraphy after anthracyclines prior to adjuvant trastuzumab potentially identifies pts susceptible for trastuzumab-related cardiotoxicity
Perik et al. 2006 [267]	17	Trastuzumab	^{111}In-DTPA-trastuzumab scintigraphy, blood test	HER2 expression, NT-proBNP, troponin I	Radiolabeled trastuzumab scintigraphy was not valuable in predicting trastuzumab-related cardiotoxicity. NT-proBNP results were promising regarding prediction of trastuzumab-related cardiotoxicity

trastuzumab scans in 10 patients shortly after anthracyclines, to reproduce the schedule of trastuzomab administration in an adjuvant setting. They used 10 patients with nonanthracycline-related HF as a control group. About 50% of the patients showed myocardial HER2 expression at levels detectable with ^{111}In-DTPA-trastuzumab SPECT imaging, whereas no myocardial ^{111}In-DTPA-trastuzumab was observed in any of the 10 patients with HF due to cardiac disease. Based on these data, it seems that trastuzumab-related cardiotoxicity occurring after anthracyclines is a two-step process. During the first step, cardiac stress induced by anthracyclines causes an increase in myocardial HER2 expression. Then, trastuzumab treatment subsequently results in cardiac dysfunction through inhibition of HER2-mediated signaling. On this basis, Korte et al. initiated a new study, still ongoing, exploring the time of occurrence and duration of myocardial HER2 expression in relation to anthracycline chemotherapy. Fig. 22.4 presents an example of the use of a ^{111}In-DTPA-trastuzumab SPECT scan in patients with cancer after chemotherapy with anthracycline.

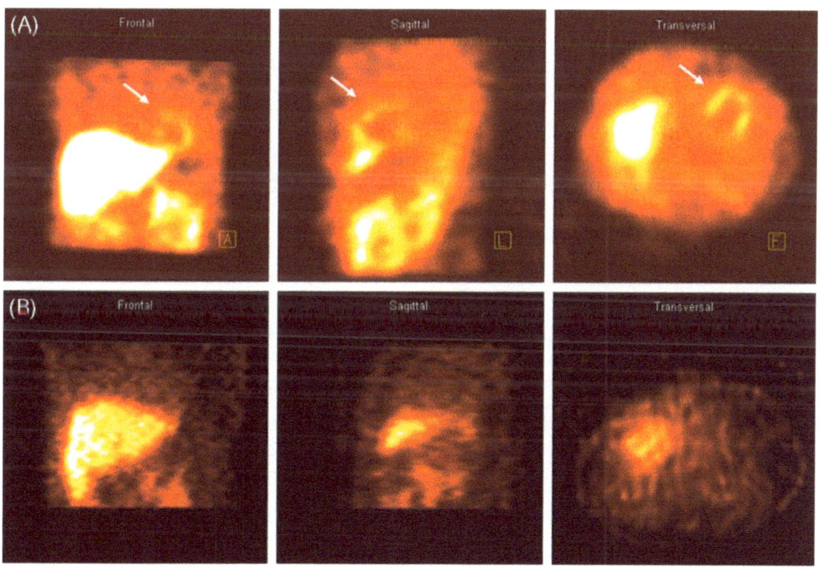

FIGURE 22.4 ^{111}In-DTPA-trastuzumab SPECT scan in patients with cancer after chemotherapy with anthracycline showing patient with myocardial uptake of ^{111}In-DTPA-trastuzumab at the left ventricle (A) or patient without myocardial uptake (B). In both patients normal uptake in the liver is present. *Adapted from de Korte MA, et al. 111Indium-trastuzumab visualises myocardial human epidermal growth factor receptor 2 expression shortly after anthracycline treatment but not during heart failure: a clue to uncover the mechanisms of trastuzumab-related cardiotoxicity. Eur J Cancer 2007;43(14):2046–51.*

Apoptosis Imaging

The term "apoptosis" refers to the biologic process of programmed cell death, an active process requiring energy and regulated by the activation of specific genes, whose transcription and translation into active proteins determine the death of the cell. The histologic changes of apoptosis are preceded by an initiation stage, the "lag or trigger phase" [269–272], whereas multiple triggers, such as withdrawal of growth factors, DNA damage, immune reactions, ionizing radiation, chemotherapy, and ischemic injury [273–276] can start a cascade of events that lead to the morphologic changes of apoptosis. The lag time between exposure to the trigger(s) and the time when morphologic signs of apoptosis can be observed is highly variable as it heavily depends on cell type, type of trigger(s), intensity and exposure, duration of trigger, and local environmental conditions [277]. The apoptotic process can be divided into four different phases: initiation, execution, recognition/phagocytosis of the apoptotic bodies, and removal [278,279]. The hallmark of the start of the execution phase is redistribution and exposure of phosphatidylserine (PS) on the outer layer of the cell membrane [280]. PS exposure is recognized as a ubiquitous phenomenon of apoptosis that is independent of cell type and of cell-death-inducing trigger [281] and is phylogenetically conserved [282]. Dysregulation of apoptosis can cause either the accumulation of unwanted cells (as may happen in cancer) or the premature removal of useful and/or essential cells (as may happen in Alzheimer's disease or in some autoimmune rheumatologic disorders). Apoptosis of myocardiocytes plays a critical role in the onset of cardiomyopathy and has been observed in several conditions (e.g., hypoxia, ischemia, anthracycline-induced cardiomyopathy, and end-stage HF). Since PS externalization represents the hallmark of apoptosis, a variety of PS-binding compounds have been extensively investigated for imaging, including proteins [283], peptides [284–287], and small chemical entities [288]. Peptides and small chemical compounds having the advantage of being quickly and efficiently cleared from the blood circulation, exhibit optimal properties as imaging probes, since their signal-to-background ratio is favorable. The main disadvantage of these compounds is their low affinity for PS. On the other hand, proteins exhibit higher affinities for PS, but due to their higher molecular weight, they are usually cleared from the blood circulation with slower kinetics [283–289]. Annexin V, a 36-kDa vesicle-associated protein, is perhaps the most widely investigated PS-targeting moiety. Annexin V binds to PS in a Ca^{2+}-dependent manner, with nanomolar affinity. The availability of recombinant annexin V, which exhibits PS binding properties identical to those of annexin V purified from human tissue, spurred synthesis of a wide range of labeled forms of annexin V to image PS expression using optical, radionuclide, and magnetic resonance imaging [18,290]. Additionally, positive or bimodal MR contrast as well as multimodal contrast agents cointaining annexin V have been developed. Radiolabeling of rh-annexin V with ^{99m}Tc-pertechnetate can be performed by the penthioate radioligand (N_2S_2) method [291], which is cumbersome presenting low labeling efficiency (30–40%), and entails a high nonspecific excretion of radioactivity into the bowel via biliary excretion. For these reasons, an improved labeling method using the bifunctional agent hydrazinonicotinamide (HYNIC) was selected for clinical trials [292].

However this method could compromise the binding of annexin V to PS [293]. Therefore, different variants of annexin V have been generated, leading to molecules successfully coupled with a number of compounds without adversely affecting its binding affinity for PS [294–300].

Both the V-117 and V-128 variants have major advantages over HYNIC-annexin V, including a 50–75% lower renal accumulation and a markedly improved in vivo localization to sites of apoptosis in animal models [293]. Annexin V has also been proven to be quite heat-labile, as it loses most of its activity with heating at 56°C for 10 min [282], thus precluding the use of many different types of labeling chemistries. Several approaches to label annexin V with fluorine-18 (^{18}F) [301] for PET imaging have been developed. One method has used N-succinimidyl 4-fluorobenzoate to synthesize F-annexin V. The fluorine-labeled agent has lower uptake in the liver, spleen, and kidney than HYNIC-annexin V. Another method involves site-specific derivatization with an ^{18}F-maleimide-labeled compound of mutant annexin V-117 or annexin V-128 [295]. However, both methods need more preclinical investigations before further development as imaging agents for apoptosis in patients. Other radionuclide derivatives of annexin V have been developed, including annexin V-labeled ^{123}I [302] or ^{124}I [303] and ^{64}Cu-labeled streptavidin for PET imaging after pretargeting of PS with biotinylated annexin V [304].

^{99m}Tc-rh-annexin V has been extensively used in patients with cancer, following a single administration of chemotherapeutic agents to predict the efficacy of chemotherapy and RT [305]. In fact, although the baseline tumor uptake of ^{99m}Tc-HYNIC annexin-V differs significantly from patient to patient, in general patients displaying tumor progression or stable disease exhibited a higher than background uptake in their tumor tissue, whereas patients responding to treatment display a comparable or lower than background uptake in their tumor.

^{99m}Tc-annexin V scintigraphy has been used to assess acute and chronic doxorubicin-induced cardiomyopathy based on early apoptosis in animal models. Increased ^{99m}Tc-annexin V uptake was observed in the myocardium of doxorubicin-treated animals and cardiac oxidative stress was confirmed by histological analysis [231,306]. Gabrielson et al. [307] introduced the use of SPECT with ^{99m}Tc-annexin V to detect early onset of adriamycin-induced cardiomyopathy. They demonstrated the ability of ^{99m}Tc-annexin V SPECT to detect myocardial cell death at a lower dose and therefore earlier stage than by echocardiography. Furthermore, this method should be suitable for detection of numerous other cardiomyopathies, including those induced by other antineoplastic agents and by radiation. A number of critical issues, however, remain to be resolved. It would clearly be desirable to detect adriamycin cardiomyopathy at an early stage before irreversible damage to the heart has occurred. Clearly, this is not being accomplished in this case since cell death is being detected. A better understanding of the mechanism underlying adriamycin cardiotoxicity might lead to the design of methods that could detect the onset of toxicity at an earlier reversible state. Thus, there has been considerable evidence that adriamycin cardiotoxicity resembles the effects of ischemia in the heart [308,309]. Evidence points to the possibility that adriamycin is producing a reversible vasoconstrictive effect, suggesting that monitoring of cardiac blood flow with ^{99m}Tc-sestamibi or by dynamic contrast-enhanced MRI or arterial spin labeling might detect cardiotoxicity at an earlier stage and that vasodilators may be effectively employed to avoid further progression of the myopathy [310].

Promising results have also been obtained in a mouse model of anthracycline cardiotoxicity using a caspase-3 substrate labeled with ^{18}F ([^{18}F]-CP18) [311]. In this animal model of cardiotoxicity, doxorubicin treatment has been to be found associated with increased myocardial caspase 3 expression and an increase in CP18 uptake quantified by microPET (Fig. 22.5A), autoradiography (Fig. 22.5B), and gamma counting, suggesting a potential role of this radiopharmaceutical to detect anthracycline-induced myocardial apoptosis. Further studies are needed of the clinical use of these radiopharmaceuticals, in particular in early identification of myocardial damage related to antineoplastic drugs.

Fatty Acid Imaging

The primary sources of energy for the fetal heart are lactate and glucose [312] while after birth, there is a rapid change, and β-oxidation of fatty acids (FAs) becomes the predominant metabolic pathway of the myocyte despite the manteinance of the ability to metabolize glucose and lactate [313]. In normal conditions, long-chain FAs represent 60–80% of the heart's energy source [314]. Several factors affect their utilization including their plasma concentration, the albumin-to-FA ratio, FA chain length, the substrate and hormonal milieu, and the availability of oxygen [315]. Under fasting conditions, when insulin levels are low and catecholamine levels rise, the plasma concentration of FAs increases, resulting in an augmentation of FA uptake by myocardial cells. When insulin levels rise (e.g., postprandially), release of FAs from adipocytes is reduced and myocardial glucose utilization increases [316,317]. Failure in storing of free-FA in the cytosol lipid pool and impairment of mitochondrial free FA uptake for β-oxidation has also been described as a consequence of impaired microtubular transport system in cardiomyocytes induced by taxanes.

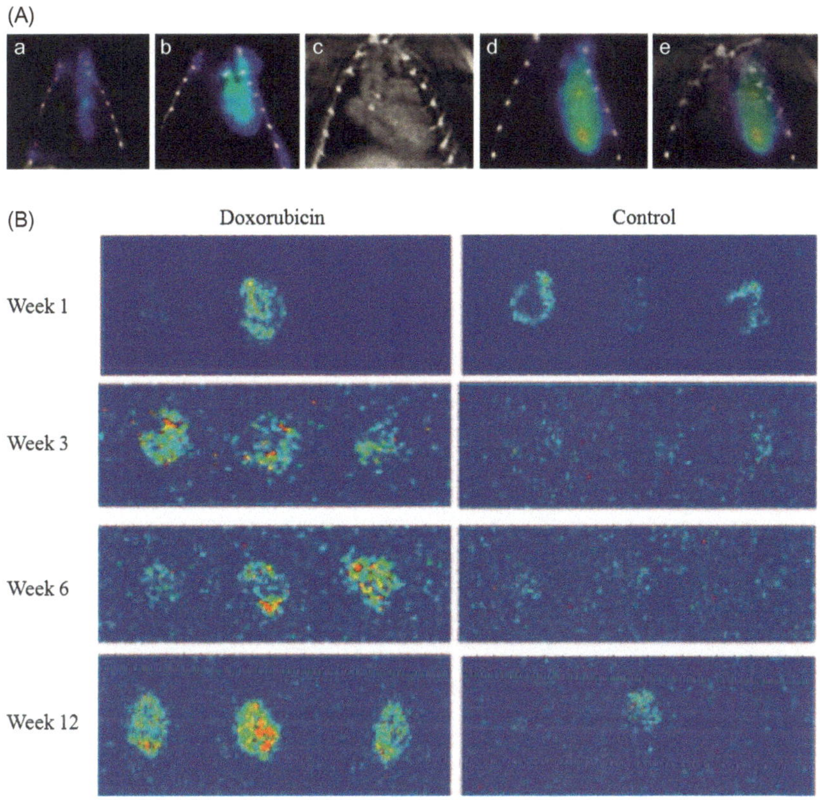

FIGURE 22.5 (A) In vivo microPET imaging of ^{18}F-CP18 performed in doxorubicin-treated mice using an INVEON Multimodality scanner at weeks 1 (a), 6 (b), and 12 (d) of treatment; CT angiogram (c) and coregistration of microPET with CT angiogram (e). Progressive increase in radiopharmaceutical uptake is evident over time. (B) Autoradiography images of heart explanted from doxorubicin-treated mice and control mice after treatment for 3, 6, and 12 weeks. Increase in ^{18}F-CP18 uptake of myocardial tissue sections evident compared with minimal ^{18}F-CP18 uptake seen in control is depicted. Regions in red represent foci with high uptake, yellow and green represent intermediate uptake, and blue represents background. Each slide contains myocardial sections from the base, mid, and distal segments of the heart from individual animal. *Adapted from Su H, et al. Noninvasive Molecular Imaging of Apoptosis in a Mouse Model of Anthracycline-Induced Cardiotoxicity. Circ Cardiovasc Imaging. 2015;8(2): e001952.*

Cardiac imaging of FAs is performed using both SPECT and PET radiopharmaceuticals (Table 22.7). The SPECT tracers include 15-(p-[^{123}I]-iodophenyl)-pentadecanoic acid and its branched-chain analogue, β-methyl-*p*-[^{123}I]-iodophenyl-pentadecanoic acid (^{123}I-BMIPP). ^{123}I-BMIPP is rapidly taken up by normally perfused myocardial tissue and is cleared at rates directly correlated with its β-oxidation. The presence of its methyl side chain sterically inhibits β-oxidation of ^{123}I-BMIPP and the tracer is shunted to the

TABLE 22.7 Summary of the Main Publications on Cardiotoxicity Imaged by Fatty Acid Imaging

References	Patients (*n*)	Treatment	Test(s)	Parameter(s) Evaluated	Main Findings
Takeishi et al. 1994 [318]	13	Anthracycline	^{123}I-BMIPP scintigraphy, ^{123}I-MIBG scintigraphy, 2D-echo	Heart-to-mediastinum ratio (H/M), LV shortening fraction, E/A ratio	Myocardial imaging with ^{123}I-MIBG could detect myocardial damage in pts treated with anthracycline in the early stage when cardiac systolic and diastolic function was still preserved potentially reducing the incidence and severity of HF
Saito et al. 2000 [319]	36	Doxorubicin	^{123}I-BMIPP scintigraphy	Uptake, time–activity curve (TAC)	^{123}I-BMIPP scintigraphy permitted early detection of doxorubicin-induced cardiomyopathy
Kitagawa et al. 2002 [320]	44	Doxorubicin	^{123}I-BMIPP scintigraphy	Uptake, time–activity curve (TAC)	Fatty acid metabolic disorder is characterized by a delay in metabolism in doxorubicin-induced myocardial damage and by increased back diffusion in ischemic heart disease
Umezawa et al. 2013 [321]	34	RT	^{123}I-BMIPP scintigraphy	Uptake	Based on dose recieved by RT, reduced uptake was detected in 43% of segment 40 Gy, 68% of segment 60 Gy and 13% of segment 0 Gy
Umezawa et al. 2015 [322]	5	RT $\pm$ cisplatin or nedplatin + 5-fluorouracil	^{123}I-BMIPP scintigraphy	Uptake	Reduced ^{123}I-BMIPP uptake in RT fields in all pts
Jingu et al. 2006 [175]	64	RT	PET ([^{18}F]FDG) $\pm$ MPI (^{201}Tl) $\pm$ ^{123}I-BMIPP scintigraphy $\pm$ MRI	Metabolism	High [^{18}F]FDG uptake in the basal myocradium corresponding to the irradiated fields compared to uptake in the myocardium outside the irradiated fields, in 20% of pts. Low ^{123}I-BMIPP and ^{201}Tl uptake (in the area corresponding to high [^{18}F]FDG uptake) respectively in 62% and 50% of pts
Nony et al. 2000 [93]	6	Doxorubicin	PET (^{11}C-acetate), RNV	Oxidative metabolism, blood flow, LVEF	Using PET to evaluate both acute and chronic toxicity, no significant effect was observed either on the flux through the tricarboxylic acid cycle or on myocardial blood flow. Systolic LV function showed a significant impairment after 300 mg/m^2 of doxorubicin

triglyceride pool, resulting in enhanced radiotracer retention that facilitates qualitative FA imaging [317]. ^{123}I-BMIPP scintigraphy has been successfully used to assess the biochemical perturbation in free fatty acid oxidation in a comparative study of MPI and ^{123}I-BMIPP SPECT in patients treated with combination of taxanes plus carboplatin [107]. Results from this study show significantly lower BMIPP uptake scores after chemotherapy as compared to those obtained at baseline, whereas MPI was not significantly affected. Moreover, patients who developed LV dysfunction also had a significant decrease in total BMIPP uptake scores. The value of ^{123}I-BMIPP in prediction of cardiotoxicity was also documented after doxorubicin treatment [319] with a significant dose-related reduction in ^{123}I-BMIPP uptake and a higher rate of late LV dysfunction development in patients presenting decreased uptake, despite preserved LVEF at echocardiography. However, in patients treated with anthracycline in the early stages of cardiotoxicity when cardiac systolic and diastolic function were still preserved, ^{123}I-MIBG was shown to be more sensitive in detecting myocardial damage as compared to ^{123}I-BMIPP that showed preserved H/M ratio and clearance [318]. Fig. 22.6 shows an example of reduced myocardial FA metabolism at ^{123}I-BMIPP SPECT after chemotherapy.

For a quantitation of myocardial FA metabolism by applying specific kinetic models to straight-chain FA labeled with ^{11}C or ^{18}F in the C1 position, at the carboxylic acid end of the FA, where β-oxidation commences are needed. In fact, only these FA derivatives accurately reflect physiologic FA

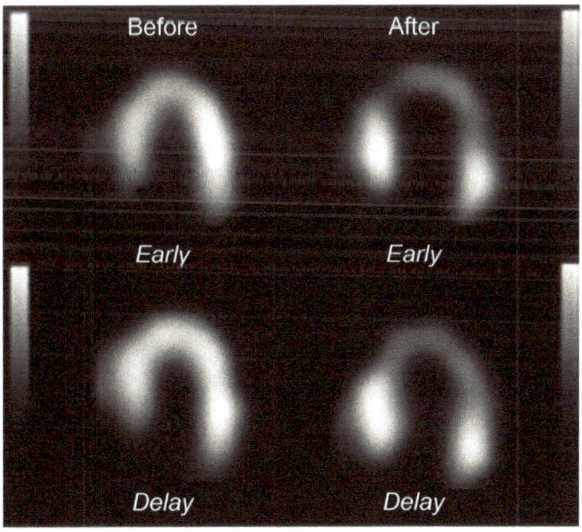

FIGURE 22.6 ^{123}I-BMIPP myocardial SPECT images in horizontal section at baseline and after chemotherapy. Decreased uptake is observed in the anterolateral wall on either the early or delayed image after chemotherapy. *Adapted from Saito K, et al. Detection of doxorubicin cardiotoxicity by using iodine-123 BMIPP early dynamic SPECT: quantitative evaluation of early abnormality of fatty acid metabolism with the Rutland method. J Nucl Cardiol 2000;7(6):553–61.*

metabolism, because all other carbons in the chain can be subject to multiple alternative metabolic fates [317,323].

Very recently, the feasibility of [^{11}C]-acetoacetate as a radiotracer for PET imaging in HF induce by doxorubicin was investigated [324]. In this model, in vivo uptake and clearance rates of the radiopharmaceutical were both reduced at an early stage in a resting state. Whereas further studies would be required to relate these uptake and clearance rate constants to the cardiac oxidative stress and ketone metabolism, results suggest [^{11}C]-acetoacetate as a potential candidate for further investigations.

Reduced myocardial FA metabolism has also been demonstrated in patients with esophageal cancer treated with mediastinal RT [175,321]. Reduced uptake was present in about 50% of segments corresponding to RT fields, with 82% of patients presenting at least one positive segment [322]. In addition, dose–effect relations for reduced uptake tended to be observed at 6 months after RT as compared to baseline with mean decreases of 9% in regions at 10–15 Gy, 12.6% in regions at 20–25 Gy, 15.6% in regions at 30–35 Gy, 19% in regions at 40–45 Gy, and 16% in regions at 50–55 Gy [322]. The only patients who did not receive concomitant chemotherapy consisting of cisplatin or nedaplatin and 5-fluorouracil presented the milder reduced uptake.

Future Perspectives

Beside the traditional approach of evaluating EF and MPI or imaging well-established targets of early myocardial damage caused by cardiotoxic agents, a high number of potential imaging targets have till now remained unexplored. For example, stromal antigens, integrins, and enzymes involved in extracellular matrix component degradation such as matrix metalloproteinases (MMP) might be additional promising targets for nuclear imaging. Indeed, increased MMP gene expression and activity have been seen after chronic doxorubicin treatment [325]. In a recent study MMP-2 has been shown to be acutely activated after doxorubicin treatment and showed that MMP-2 activation is combined with in vivo LV systolic dysfunction and increased in vitro passive myocardial stiffness in rats [326]. Therefore efforts in the large-scale clinical application of novel radiopharmaceuticals is warranted.

Furthermore, multimodality imaging may be improved by the combination of PET or SPECT imaging with MRI. Cardiac MR can be used to evaluate ventricular structure and function, which is important for management decisions to prevent further cardiac injury. For example, in patients with a drop in systolic function at standard surveillance imaging with/without symptoms, the use of cardiac MR is considered an appropriate next step for further evaluation due to accuracy and reproducibility of measurement of function and volumes [327]. The great advantage of MR in terms of differentiate soft-tissue boundaries [328] and of the addition of a molecular MR agent to trace two biological targets simultaneously [329] would impact significantly in research on cardiotoxicity. Particularly, the combination of the different PET radiopharmaceuticals to MRI imaging could significantly improve the sensitivity in the early diagnosis and monitoring of chemotherapy- and RT-induced cardiac toxicity.

Preliminary results in cardiac PET/MR imaging, despite being limited to a few centers and only to specific clinical applications (i.e., perfusion, viability, atherosclerosis, myocarditis, sarcoidosis, and amyloidosis), support the advantages of PET/MR as compared to other hybrid techniques [330] not only in terms of more accurate assessment and better anatomical localization of lesions in soft tissues. In fact, MR offers the opportunity to gather functional MRI (fMRI), which includes diffusion-weighted imaging (DWI), magnetic resonance spectroscopy (MRS), and perfusion imaging, eventually providing significant advantages in understanding the basis of cardiotoxic related myocardial injury.

REFERENCES

[1] Yeh ETH, Bickford CL. Cardiovascular complications of cancer therapy: incidence, pathogenesis, diagnosis, and management. J Am Coll Cardiol 2009;53:2231–47. [cited 2015 Aug 17] Available from: http://www.ncbi.nlm.nih.gov/pubmed/19520246.

[2] Curigliano G, Mayer EL, Burstein HJ, Winer EP, Goldhirsch A. Cardiac toxicity from systemic cancer therapy: a comprehensive review. Prog Cardiovasc Dis 2010;53:94–104. [cited 2015 Aug 17] Available from: http://www.ncbi.nlm.nih.gov/pubmed/20728696.

[3] Lancellotti P, Nkomo VT, Badano LP, Bergler-Klein J, Bergler J, Bogaert J, et al. Expert consensus for multi-modality imaging evaluation of cardiovascular complications of radiotherapy in adults: a report from the European Association of Cardiovascular Imaging and the American Society of Echocardiography. J Am Soc Echocardiogr 2013;26:1013–32. [cited 2015 Aug 17] Available from: http://www.ncbi.nlm.nih.gov/pubmed/23998694.

[4] Hendel RC, Patel MR, Kramer CM, Poon M, Carr JC, Gerstad NA, et al. ACCF/ACR/SCCT/SCMR/ASNC/NASCI/SCAI/SIR 2006 appropriateness criteria for cardiac computed tomography and cardiac magnetic resonance imaging: a report of the American College of Cardiology Foundation Quality Strategic Directions Committee Appropriateness C. J Am Coll Cardiol 2006;48:1475–97. [cited 2015 Aug 18] Available from: http://www.ncbi.nlm.nih.gov/pubmed/17010819.

[5] Martín M, Esteva FJ, Alba E, Khandheria B, Pérez-Isla L, García-Sáenz JA, et al. Minimizing cardiotoxicity while optimizing treatment efficacy with trastuzumab: review and expert recommendations. Oncologist 2009;14:1–11. [cited 2015 Aug 18] Available from: http://www.ncbi.nlm.nih.gov/pubmed/19147689.

[6] Bovelli D, Plataniotis G, Roila F. Cardiotoxicity of chemotherapeutic agents and radiotherapy-related heart disease: ESMO Clinical Practice Guidelines. Ann Oncol 2010;21(Suppl. 5):v277–82. [cited 2015 Aug 18] Available from: http://www.ncbi.nlm.nih.gov/pubmed/20555097.

[7] Chanan-Khan A, Srinivasan S, Czuczman MS. Prevention and management of cardiotoxicity from antineoplastic therapy. J Support Oncol 2004;2:251–6. discussion 259–261, 264–266. [cited 2015 Aug 18] Available from: http://www.ncbi.nlm.nih.gov/pubmed/15328825.

[8] Steinherz LJ, Graham T, Hurwitz R, Sondheimer HM, Schwartz RG, Shaffer EM, et al. Guidelines for cardiac monitoring of children during and after anthracycline therapy: report of the Cardiology Committee of the Childrens Cancer Study Group. Pediatrics 1992;89:942–9. [cited 2015 Aug 18] Available from: http://www.ncbi.nlm.nih.gov/pubmed/1579408.

[9] Hunt SA. ACC/AHA 2005 guideline update for the diagnosis and management of chronic heart failure in the adult: a report of the American College of Cardiology/American Heart Association Task Force on Practice Guidelines (Writing Committee to Update the 2001 Guideli). J Am Coll Cardiol. 2005;46:e1–82. [cited 2015 Aug 18] Available from: http://www.ncbi.nlm.nih.gov/pubmed/16168273.

[10] Jones AL, Barlow M, Barrett-Lee PJ, Canney PA, Gilmour IM, Robb SD, et al. Management of cardiac health in trastuzumab-treated patients with breast cancer: updated United Kingdom National Cancer Research Institute recommendations for monitoring. Br J Cancer 2009;100:684–92. [cited 2015 Jun 5] Available from: http://www.pubmedcentral.nih.gov/articlerender.fcgi?artid=2653760&tool=pmcentrez&rendertype=abstract.

[11] Mason JW, Bristow MR, Billingham ME, Daniels JR. Invasive and noninvasive methods of assessing adriamycin cardiotoxic effects in man: superiority of histopathologic assessment using endomyocardial biopsy. Cancer Treat Rep. 1978;62:857–64. [cited 2015 Aug 18] Available from: http://www.ncbi.nlm.nih.gov/pubmed/667859.

[12] Seidman A, Hudis C, Pierri MK, Shak S, Paton V, Ashby M, et al. Cardiac dysfunction in the trastuzumab clinical trials experience. J Clin Oncol 2002;20:1215–21. [cited 2015 Aug 1] Available from: http://www.ncbi.nlm.nih.gov/pubmed/11870163.

[13] D'Amore C, Gargiulo P, Paolillo S, Pellegrino AM, Formisano T, Mariniello A, et al. Nuclear imaging in detection and monitoring of cardiotoxicity. World J Radiol 2014;6:486–92. [cited 2015 Aug 18] Available from: http://www.pubmedcentral.nih.gov/articlerender.fcgi?artid=4109100&tool=pmcentrez&rendertype=abstract.

[14] Hesse B, Lindhardt TB, Acampa W, Anagnostopoulos C, Ballinger J, Bax JJ, et al. EANM/ESC guidelines for radionuclide imaging of cardiac function. Eur J Nucl Med Mol Imaging 2008;35:851–85. [cited 2015 Aug 18] Available from: http://www.ncbi.nlm.nih.gov/pubmed/18224320.

[15] Nichols K, DePuey EG, Gooneratne N, Salensky H, Friedman M, Cochoff S. First-pass ventricular ejection fraction using a single-crystal nuclear camera. J Nucl Med 1994;35:1292–300. [cited 2015 Aug 18] Available from: http://www.ncbi.nlm.nih.gov/pubmed/8046481.

[16] Marving J, Høilund-Carlsen PF, Chraemmer-Jørgensen B, Gadsbøll N. Are right and left ventricular ejection fractions equal? Ejection fractions in normal subjects and in patients with first acute myocardial infarction. Circulation 1985;72:502–14. [cited 2015 Aug 18] Available from: http://www.ncbi.nlm.nih.gov/pubmed/4017205.

[17] Friedman JD, Berman DS, Borges-Neto S, Hayes SW, Johnson LL, Nichols KJ, et al. First-pass radionuclide angiography. J Nucl Cardiol 2006;13:e42–55. [cited 2015 Aug 18] Available from: http://www.ncbi.nlm.nih.gov/pubmed/17174796.

[18] Maurer AH, Urbain JL, Krevsky B, Knight LC, Revesz G, Brown K. Effects of in vitro versus in vivo red cell labeling on image quality in gastrointestinal bleeding studies. J Nucl Med Technol 1998;26:87–90. [cited 2015 Aug 18] Available from: http://www.ncbi.nlm.nih.gov/pubmed/9604828.

[19] Patrick ST, Glowniak JV, Turner FE, Robbins MS, Wolfangel RG. Comparison of in vitro RBC labeling with the UltraTag RBC kit versus in vivo labeling. J Nucl Med 1991;32:242–4. [cited 2015 Aug 18] Available from: http://www.ncbi.nlm.nih.gov/pubmed/1992026.

[20] Ponto JA. Salvage of substandard in vitro technetium Tc-99m-labeled red blood cells. J Am Pharm Assoc 2003;46:401–2. [cited 2015 Aug 18] Available from: http://www.ncbi.nlm.nih.gov/pubmed/16739764.

[21] Callahan RJ, Froelich JW, McKusick KA, Leppo J, Strauss HW. A modified method for the in vivo labeling of red blood cells with Tc-99m: concise communication. J Nucl Med 1982;23:315–18. [cited 2015 Aug 18] Available from: http://www.ncbi.nlm.nih.gov/pubmed/6279801.

[22] Kuehne R, Reuter E. High RBC labeling efficiency by controlling pretinning with the modified in vivo/in vitro labeling method. J Nucl Med Technol 1999;27:222–6. [cited 2015 Aug 18] Available from: http://www.ncbi.nlm.nih.gov/pubmed/10512479.

[23] Calculation of the administered activity in [MBq] and [mCi]. European Association of Nuclear Medicine. http://www.eanm.org/publications/dosage_calculator.php?navId5285; [cited 2015 Aug 18]. Available from: http://www.eanm.org/publications/dosage_calculator.php?navId = 285.

[24] Lassmann M, Treves ST. Paediatric radiopharmaceutical administration: harmonization of the 2007 EANM paediatric dosage card (version 1.5.2008) and the 2010 North American consensus guidelines. Eur J Nucl Med Mol Imaging 2014;41:1036–41. [cited 2015 Aug 18] Available from: http://www.ncbi.nlm.nih.gov/pubmed/24599377.

[25] Vasculocis, Summary of product characteristics. CIS Biointernational. Available from: http://www.ibamolecular.eu/sites/default/files/TL-201-S-1SPC.pdf.

[26] Mps S. Technescan HSA, Summary of product characteristics. Mallinckrodt; 2000.

[27] International Atomic Energy Agency. Applying radiation safety standards in nuclear medicine no. 40. IAEA safety related publications. Appendix VI: guidance levels for diagnostic procedures. Vienna: IAEA; 2005.

[28] Wackers FJTh, Bruni W, Zaret BL. Nuclear Cardiology: The Basics. How to Set Up and Maintain a Laboratory, 2nd ed. Contemporary Cardiology series. Humana Press: Totowa, NJ. 2003.

[29] Hecht HS, Josephson MA, Hopkins JM, Singh BN. Reproducibility of equilibrium radionuclide ventriculography in patients with coronary artery disease: response of left ventricular ejection fraction and regional wall motion to supine bicycle exercise. Am Heart J 1982;104:567–74. [cited 2015 Aug 18] Available from: http://www.ncbi.nlm.nih.gov/pubmed/7113897.

[30] Schwartz RG, McKenzie WB, Alexander J, Sager P, D'Souza A, Manatunga A, et al. Congestive heart failure and left ventricular dysfunction complicating doxorubicin therapy. Seven-year experience using serial radionuclide angiocardiography. Am J Med 1987;82:1109–18. [cited 2015 Aug 1] Available from: http://www.ncbi.nlm.nih.gov/pubmed/3605130.

[31] Mitani I, Jain D, Joska TM, Burtness B, Zaret BL. Doxorubicin cardiotoxicity: prevention of congestive heart failure with serial cardiac function monitoring with equilibrium

radionuclide angiocardiography in the current era. J Nucl Cardiol 2003;10:132–9. [cited 2015 Aug 18] Available from: http://www.ncbi.nlm.nih.gov/pubmed/12673177.

[32] Ewer MS, Ali MK, Mackay B, Wallace S, Valdivieso M, Legha SS, et al. A comparison of cardiac biopsy grades and ejection fraction estimations in patients receiving Adriamycin. J Clin Oncol 1984;2:112–17. [cited 2015 Aug 18] Available from: http://www.ncbi.nlm.nih.gov/pubmed/6699662.

[33] Gottdiener JS, Mathisen DJ, Borer JS, Bonow RO, Myers CE, Barr LH, et al. Doxorubicin cardiotoxicity: assessment of late left ventricular dysfunction by radionuclide cineangiography. Ann Intern Med 1981;94:430–5. [cited 2015 Aug 18] Available from: http://www.ncbi.nlm.nih.gov/pubmed/7212498.

[34] McKillop JH, Bristow MR, Goris ML, Billingham ME, Bockemuehl K. Sensitivity and specificity of radionuclide ejection fractions in doxorubicin cardiotoxicity. Am Heart J 1983;106:1048–56. [cited 2015 Aug 18] Available from: http://www.ncbi.nlm.nih.gov/pubmed/6637763.

[35] Muntinga HJ, van den Berg F, Knol HR, Niemeyer MG, Blanksma PK, Louwes H, et al. Normal values and reproducibility of left ventricular filling parameters by radionuclide angiography. Int J Card Imaging 1997;13:165–71. discussion 173 [cited 2015 Aug 18] Available from: http://www.ncbi.nlm.nih.gov/pubmed/9110196.

[36] Kusuoka H, Futaki S, Koretsune Y, Kitabatake A, Suga H, Kamada T, et al. Alterations of intracellular calcium homeostasis and myocardial energetics in acute adriamycin-induced heart failure. J Cardiovasc Pharmacol 1991;18:437–44. [cited 2015 Aug 18] Available from: http://www.ncbi.nlm.nih.gov/pubmed/1720844.

[37] Pelikan PC, Weisfeldt ML, Jacobus WE, Miceli MV, Bulkley BH, Gerstenblith G. Acute doxorubicin cardiotoxicity: functional, metabolic, and morphologic alterations in the isolated, perfused rat heart. J Cardiovasc Pharmacol 1986;8:1058–66. [cited 2015 Aug 18] Available from: http://www.ncbi.nlm.nih.gov/pubmed/2429080.

[38] Cottin Y, Touzery C, Coudert B, Gilles A, Walker P, Massing JL, et al. Impairment of diastolic function during short-term anthracycline chemotherapy. Br Heart J 1995;73:61–4. [cited 2015 Aug 18] Available from: http://www.pubmedcentral.nih.gov/articlerender.fcgi?artid=483757&tool=pmcentrez&rendertype=abstract.

[39] Lapińska G, Kozłowicz-Gudzińska I, Sackiewicz-Słaby A. Equilibrium radionuclide ventriculography in the assessment of cardiotoxicity of chemotherapy and chemoradiotherapy in patients with breast cancer. Nucl Med Rev Cent East Eur 2012;15:26–30. [cited 2015 Aug 18] Available from: http://www.ncbi.nlm.nih.gov/pubmed/23047570.

[40] Nousiainen T, Jantunen E, Vanninen E, Hartikainen J. Early decline in left ventricular ejection fraction predicts doxorubicin cardiotoxicity in lymphoma patients. Br J Cancer 2002;86:1697–700. [cited 2015 Aug 18] Available from: http://www.pubmedcentral.nih.gov/articlerender.fcgi?artid=2375393&tool=pmcentrez&rendertype=abstract.

[41] Swain SM, Whaley FS, Ewer MS. Congestive heart failure in patients treated with doxorubicin: a retrospective analysis of three trials. Cancer 2003;97:2869–79. [cited 2015 Aug 18] Available from: http://www.ncbi.nlm.nih.gov/pubmed/12767102.

[42] Fatima N, Zaman MU, Hashmi A, Kamal S, Hameed A. Assessing adriamycin-induced early cardiotoxicity by estimating left ventricular ejection fraction using technetium-99m multiple-gated acquisition scan and echocardiography. Nucl Med Commun 2011;32:381–5. [cited 2015 Aug 20] Available from: http://www.ncbi.nlm.nih.gov/pubmed/21346663.

[43] Skovgaard D, Hasbak P, Kjaer A, D'Amore C, Gargiulo P, Paolillo S, et al. BNP predicts chemotherapy-related cardiotoxicity and death: comparison with gated equilibrium radionuclide ventriculography. World J Radiol 2014;6:486–92. [cited 2015 Aug 18] Available from: http://dx.doi.org/10.1016/j.nucmedbio.2014.08.006.

[44] Tantawy AAG, Elmasry OA, Shaaban M, Toaima DN, El Shahat AM. Radionuclide ventriculography detects early anthracycline cardiotoxicity in children with Hodgkin lymphoma. J Pediatr Hematol Oncol 2011;33:e132–7. [cited 2015 Aug 18] Available from: http://www.ncbi.nlm.nih.gov/pubmed/21516011.

[45] Aapro MS, Alberts DS, Woolfenden JM, Mackel C. Prospective study of left ventricular function using radionuclide scans in patients receiving mitoxantrone. Invest New Drugs 1983;1:341–7. [cited 2015 Aug 25] Available from: http://www.ncbi.nlm.nih.gov/pubmed/6678882.

[46] Abu-Khalaf MM, Juneja V, Chung GG, DiGiovanna MP, Sipples R, McGurk M, et al. Long-term assessment of cardiac function after dose-dense and -intense sequential doxorubicin (A), paclitaxel (T), and cyclophosphamide (C) as adjuvant therapy for high risk breast cancer. Breast Cancer Res Treat 2007;104:341–9. [cited 2015 Aug 25] Available from: http://www.ncbi.nlm.nih.gov/pubmed/17051423.

[47] Agarwala S, Kumar R, Bhatnagar V, Bajpai M, Gupta DK, Mitra DK. High incidence of adriamycin cardiotoxicity in children even at low cumulative doses: role of radionuclide cardiac angiography. J Pediatr Surg 2000;35:1786–9. [cited 2015 Aug 20] Available from: http://www.ncbi.nlm.nih.gov/pubmed/11101737.

[48] Alcan KE, Robeson W, Graham MC, Palestro C, Oliver FH, Benua RS. Early detection of anthracycline-induced cardiotoxicity by stress radionuclide cineangiography in conjunction with Fourier amplitude and phase analysis. Clin Nucl Med 1985;10:160–6. [cited 2015 Aug 25] Available from: http://www.ncbi.nlm.nih.gov/pubmed/2985319.

[49] Alexander J, Dainiak N, Berger HJ, Goldman L, Johnstone D, Reduto L, et al. Serial assessment of doxorubicin cardiotoxicity with quantitative radionuclide angiocardiography. N Engl J Med 1979;300:278–83. [cited 2015 Aug 25] Available from: http://www.ncbi.nlm.nih.gov/pubmed/759880.

[50] Appel JM, Zerahn B, Møller S, Christensen HM, Søgaard P, Ejlertsen B, et al. Long-term heart function after adjuvant epirubicin chemotherapy for breast cancer. Acta Oncol 1990;51:1054–61. [cited 2015 Aug 22] Available from: http://www.ncbi.nlm.nih.gov/pubmed/22909389.

[51] Barendswaard EC, Prpic H, Van der Wall EE, Camps JA, Keizer HJ, Pauwels EK. Right ventricle wall motion abnormalities in patients treated with chemotherapy. Clin Nucl Med 1991;16:513–16. [cited 2015 Aug 22] Available from: http://www.ncbi.nlm.nih.gov/pubmed/1934797.

[52] Basar EZ, Corapcioglu F, Babaoglu K, Anik Y, Gorur Daglioz G, Dedeoglu R. Are cardiac magnetic resonance imaging and radionuclide ventriculography good options against echocardiography for evaluation of anthracycline induced chronic cardiotoxicity in childhood cancer survivors? Pediatr Hematol 2014;31:237–52. [cited 2015 Aug 25] Available from: http://www.ncbi.nlm.nih.gov/pubmed/24499452.

[53] Carrió I, Lopez-Pousa A, Estorch M, Duncker D, Berná L, Torres G, et al. Detection of doxorubicin cardiotoxicity in patients with sarcomas by indium-111-antimyosin monoclonal antibody studies. J Nucl Med 1993;34:1503–7. [cited 2015 Aug 22] Available from: http://www.ncbi.nlm.nih.gov/pubmed/8355070.

[54] Carrió I, Estorch M, Berná L, López-Pousa J, Tabernero J, Torres G. Indium-111-antimyosin and iodine-123-MIBG studies in early assessment of doxorubicin cardiotoxicity. J Nucl Med 1995;36:2044–9. [cited 2015 Aug 22] Available from: http://www.ncbi.nlm.nih.gov/pubmed/7472595.

[55] Cassidy J, Merrick MV, Smyth JF, Leonard RC. Cardiotoxicity of mitoxantrone assessed by stress and resting nuclear ventriculography. Eur J Cancer Clin Oncol 1988;24:935–8. [cited 2015 Aug 22] Available from: http://www.ncbi.nlm.nih.gov/pubmed/3169098.

[56] Choi BW, Berger HJ, Schwartz PE, Alexander J, Wackers FJ, Gottschalk A, et al. Serial radionuclide assessment of doxorubicin cardiotoxicity in cancer patients with abnormal baseline resting left ventricular performance. Am Heart J 1983;106:638–43. [cited 2015 Aug 25] Available from: http://www.ncbi.nlm.nih.gov/pubmed/6613807.

[57] Cochet A, Quilichini G, Dygai-Cochet I, Touzery C, Toubeau M, Berriolo-Riedinger A, et al. Baseline diastolic dysfunction as a predictive factor of trastuzumab-mediated cardiotoxicity after adjuvant anthracycline therapy in breast cancer. Breast Cancer Res Treat 2011;130:845–54. [cited 2015 Aug 25] Available from: http://www.ncbi.nlm.nih.gov/pubmed/21918836.

[58] Coleman RE, Maisey MN, Knight RK, Rubens RD. Mitoxantrone in advanced breast cancer—a phase II study with special attention to cardiotoxicity. Eur J Cancer Clin Oncol 1984;20:771–6. [cited 2015 Aug 25] Available from: http://www.ncbi.nlm.nih.gov/pubmed/6540179.

[59] Constine LS, Schwartz RG, Savage DE, King V, Muhs A. Cardiac function, perfusion, and morbidity in irradiated long-term survivors of Hodgkin's disease. Int J Radiat Oncol Biol Phys 1997;39:897–906. [cited 2015 Aug 23] Available from: http://www.ncbi.nlm.nih.gov/pubmed/9369139.

[60] Cottin Y, Touzery C, Dalloz F, Coudert B, Toubeau M, Riedinger A, et al. Comparison of epirubicin and doxorubicin cardiotoxicity induced by low doses: evolution of the diastolic and systolic parameters studied by radionuclide angiography. Clin Cardiol 1998;21:665–70. [cited 2015 Aug 22] Available from: http://www.ncbi.nlm.nih.gov/pubmed/9755384.

[61] De Bree E, van Ruth S, Schotborgh CE, Baas P, Zoetmulder FAN. Limited cardiotoxicity after extensive thoracic surgery and intraoperative hyperthermic intrathoracic chemotherapy with doxorubicin and cisplatin. Ann Surg Oncol 2007;14:3019–26. [cited 2015 Aug 22] Available from: http://www.ncbi.nlm.nih.gov/pubmed/17638057.

[62] De Leonardis V, Bartalucci S, Cinelli P, De Scalzi M, Becucci A, Lottini G, et al. Ventricular late potentials in the assessment of mitoxantrone cardiotoxicity. Cardiology 1991;79:110–15. [cited 2015 Aug 25] Available from: http://www.ncbi.nlm.nih.gov/pubmed/1933962.

[63] Dresdale A, Bonow RO, Wesley R, Palmeri ST, Barr L, Mathison D, et al. Prospective evaluation of doxorubicin-induced cardiomyopathy resulting from postsurgical adjuvant treatment of patients with soft tissue sarcomas. Cancer 1983;52:51–60. [cited 2015 Aug 25] Available from: http://www.ncbi.nlm.nih.gov/pubmed/6850545.

[64] Druck MN, Gulenchyn KY, Evans WK, Gotlieb A, Srigley JR, Bar-Shlomo BZ, et al. Radionuclide angiography and endomyocardial biopsy in the assessment of doxorubicin cardiotoxicity. Cancer 1984;53:1667–74. [cited 2015 Aug 25] Available from: http://www.ncbi.nlm.nih.gov/pubmed/6697304.

[65] Duan H, Liang C, Deng H. [99mTc-MIBI myocardial perfusion tomography for monitoring the anthracycline cardiotoxicity]. Hunan Yi Ke Da Xue Xue Bao 2003;28:167–70. [cited 2015 Aug 20] Available from: http://www.ncbi.nlm.nih.gov/pubmed/12934369.

[66] Eising EG, Gries P, Eggert J, Scheulen ME. Does the multidrug-resistance modulator cyclosporin A increase the cardiotoxicity of high-dose anthracycline chemotherapy? Acta Oncol 1997;36:735–40. [cited 2015 Aug 22] Available from: http://www.ncbi.nlm.nih.gov/pubmed/9490093.

[67] Estabragh ZR, Knight K, Watmough SJ, Lane S, Vinjamuri S, Hart G, et al. A prospective evaluation of cardiac function in patients with chronic myeloid leukaemia treated with imatinib. Leuk Res 2011;35:49–51. [cited 2015 Aug 23] Available from: http://www.ncbi.nlm.nih.gov/pubmed/21030079.

[68] Ettinghausen SE, Bonow RO, Palmeri ST, Seipp CA, Steinberg SM, White DE, et al. Prospective study of cardiomyopathy induced by adjuvant doxorubicin therapy in patients with soft-tissue sarcomas. Arch Surg 1986;121:1445–51. [cited 2015 Aug 25] Available from: http://www.ncbi.nlm.nih.gov/pubmed/3789915.

[69] Feola M, Garrone O, Occelli M, Francini A, Biggi A, Visconti G, et al. Cardiotoxicity after anthracycline chemotherapy in breast carcinoma: effects on left ventricular ejection fraction, troponin I and brain natriuretic peptide. Int J Cardiol 2011;148:194–8. [cited 2015 Aug 22] Available from: http://www.ncbi.nlm.nih.gov/pubmed/19945181.

[70] Geidel S, Garn M, Grävinghoff L, Hausdorf G, Morf G, Bielack S, et al. [Cardiomyopathy after osteosarcoma treatment: a contribution to the cardiotoxicity of adriamycin]. Klin Padiatr 1991;203:257–61. [cited 2015 Aug 25] Available from: http://www.ncbi.nlm.nih.gov/pubmed/?term=Cardiomyopathy+after+osteosarcoma+treatment%3A+a+contribution+to+the+cardiotoxicity+of+adriamycin.

[71] Gill SE, Savage K, Wysham WZ, Blackhurst DW, Winter WE, Puls LE. Continuing routine cardiac surveillance in long-term use of pegylated liposomal doxorubicin: is it necessary?. Gynecol Oncol 2013;129:544–7. [cited 2015 Aug 23] Available from: http://www.ncbi.nlm.nih.gov/pubmed/23523653.

[72] Goffette S, van Pesch V, Vanoverschelde JL, Morandini E, Sindic CJM. Severe delayed heart failure in three multiple sclerosis patients previously treated with mitoxantrone. J Neurol 2005;252:1217–22. [cited 2015 Aug 23] Available from: http://www.ncbi.nlm.nih.gov/pubmed/15834643.

[73] Haas NB, Manola J, Ky B, Flaherty KT, Uzzo RG, Kane CJ, et al. Effects of Adjuvant Sorafenib and Sunitinib on Cardiac Function in Renal Cell Carcinoma Patients without Overt Metastases: results from ASSURE, ECOG 2805. Clin Cancer Res 2015; [cited 2015 Aug 25]; Available from: http://www.ncbi.nlm.nih.gov/pubmed/25967143.

[74] Harris L, Batist G, Belt R, Rovira D, Navari R, Azarnia N, et al. Liposome-encapsulated doxorubicin compared with conventional doxorubicin in a randomized multicenter trial as first-line therapy of metastatic breast carcinoma. Cancer 2002;94:25–36. [cited 2015 Aug 25] Available from: http://www.ncbi.nlm.nih.gov/pubmed/11815957.

[75] Hofheinz R-D, Porta C, Hartung G, Santoro A, Hanauske A-R, Kutz K, et al. BBR 3438, a novel 9-aza-anthrapyrazole, in patients with advanced gastric cancer: a phase II study group trial of the central European Society of Anticancer-Drug Research (CESAR). Invest New Drugs 2005;23:363–8. [cited 2015 Aug 25] Available from: http://www.ncbi.nlm.nih.gov/pubmed/16012796.

[76] Jain KK, Casper ES, Geller NL, Hakes TB, Kaufman RJ, Currie V, et al. A prospective randomized comparison of epirubicin and doxorubicin in patients with advanced breast cancer. J Clin Oncol 1985;3:818–26. [cited 2015 Aug 3] Available from: http://www.ncbi.nlm.nih.gov/pubmed/3859587.

[77] Jensen SA, Hasbak P, Mortensen J, Sørensen JB. Fluorouracil induces myocardial ischemia with increases of plasma brain natriuretic peptide and lactic acid but without

dysfunction of left ventricle. J Clin Oncol 2010;28:5280–6. [cited 2015 Aug 22] Available from: http://www.ncbi.nlm.nih.gov/pubmed/21079148.

[78] Kingwell E, Koch M, Leung B, Isserow S, Geddes J, Rieckmann P, et al. Cardiotoxicity and other adverse events associated with mitoxantrone treatment for MS. Neurology 2010;74:1822–6. [cited 2015 Aug 23] Available from: http://www.pubmedcentral.nih.gov/articlerender.fcgi?artid=2882218&tool=pmcentrez&rendertype=abstract.

[79] Knesewitsch P, Göldel NH, Fritsch S, Moser E. Evaluation of adriamycin cardiotoxicity using equilibrium radionuclide ventriculography. I. Results at rest. Nuklearmedizin 1987;26:206–11. [cited 2015 Aug 25] Available from: http://www.ncbi.nlm.nih.gov/pubmed/3432064.

[80] Knesewitsch P, Göldel NH, Fritsch S, Moser E. Evaluation of adriamycin cardiotoxicity using equilibrium radionuclide ventriculography. II. Results during exercise. Nuklearmedizin 1987;26:212–19. [cited 2015 Aug 25] Available from: http://www.ncbi.nlm.nih.gov/pubmed/3432065.

[81] Lahtinen R, Kuikka J, Nousiainen T, Uusitupa M, Länsimies E. Cardiotoxicity of epirubicin and doxorubicin: a double-blind randomized study. Eur J Haematol 1991;46:301–5. [cited 2015 Aug 25] Available from: http://www.ncbi.nlm.nih.gov/pubmed/2044726.

[82] Landys K, Borgstrom S, Andersson T, Noppa H. Mitoxantrone as a first-line treatment of advanced breast cancer. Invest New Drugs 1985;3:133–7. [cited 2015 Aug 25] Available from: http://www.ncbi.nlm.nih.gov/pubmed/4019117.

[83] Lee BH, Goodenday LS, Muswick GJ, Yasnoff WA, Leighton RF, Skeel RT. Alterations in left ventricular diastolic function with doxorubicin therapy. J Am Coll Cardiol 1987;9:184–8. [cited 2015 Aug 25] Available from: http://www.ncbi.nlm.nih.gov/pubmed/3794095.

[84] Lekakis J, Prassopoulos V, Athanassiadis P, Kostamis P, Moulopoulos S. Doxorubicin-induced cardiac neurotoxicity: study with iodine 123-labeled metaiodobenzylguanidine scintigraphy. J Nucl Cardiol 1996;3:37–41. [cited 2015 Aug 25] Available from: http://www.ncbi.nlm.nih.gov/pubmed/8799226.

[85] Lopez M, Vici P, Di Lauro K, Conti F, Paoletti G, Ferraironi A, et al. Randomized prospective clinical trial of high-dose epirubicin and dexrazoxane in patients with advanced breast cancer and soft tissue sarcomas. J Clin Oncol 1998;16:86–92. [cited 2015 Aug 22] Available from: http://www.ncbi.nlm.nih.gov/pubmed/9440727.

[86] Lu CY, Srasuebkul P, Drew AK, Ward RL, Pearson S-A. Positive spillover effects of prescribing requirements: increased cardiac testing in patients treated with trastuzumab for HER2+ metastatic breast cancer. Intern Med J 2012;42:1229–35. [cited 2015 Aug 23] Available from: http://www.ncbi.nlm.nih.gov/pubmed/21981464.

[87] Luk WH, Au-Yeung AWS, Lo AXN, Loke TKL, Ng TW. Comparing left ventricular ejection fraction measurement using cardiovascular magnetic resonance imaging. Radiol Technol 2014;85:494–9. [cited 2015 Aug 18] Available from: http://www.ncbi.nlm.nih.gov/pubmed/24806052.

[88] Maini CL, Sciuto R, Ferraironi A, Vici P, Tofani A, Festa A, et al. Clinical relevance of radionuclide angiography and antimyosin immunoscintigraphy for risk assessment in epirubicin cardiotoxicity. J Nucl Cardiol 1997;4:502–8. [cited 2015 Aug 22] Available from: http://www.ncbi.nlm.nih.gov/pubmed/9456190.

[89] Morgan GW, McIlveen BM, Freedman A, Murray IP. Radionuclide ejection fraction in doxorubicin cardiotoxicity. Cancer Treat Rep 1981;65:629–38. [cited 2015 Aug 25] Available from: http://www.ncbi.nlm.nih.gov/pubmed/7248982.

[90] Morgan GW, Freeman AP, McLean RG, Jarvie BH, Giles RW. Late cardiac, thyroid, and pulmonary sequelae of mantle radiotherapy for Hodgkin's disease. Int J Radiat Oncol Biol Phys 1985;11:1925–31. [cited 2015 Aug 24] Available from: http://www.ncbi.nlm.nih.gov/pubmed/3932270.

[91] Neri B, Pacini P, Bartolucci S, Moroni F, Menchi I, Cappellini MC. Epirubicin high-dose therapy in advanced breast cancer: preliminary clinical data. Epirubicin as a single agent in breast cancer. Int J Clin Pharmacol Ther Toxicol 1989;27:388–91. [cited 2015 Aug 25] Available from: http://www.ncbi.nlm.nih.gov/pubmed/?term=Epirubicin+high-dose+therapy+in+advanced+breast+cancer%3A+preliminary+clinical+data.+Epirubicin+as+a+single+agent+in+breast+cancer.

[92] Neri B, De Scalzi M, De Leonardis V, Gemelli MT, Ghezzi P, Pacini P. Preliminary study on behaviour of atrial natriuretic factor in anthracycline-related cardiac toxicity. Int J Clin Pharmacol Res 1991;11:75–81. [cited 2015 Aug 20] Available from: http://www.ncbi.nlm.nih.gov/pubmed/1831809.

[93] Nony P, Guastalla JP, Rebattu P, Landais P, Lievre M, Bontemps L, et al. In vivo measurement of myocardial oxidative metabolism and blood flow does not show changes in cancer patients undergoing doxorubicin therapy. Cancer Chemother Pharmacol 2000;45:375–80. [cited 2015 Aug 25] Available from: http://www.ncbi.nlm.nih.gov/pubmed/10803920.

[94] Nousiainen T, Vanninen E, Jantunen E, Remes J, Ritanen E, Vuolteenaho O, et al. Neuroendocrine changes during the evolution of doxorubicin-induced left ventricular dysfunction in adult lymphoma patients. Clin Sci (Lond) 2001;101:601–7. [cited 2015 Aug 22] Available from: http://www.ncbi.nlm.nih.gov/pubmed/11724646.

[95] Parmentier S, Melin JA, Piret L, Beckers C. Assessment of left ventricular diastolic function in patients receiving anthracycline therapy. Eur J Nucl Med 1988;13:563–7. [cited 2015 Aug 20] Available from: http://www.ncbi.nlm.nih.gov/pubmed/3162416.

[96] Pauwels EK, Horning SJ, Goris ML. Sequential equilibrium gated radionuclide angiocardiography for the detection of doxorubicin cardiotoxicity. Radiother Oncol 1983;1:83–7. [cited 2015 Aug 25] Available from: http://www.ncbi.nlm.nih.gov/pubmed/6095370.

[97] Pichon MF, Cvitkovic F, Hacene K, Delaunay J, Lokiec F, Collignon MA, et al. Drug-induced cardiotoxicity studied by longitudinal B-type natriuretic peptide assays and radionuclide ventriculography. In Vivo 2005;19:567–76. [cited 2015 Aug 25] Available from: http://www.ncbi.nlm.nih.gov/pubmed/15875778.

[98] Pihkala J, Saarinen UM, Lundström U, Virtanen K, Virkola K, Siimes MA, et al. Myocardial function in children and adolescents after therapy with anthracyclines and chest irradiation. Eur J Cancer 1996;32A:97–103. [cited 2015 Aug 22] Available from: http://www.ncbi.nlm.nih.gov/pubmed/8695252.

[99] Piver MS, Marchetti DL, Parthasarathy KL, Bakshi S, Reese P. Doxorubicin hydrochloride (Adriamycin) cardiotoxicity evaluated by sequential radionuclide angiocardiography. Cancer 1985;56:76–80. [cited 2015 Aug 25] Available from: http://www.ncbi.nlm.nih.gov/pubmed/2988739.

[100] Rabinovitch M, Suissa S, Stern J, Adam J, Mettauer B, Boileau G, et al. Prediction of the left ventricular ejection fraction response to doxorubicin using a multiple linear regression model. Can J Cardiol 1989;5:382–8. [cited 2015 Aug 22] Available from: http://www.ncbi.nlm.nih.gov/pubmed/2605548.

[101] Reuvekamp EJ, Bulten BF, Nieuwenhuis AA, Meekes MRA, de Haan AFJ, Tol J, et al. Does diastolic dysfunction precede systolic dysfunction in trastuzumab-induced

cardiotoxicity? Assessment with multigated radionuclide angiography (MUGA). J Nucl Cardiol 2015; [cited 2015 Aug 23] Available from: http://www.ncbi.nlm.nih.gov/pubmed/26048264.

[102] Ritchie JL, Singer JW, Thorning D, Sorensen SG, Hamilton GW. Anthracycline cardiotoxicity: clinical and pathologic outcomes assessed by radionuclide ejection fraction. Cancer 1980;46:1109–16. [cited 2015 Aug 25] Available from: http://www.ncbi.nlm.nih.gov/pubmed/6938301.

[103] Robinson BA, Colls BM, Turner JG. Adriamycin cardiotoxicity monitoring by radionuclide scan. Br J Cancer 1983;48:315–17. [cited 2015 Aug 25] Available from: http://www.pubmedcentral.nih.gov/articlerender.fcgi?artid=2011444&tool=pmcentrez&rendertype=abstract.

[104] Rohde LE, Belló-Klein A, Pereira RP, Mazzotti NG, Geib G, Weber C, et al. Superoxide dismutase activity in adriamycin-induced cardiotoxicity in humans: a potential novel tool for risk stratification. J Card Fail 2005;11:220–6. [cited 2015 Aug 20] Available from: http://www.ncbi.nlm.nih.gov/pubmed/15812751.

[105] Rohde LE, Baldi A, Weber C, Geib G, Mazzotti NG, Fiorentini M, et al. Tei index in adult patients submitted to adriamycin chemotherapy: failure to predict early systolic dysfunction. Diagnosis of adriamycin cardiotoxicity. Int J Cardiovasc Imaging 2007;23:185–91. [cited 2015 Aug 20] Available from: http://www.ncbi.nlm.nih.gov/pubmed/16972144.

[106] Safra T, Muggia F, Jeffers S, Tsao-Wei DD, Groshen S, Lyass O, et al. Pegylated liposomal doxorubicin (doxil): reduced clinical cardiotoxicity in patients reaching or exceeding cumulative doses of 500 mg/m^2. Ann Oncol 2000;11:1029–33. [cited 2015 Aug 25] Available from: http://www.ncbi.nlm.nih.gov/pubmed/11038041.

[107] Saito K, Takeda K, Imanaka-Yoshida K, Imai H, Sekine T, Kamikura Y. Assessment of fatty acid metabolism in taxan-induced myocardial damage with iodine-123 BMIPP SPECT: comparative study with myocardial perfusion, left ventricular function, and histopathological findings. Ann Nucl Med 2003;17:481–8. [cited 2015 Aug 23] Available from: http://www.ncbi.nlm.nih.gov/pubmed/14575384.

[108] Sartori M, Andorno S, La Terra G, Pozzoli G, Rudoni M, Sacchetti GM, et al. Assessment of interferon cardiotoxicity with quantitative radionuclide angiocardiography. Eur J Clin Invest 1995;25:68–70. [cited 2015 Aug 23] Available from: http://www.ncbi.nlm.nih.gov/pubmed/7705390.

[109] Savage DE, Constine LS, Schwartz RG, Rubin P. Radiation effects on left ventricular function and myocardial perfusion in long term survivors of Hodgkin's disease. Int J Radiat Oncol Biol Phys 1990;19:721–7. [cited 2015 Aug 24] Available from: http://www.ncbi.nlm.nih.gov/pubmed/2211221.

[110] Scopinaro F, Banci M, Vania A, Tavolaro R, Schillaci O, Tisei A, et al. Radioisotope assessment of heart damage in hypertransfused thalassaemic patients. Eur J Nucl Med 1993;20:603–8. [cited 2015 Aug 23] Available from: http://www.ncbi.nlm.nih.gov/pubmed/8370381.

[111] Shpall EJ, Jones RB, Holland JF, Bhardwaj S, Paciucci PA, Wilfinger CL, et al. Intensive single-agent mitoxantrone for metastatic breast cancer. J Natl Cancer Inst 1988;80:204–8. [cited 2015 Aug 23] Available from: http://www.ncbi.nlm.nih.gov/pubmed/3279218.

[112] Sobić-Saranović D, Pavlović S, Susnjar S, Neskovi c-Konstantinović Z, Jelić S. Assessment of early epirubicin cardiotoxicity in women with breast cancer. Anticancer

Res 1997;17:3889–91. [cited 2015 Aug 22] Available from: http://www.ncbi.nlm.nih.gov/pubmed/9427798.

[113] Steinherz LJ, Steinherz PG, Tan C. Cardiac failure and dysrhythmias 6–19 years after anthracycline therapy: a series of 15 patients. Med Pediatr Oncol 1995;24:352–61. [cited 2015 Aug 20] Available from: http://www.ncbi.nlm.nih.gov/pubmed/7715541.

[114] Strashun AM, Goldsmith SJ, Horowitz SF. Gated blood pool scintigraphic monitoring of doxorubicin cardiomyopathy: comparison of camera and computerized probe results in 101 patients. J Am Coll Cardiol 1986;8:1082–7. [cited 2015 Aug 25] Available from: http://www.ncbi.nlm.nih.gov/pubmed/3760382.

[115] Suzuki J, Yanagisawa A, Shigeyama T, Tsubota J, Yasumura T, Shimoyama K, et al. Early detection of anthracycline-induced cardiotoxicity by radionuclide angiocardiography. Angiology 1999;50:37–45. [cited 2015 Aug 25] Available from: http://www.ncbi.nlm.nih.gov/pubmed/9924887.

[116] Trappolini M, Matteoli S, Galli V, Grego V. Evaluation of peak filling rate for the early identification of daunorubicin cardiotoxicity. G Ital Cardiol 1988;18:55–60. [cited 2015 Aug 22] Available from: http://www.ncbi.nlm.nih.gov/pubmed/3384249.

[117] Valdés Olmos RA, ten Bokkel Huinink WW, Greve JC, Hoefnagel CA. I-123 MIBG and serial radionuclide angiocardiography in doxorubicin-related cardiotoxicity. Clin Nucl Med 1992;17:163–7. [cited 2015 Aug 25] Available from: http://www.ncbi.nlm.nih.gov/pubmed/1611784.

[118] Vici P, Ferraironi A, Di Lauro L, Carpano S, Conti F, Belli F, et al. Dexrazoxane cardioprotection in advanced breast cancer patients undergoing high-dose epirubicin treatment. Clin Ter 1998;149:15–20. [cited 2015 Aug 22] Available from: http://www.ncbi.nlm.nih.gov/pubmed/9621483.

[119] Vorobiof DA, Iturralde M, Falkson G. Amsacrine cardiotoxicity: assessment of ventricular function by radionuclide angiography. Cancer Treat Rep 1983;67:1115–17. [cited 2015 Aug 25] Available from: http://www.ncbi.nlm.nih.gov/pubmed/6689141.

[120] Vorobiof DA, Iturralde M, Falkson G. Assessment of ventricular function by radionuclide angiography in patients receiving 4′-epidoxorubicin and mitoxantrone. Cancer Chemother Pharmacol 1985;15:253–7. [cited 2015 Aug 25] Available from: http://www.ncbi.nlm.nih.gov/pubmed/3863718.

[121] Wachters FM, Van Der Graaf WTA, Groen HJM. Cardiotoxicity in advanced non-small cell lung cancer patients treated with platinum and non platinum based combinations as first-line treatment. Anticancer Res 2004;24:2079–83. [cited 2015 Aug 23] Available from: http://www.ncbi.nlm.nih.gov/pubmed/15274404.

[122] Walker J, Bhullar N, Fallah-Rad N, Lytwyn M, Golian M, Fang T, et al. Role of three-dimensional echocardiography in breast cancer: comparison with two-dimensional echocardiography, multiple-gated acquisition scans, and cardiac magnetic resonance imaging. J Clin Oncol 2010;28:3429–36. [cited 2015 Aug 25] Available from: http://www.ncbi.nlm.nih.gov/pubmed/20530277.

[123] Wheeler RH, Ensminger WD, Thrall JH, Anderson JL. High-dose doxorubicin: an exploration of the dose-response curve in human neoplasia. Cancer Treat Rep 1982;66:493–8. [cited 2015 Aug 22] Available from: http://www.ncbi.nlm.nih.gov/pubmed/7060037.

[124] Yabuta M. Evaluation of cardiotoxicity by radionuclide angiocardiography in the chemotherapy of gynecologic malignancies. Nihon Gan Chiryo Gakkai Shi 1990;25:1146–56. [cited 2015 Aug 20] Available from: http://www.ncbi.nlm.nih.gov/pubmed/2398300.

[125] Calnon DA, Kastner RJ, Smith WH, Segalla D, Beller GA, Watson DD. Validation of a new counts-based gated single photon emission computed tomography method for quantifying left ventricular systolic function: comparison with equilibrium radionuclide angiography. J Nucl Cardiol 1997;4:464–71. [cited 2015 Aug 18] Available from: http://www.ncbi.nlm.nih.gov/pubmed/9456185.

[126] Groch MW, Marshall RC, Erwin WD, Schippers DJ, Barnett CA, Leidholdt EM. Quantitative gated blood pool SPECT for the assessment of coronary artery disease at rest. J Nucl Cardiol 1998;5:567–73. [cited 2015 Aug 18] Available from: http://www.ncbi.nlm.nih.gov/pubmed/9869478.

[127] Groch MW, DePuey EG, Belzberg AC, Erwin WD, Kamran M, Barnett CA, et al. Planar imaging versus gated blood-pool SPECT for the assessment of ventricular performance: a multicenter study. J Nucl Med 2001;42:1773–9. [cited 2015 Aug 18] Available from: http://www.ncbi.nlm.nih.gov/pubmed/11752072.

[128] Hacker M, Hoyer X, Kupzyk S, La Fougere C, Kois J, Stempfle H-U, et al. Clinical validation of the gated blood pool SPECT QBS processing software in congestive heart failure patients: correlation with MUGA, first-pass RNV and 2D-echocardiography. Int J Cardiovasc Imaging 2006;22:407–16. [cited 2015 Aug 18] Available from: http://www.ncbi.nlm.nih.gov/pubmed/16328851.

[129] Odagiri K, Wakabayashi Y, Tawarahara K, Kurata C, Urushida T, Katoh H, et al. Evaluation of right and left ventricular function by quantitative blood-pool SPECT (QBS): comparison with conventional methods and quantitative gated SPECT (QGS). Ann Nucl Med 2006;20:519–26. [cited 2015 Aug 18] Available from: http://www.ncbi.nlm.nih.gov/pubmed/17134018.

[130] Massardo T, Jaimovich R, Lavados H, Gutiérrez D, Rodríguez JC, Saavedra JM, et al. Comparison of radionuclide ventriculography using SPECT and planar techniques in different cardiac conditions. Eur J Nucl Med Mol Imaging 2007;34:1735–46. [cited 2015 Aug 18] Available from: http://www.ncbi.nlm.nih.gov/pubmed/17579852.

[131] Maurea S, Cuocolo A, Soricelli A, Castelli L, Nappi A, Squame F, et al. Enhanced detection of viable myocardium by technetium-99m-MIBI imaging after nitrate administration in chronic coronary artery disease. J Nucl Med 1995;36:1945–52. [cited 2015 Aug 18] Available from: http://www.ncbi.nlm.nih.gov/pubmed/7472580.

[132] Verberne HJ, Acampa W, Anagnostopoulos C, Ballinger J, De Bondt P, Buechel RR, et al. EANM procedural guidelines for radionuclide myocardial perfusion imaging with SPECT and SPECT/CT: 2015 revision. Eur J Nucl Med Mol Imaging. 2015;42(12):1929–40.

[133] Nkoulou R, Pazhenkottil AP, Kuest SM, Ghadri JR, Wolfrum M, Husmann L, et al. Semiconductor detectors allow low-dose-low-dose 1-day SPECT myocardial perfusion imaging. J Nucl Med 2011;52:1204–9. [cited 2015 Aug 24] Available from: http://www.ncbi.nlm.nih.gov/pubmed/21810589.

[134] Duvall WL, Croft LB, Ginsberg ES, Einstein AJ, Guma KA, George T, et al. Reduced isotope dose and imaging time with a high-efficiency CZT SPECT camera. J Nucl Cardiol 2011;18:847–57. [cited 2015 Aug 24] Available from: http://www.ncbi.nlm.nih.gov/pubmed/21528422.

[135] Oddstig J, Hedeer F, Jögi J, Carlsson M, Hindorf C, Engblom H. Reduced administered activity, reduced acquisition time, and preserved image quality for the new CZT camera. J Nucl Cardiol 2013;20:38–44. [cited 2015 Aug 24] Available from: http://www.ncbi.nlm.nih.gov/pubmed/23143809.

[136] Slomka PJ, Nishina H, Abidov A, Hayes SW, Friedman JD, Berman DS, et al. Combined quantitative supine-prone myocardial perfusion SPECT improves detection of coronary artery disease and normalcy rates in women. J Nucl Cardiol 2007;14:44–52. [cited 2015 Aug 24] Available from: http://www.ncbi.nlm.nih.gov/pubmed/17276305.

[137] Sharir T, Bacher-Stier C, Dhar S, Lewin HC, Miranda R, Friedman JD, et al. Identification of severe and extensive coronary artery disease by postexercise regional wall motion abnormalities in Tc-99m sestamibi gated single-photon emission computed tomography. Am J Cardiol 2000;86:1171–5. [cited 2015 Aug 25] Available from: http://www.ncbi.nlm.nih.gov/pubmed/11090786.

[138] Yamagishi H, Shirai N, Yoshiyama M, Teragaki M, Akioka K, Takeuchi K, et al. Incremental value of left ventricular ejection fraction for detection of multivessel coronary artery disease in exercise (201)Tl gated myocardial perfusion imaging. J Nucl Med 2002;43:131–9. [cited 2015 Aug 25] Available from: http://www.ncbi.nlm.nih.gov/pubmed/11850475.

[139] DePuey EG, Rozanski A. Using gated technetium-99m-sestamibi SPECT to characterize fixed myocardial defects as infarct or artifact. J Nucl Med 1995;36:952–5. [cited 2015 Aug 25] Available from: http://www.ncbi.nlm.nih.gov/pubmed/7769451.

[140] Sharir T, Germano G, Kavanagh PB, Lai S, Cohen I, Lewin HC, et al. Incremental prognostic value of post-stress left ventricular ejection fraction and volume by gated myocardial perfusion single photon emission computed tomography. Circulation 1999;100:1035–42. [cited 2015 Jul 18] Available from: http://www.ncbi.nlm.nih.gov/pubmed/10477527.

[141] Vavere AL, Arbab-Zadeh A, Rochitte CE, Dewey M, Niinuma H, Gottlieb I, et al. Coronary artery stenoses: accuracy of 64-detector row CT angiography in segments with mild, moderate, or severe calcification—a subanalysis of the CORE-64 trial. Radiology 2011;261:100–8. [cited 2015 Aug 24] Available from: http://www.pubmedcentral.nih.gov/articlerender.fcgi?artid=3176425&tool=pmcentrez&rendertype=abstract.

[142] Lembcke A, Schwenke C, Hein PA, Knobloch G, Durmus T, Hamm B, et al. High-pitch dual-source CT coronary angiography with low volumes of contrast medium. Eur Radiol 2014;24:120–7. [cited 2015 Aug 24] Available from: http://www.ncbi.nlm.nih.gov/pubmed/23949727.

[143] Budoff MJ, Dowe D, Jollis JG, Gitter M, Sutherland J, Halamert E, et al. Diagnostic performance of 64-multidetector row coronary computed tomographic angiography for evaluation of coronary artery stenosis in individuals without known coronary artery disease: results from the prospective multicenter ACCURACY (Assessment by Coro). J Am Coll Cardiol 2008;52:1724–32. [cited 2015 Jun 22] Available from: http://www.ncbi.nlm.nih.gov/pubmed/19007693.

[144] Glanzmann C, Kaufmann P, Jenni R, Hess OM, Huguenin P. Cardiac risk after mediastinal irradiation for Hodgkin's disease. Radiother Oncol 1998;46:51–62. [cited 2015 Aug 24] Available from: http://www.ncbi.nlm.nih.gov/pubmed/9488128.

[145] Gustavsson A, Eskilsson J, Landberg T, Svahn-Tapper G, White T, Wollmer P, et al. Late cardiac effects after mantle radiotherapy in patients with Hodgkin's disease. Ann Oncol 1990;1:355–63. [cited 2015 Aug 18] Available from: http://www.ncbi.nlm.nih.gov/pubmed/2261376.

[146] Maunoury C, Pierga JY, Valette H, Tchernia G, Cosset JM, Desgrez A. Myocardial perfusion damage after mediastinal irradiation for Hodgkin's disease: a thallium-201 single photon emission tomography study. Eur J Nucl Med 1992;19:871–3. [cited 2015 Aug 18] Available from: http://www.ncbi.nlm.nih.gov/pubmed/1451703.

[147] Pierga JY, Maunoury C, Valette H, Socie G, Girinski T, Tchernia G, et al. Follow-up thallium-201 scintigraphy after mantle field radiotherapy for Hodgkin's disease. Int J Radiat Oncol Biol Phys 1993;25:871–6. [cited 2015 Aug 18] Available from: http://www.ncbi.nlm.nih.gov/pubmed/8478238.

[148] Girinsky T, Cordova A, Rey A, Cosset JM, Tertian G, Pierga JY. Thallium-201 scintigraphy is not predictive of late cardiac complications in patients with Hodgkin's disease treated with mediastinal radiation. Int J Radiat Oncol Biol Phys 2000;48:1503–6. [cited 2015 Aug 18] Available from: http://www.ncbi.nlm.nih.gov/pubmed/11121655.

[149] Cowen D, Gonzague-Casabianca L, Brenot-Rossi I, Viens P, Mace L, Hannoun-Levi JM, et al. Thallium-201 perfusion scintigraphy in the evaluation of late myocardial damage in left-side breast cancer treated with adjuvant radiotherapy. Int J Radiat Oncol Biol Phys 1998;41:809–15. [cited 2015 Aug 18] Available from: http://www.ncbi.nlm.nih.gov/pubmed/9652842.

[150] Gyenes G, Fornander T, Carlens P, Glas U, Rutqvist LE. Myocardial damage in breast cancer patients treated with adjuvant radiotherapy: a prospective study. Int J Radiat Oncol Biol Phys 1996;36:899–905. [cited 2015 Aug 18] Available from: http://www.ncbi.nlm.nih.gov/pubmed/8960519.

[151] Gyenes G, Fornander T, Carlens P, Glas U, Rutqvist LE. Detection of radiation-induced myocardial damage by technetium-99m sestamibi scintigraphy. Eur J Nucl Med 1997;24:286–92. [cited 2015 Aug 18] Available from: http://www.ncbi.nlm.nih.gov/pubmed/9143466.

[152] Gustavsson A, Bendahl PO, Cwikiel M, Eskilsson J, Thapper KL, Pahlm O. No serious late cardiac effects after adjuvant radiotherapy following mastectomy in premenopausal women with early breast cancer. Int J Radiat Oncol Biol Phys 1999;43:745–54. [cited 2015 Aug 18] Available from: http://www.ncbi.nlm.nih.gov/pubmed/10098429.

[153] Seddon B, Cook A, Gothard L, Salmon E, Latus K, Underwood SR, et al. Detection of defects in myocardial perfusion imaging in patients with early breast cancer treated with radiotherapy. Radiother Oncol 2002;64:53–63. [cited 2015 Aug 18] Available from: http://www.ncbi.nlm.nih.gov/pubmed/12208576.

[154] Pistevou-Gompaki K, Eleftheriadis D, Trontzos C, Goutzioulis M, Kouloulias V, Eleftheriadis N, et al. Technetium-99m-tetrofosmin myocardial imaging in cardiotoxicity screening for left-sided breast cancer irradiation. Acta Oncol 2003;42:349–51. [cited 2015 Aug 18] Available from: http://www.ncbi.nlm.nih.gov/pubmed/12899510.

[155] Tzonevska A, Tzvetkov K, Parvanova V, Dimitrova M. 99mTc-MIBI myocardial perfusion scintigraphy for assessment of myocardial damage after radiotherapy in patients with breast cancer. J BUON 2006;11:505–9. [cited 2015 Aug 18] Available from: http://www.ncbi.nlm.nih.gov/pubmed/17309185.

[156] Marks LB, Yu X, Prosnitz RG, Zhou S-M, Hardenbergh PH, Blazing M, et al. The incidence and functional consequences of RT-associated cardiac perfusion defects. Int J Radiat Oncol Biol Phys 2005;63:214–23. [cited 2015 Aug 18] Available from: http://www.ncbi.nlm.nih.gov/pubmed/16111592.

[157] Prosnitz RG, Hubbs JL, Evans ES, Zhou S-M, Yu X, Blazing MA, et al. Prospective assessment of radiotherapy-associated cardiac toxicity in breast cancer patients: analysis of data 3 to 6 years after treatment. Cancer 2007;110:1840–50. [cited 2015 Aug 18] Available from: http://www.ncbi.nlm.nih.gov/pubmed/17763369.

[158] HŁjris I, Sand NP, Andersen J, Rehling M, Overgaard M. Myocardial perfusion imaging in breast cancer patients treated with or without post-mastectomy radiotherapy.

Radiother Oncol 2000;55:163–72. [cited 2015 Aug 18] Available from: http://www.ncbi.nlm.nih.gov/pubmed/10799728.

[159] Hardenbergh PH, Munley MT, Bentel GC, Kedem R, Borges-Neto S, Hollis D, et al. Cardiac perfusion changes in patients treated for breast cancer with radiation therapy and doxorubicin: preliminary results. Int J Radiat Oncol Biol Phys 2001;49:1023–8. [cited 2015 Aug 18] Available from: http://www.ncbi.nlm.nih.gov/pubmed/11240243.

[160] Gallucci G, Coccaro M, Storto G, Lapadula L, Tartarone A, Nappi A, et al. The clinical impact of a cardiologic follow-up in breast cancer survivors: an observational study. Int J Immunopathol Pharmacol 2010;23:1221–7. [cited 2015 Aug 18] Available from: http://www.ncbi.nlm.nih.gov/pubmed/21244771.

[161] Tzonevska A, Chakarova A, Tzvetkov K. GSPECT-CT myocardial scintigraphy plus calcium scores as screening tool for prevention of cardiac side effects in leftsided breast cancer radiotherapy. J BUON 2014;19:667–72. [cited 2015 Aug 22] Available from: http://www.ncbi.nlm.nih.gov/pubmed/25261650.

[162] Levitt SH, Fletcher GH. Trials and tribulations: do clinical trials prove that irradiation increases cardiac and secondary cancer mortality in the breast cancer patient? Int J Radiat Oncol Biol Phys 1991;21:523–7. [cited 2015 Aug 24] Available from: http://www.ncbi.nlm.nih.gov/pubmed/2061131.

[163] Gayed IW, Liu HH, Yusuf SW, Komaki R, Wei X, Wang X, et al. The prevalence of myocardial ischemia after concurrent chemoradiation therapy as detected by gated myocardial perfusion imaging in patients with esophageal cancer. J Nucl Med 2006;47:1756–62. [cited 2015 Aug 23] Available from: http://www.ncbi.nlm.nih.gov/pubmed/17079807.

[164] Yu X, Prosnitz RR, Zhou S, Hardenberg PH, Tisch A, Blazing MA, et al. Symptomatic cardiac events following radiation therapy for left-sided breast cancer: possible association with radiation therapy-induced changes in regional perfusion. Clin Breast Cancer 2003;4:193–7. [cited 2015 Aug 23] Available from: http://www.ncbi.nlm.nih.gov/pubmed/14499012.

[165] Hutchins GD, Schwaiger M, Rosenspire KC, Krivokapich J, Schelbert H, Kuhl DE. Noninvasive quantification of regional blood flow in the human heart using N-13 ammonia and dynamic positron emission tomographic imaging. J Am Coll Cardiol 1990;15:1032–42. [cited 2015 Aug 25] Available from: http://www.ncbi.nlm.nih.gov/pubmed/2312957.

[166] Hickey KT, Sciacca RR, Bokhari S, Rodriguez O, Chou R-L, Faber TL, et al. Assessment of cardiac wall motion and ejection fraction with gated PET using N-13 ammonia. Clin Nucl Med 2004;29:243–8. [cited 2015 Aug 25] Available from: http://www.ncbi.nlm.nih.gov/pubmed/15096971.

[167] Di Carli MF, Dorbala S, Meserve J, El Fakhri G, Sitek A, Moore SC. Clinical myocardial perfusion PET/CT. J Nucl Med 2007;48:783–93. [cited 2015 Aug 25] Available from: http://www.ncbi.nlm.nih.gov/pubmed/17475968.

[168] Selwyn AP, Allan RM, L'Abbate A, Horlock P, Camici P, Clark J, et al. Relation between regional myocardial uptake of rubidium-82 and perfusion: absolute reduction of cation uptake in ischemia. Am J Cardiol 1982;50:112–21. [cited 2015 Aug 18] Available from: http://www.ncbi.nlm.nih.gov/pubmed/6979917.

[169] Mullani NA, Goldstein RA, Gould KL, Marani SK, Fisher DJ, O'Brien HA, et al. Myocardial perfusion with rubidium-82. I. Measurement of extraction fraction and flow with external detectors. J Nucl Med 1983;24:898–906. [cited 2015 Aug 18] Available from: http://www.ncbi.nlm.nih.gov/pubmed/6619960.

[170] Hoffmann U, Ferencik M, Cury RC, Pena AJ. Coronary CT angiography. J Nucl Med 2006;47:797–806. [cited 2015 Aug 18] Available from: http://www.ncbi.nlm.nih.gov/pubmed/16644750.

[171] Bax JJ, Wijns W, Cornel JH, Visser FC, Boersma E, Fioretti PM. Accuracy of currently available techniques for prediction of functional recovery after revascularization in patients with left ventricular dysfunction due to chronic coronary artery disease: comparison of pooled data. J Am Coll Cardiol 1997;30:1451–60. [cited 2015 Aug 18] Available from: http://www.ncbi.nlm.nih.gov/pubmed/9362401.

[172] Di Carli MF, Davidson M, Little R, Khanna S, Mody FV, Brunken RC, et al. Value of metabolic imaging with positron emission tomography for evaluating prognosis in patients with coronary artery disease and left ventricular dysfunction. Am J Cardiol 1994;73:527–33. [cited 2015 Aug 18] Available from: http://www.ncbi.nlm.nih.gov/pubmed/8147295.

[173] Borde C, Kand P, Basu S. Enhanced myocardial fluorodeoxyglucose uptake following Adriamycin-based therapy: evidence of early chemotherapeutic cardiotoxicity? World J Radiol 2012;4:220–3. [cited 2015 Aug 25] Available from: http://www.pubmedcentral.nih.gov/articlerender.fcgi?artid=3386534&tool=pmcentrez&rendertype=abstract.

[174] Basu S, Borde C, Kand P. Increasing cardiac ^{18}F-fluorodeoxyglucose (FDG) uptake on PET-CT as a biomarker for cardiotoxicity of chemo-radiotherapy in cancer: a myth or a reality? Radiother Oncol 2014;112:451–2. [cited 2015 Aug 25] Available from: http://www.ncbi.nlm.nih.gov/pubmed/25017999.

[175] Jingu K, Kaneta T, Nemoto K, Ichinose A, Oikawa M, Takai Y, et al. The utility of 18F-fluorodeoxyglucose positron emission tomography for early diagnosis of radiation-induced myocardial damage. Int J Radiat Oncol 2006;66:845–51. [cited 2015 Aug 25] Available from: http://www.ncbi.nlm.nih.gov/pubmed/17011456.

[176] Zöphel K, Hölzel C, Dawel M, Hölscher T, Evers C, Kotzerke J. PET/CT demonstrates increased myocardial FDG uptake following irradiation therapy. Eur J Nucl Med Mol Imaging 2007;34:1322–3. [cited 2015 Aug 25] Available from: http://www.ncbi.nlm.nih.gov/pubmed/17546454.

[177] Unal K, Unlu M, Akdemir O, Akmansu M. 18F-FDG PET/CT findings of radiotherapy-related myocardial changes in patients with thoracic malignancies. Nucl Med Commun 2013;34:855–9. [cited 2015 Aug 25] Available from: http://www.ncbi.nlm.nih.gov/pubmed/23728520.

[178] Shreve PD, Anzai Y, Wahl RL. Pitfalls in oncologic diagnosis with FDG PET imaging: physiologic and benign variants. Radiographics 1999;19:61–77. quiz 150–1 [cited 2015 Jul 9] Available from: http://www.ncbi.nlm.nih.gov/pubmed/9925392.

[179] De Groot M, Meeuwis APW, Kok PJM, Corstens FHM, Oyen WJG. Influence of blood glucose level, age and fasting period on non-pathological FDG uptake in heart and gut. Eur J Nucl Med Mol Imaging 2005;32:98–101. [cited 2015 Aug 25] Available from: http://www.ncbi.nlm.nih.gov/pubmed/15605289.

[180] Lum D, Wandell S, Ko J, Coel M. 1. Positron Emission Tomography of Thoracic Malignancies. Reduction of Myocardial Fluorodeoxyglucose Uptake Artifacts With a Carbohydrate Restricted Diet. Clin Positron Imaging 2000;3:155. [cited 2015 Aug 25] Available from: http://www.ncbi.nlm.nih.gov/pubmed/11150758.

[181] Williams G, Kolodny GM. Suppression of myocardial 18F-FDG uptake by preparing patients with a high-fat, low-carbohydrate diet. AJR Am J Roentgenol 2008;190:W151–6. [cited 2015 Aug 25] Available from: http://www.ncbi.nlm.nih.gov/pubmed/18212199.

[182] Minamimoto R, Morooka M, Kubota K, Ito K, Masuda-Miyata Y, Mitsumoto T, et al. Value of FDG-PET/CT using unfractionated heparin for managing primary cardiac lymphoma and several key findings. J Nucl Cardiol 2011;18:516–20. [cited 2015 Aug 25] Available from: http://www.ncbi.nlm.nih.gov/pubmed/21394554.

[183] Persson E. Lipoprotein lipase, hepatic lipase and plasma lipolytic activity. Effects of heparin and a low molecular weight heparin fragment (Fragmin). Acta Med Scand Suppl 1988;724:1–56. [cited 2015 Aug 25] Available from: http://www.ncbi.nlm.nih.gov/pubmed/2843005.

[184] Fan C-M, Fischman AJ, Kwek BH, Abbara S, Aquino SL. Lipomatous hypertrophy of the interatrial septum: increased uptake on FDG PET. AJR Am J Roentgenol 2005;184:339–42. [cited 2015 Aug 25] Available from: http://www.ncbi.nlm.nih.gov/pubmed/15615998.

[185] Erba PA, Sollini M, Lazzeri E, Mariani G. FDG-PET in cardiac infections. Semin Nucl Med 2013;43:377–95. [cited 2015 Aug 23] Available from: http://www.ncbi.nlm.nih.gov/pubmed/23905619.

[186] Yan R, Song J, Wu Z, Guo M, Liu J, Li J, et al. Detection of myocardial metabolic abnormalities by 18F-FDG PET/CT and corresponding pathological changes in beagles with local heart irradiation. Korean J Radiol 2015;16:919–28. [cited 2015 Aug 25] Available from: http://www.pubmedcentral.nih.gov/articlerender.fcgi?artid=4499559&tool=pmcentrez&rendertype=abstract.

[187] Gardner SF, Lazarus HM, Bednarczyk EM, Creger RJ, Miraldi FD, Leisure G, et al. High-dose cyclophosphamide-induced myocardial damage during BMT: assessment by positron emission tomography. Bone Marrow Transplant 1993;12:139–44. [cited 2015 Aug 23] Available from: http://www.ncbi.nlm.nih.gov/pubmed/8401360.

[188] Gayed IW, Liu HH, Wei X, Liao Z, Yusuf SW, Chang JY, et al. Patterns of cardiac perfusion abnormalities after chemoradiotherapy in patients with lung cancer. J Thorac Oncol 2009;4:179–84. [cited 2015 Jul 14] Available from: http://www.ncbi.nlm.nih.gov/pubmed/19179893.

[189] Pach J, Pach D, Hubalewska-Hoła A, Kroch S, Targosz D. Evaluation of carbon monoxide cardiotoxicity in group poisonings. Przegląd Lek 1998;55:505–7. [cited 2015 Aug 25] Available from: http://www.ncbi.nlm.nih.gov/pubmed/10224861.

[190] Pach J, Hubalewska-Hoła A, Pach D, Szpak D. Usefulness of rest and forced perfusion scintigraphy (SPECT) to evaluate cardiotoxicity in acute carbon monoxide poisoning. Przegląd Lek 2001;58:297–300. [cited 2015 Aug 25] Available from: http://www.ncbi.nlm.nih.gov/pubmed/11450357.

[191] Tzonevska A, Tzvetkov K, Atanasova M, Chakarova A, Piperkova E. Myocardial scintigraphy, echocardiography and proBNP for early detection of myocardial cardiotoxicity in breast cancer patients after chemo-radiotherapy. Hell J Nucl Med 2011;14:269–73. [cited 2015 Aug 25] Available from: http://www.ncbi.nlm.nih.gov/pubmed/22087448.

[192] Lautamäki R, Tipre D, Bengel FM. Cardiac sympathetic neuronal imaging using PET. Eur J Nucl Med Mol Imaging 2007;34(Suppl. 1):S74–85. [cited 2015 Aug 24] Available from: http://www.ncbi.nlm.nih.gov/pubmed/17479262.

[193] Stiles GL, Lefkowitz RJ. Cardiac adrenergic receptors. Annu Rev Med 1984;35:149–64. [cited 2015 Aug 25] Available from: http://www.ncbi.nlm.nih.gov/pubmed/6144285.

[194] Brodde OE, Michel MC. Adrenergic and muscarinic receptors in the human heart. Pharmacol Rev 1999;51:651–90. [cited 2015 Aug 25] Available from: http://www.ncbi.nlm.nih.gov/pubmed/10581327.

[195] De Geus-Oei L-F, Mavinkurve-Groothuis AMC, Bellersen L, Gotthardt M, Oyen WJG, Kapusta L, et al. Scintigraphic techniques for early detection of cancer treatment-induced cardiotoxicity. J Nucl Med 2011;52:560–71. [cited 2015 Aug 24] Available from: http://www.ncbi.nlm.nih.gov/pubmed/21421717.

[196] Francis GS, Cohn JN. The autonomic nervous system in congestive heart failure. Annu Rev Med 1986;37:235–47. [cited 2015 Aug 25] Available from: http://www.ncbi.nlm.nih.gov/pubmed/2871803.

[197] Triposkiadis F, Karayannis G, Giamouzis G, Skoularigis J, Louridas G, Butler J. The sympathetic nervous system in heart failure. J Am Coll Cardiol 2009;54:1747–62. [cited 2015 Jun 16] Available from: http://www.ncbi.nlm.nih.gov/pubmed/19874988.

[198] Delforge J, Syrota A, Lançon JP, Nakajima K, Loc'h C, Janier M, et al. Cardiac beta-adrenergic receptor density measured in vivo using PET, CGP 12177, and a new graphical method. J Nucl Med 1991;32:739–48. [cited 2015 Aug 25] Available from: http://www.ncbi.nlm.nih.gov/pubmed/1672889.

[199] Elsinga PH, Doze P, van Waarde A, Pieterman RM, Blanksma PK, Willemsen AT, et al. Imaging of beta-adrenoceptors in the human thorax using (S)-[(11)C]CGP12388 and positron emission tomography. Eur J Pharmacol 2001;433:173–6. [cited 2015 Aug 25] Available from: http://www.ncbi.nlm.nih.gov/pubmed/11755150.

[200] Law MP, Osman S, Pike VW, Davenport RJ, Cunningham VJ, Rimoldi O, et al. Evaluation of [11C]GB67, a novel radioligand for imaging myocardial alpha 1-adrenoceptors with positron emission tomography. Eur J Nucl Med 2000;27:7–17. [cited 2015 Aug 25] Available from: http://www.ncbi.nlm.nih.gov/pubmed/10654141.

[201] Lourenco CM, Kenk M, Beanlands RS, DaSilva JN. Increasing synaptic noradrenaline, serotonin and histamine enhances in vivo binding of phosphodiesterase-4 inhibitor (R)-[11C]rolipram in rat brain, lung and heart. Life Sci 2006;79:356–64. [cited 2015 Aug 25] Available from: http://www.ncbi.nlm.nih.gov/pubmed/16499932.

[202] Sasaki T, Enta A, Nozaki T, Ishii S, Senda M. Carbon-11-forskolin: a ligand for visualization of the adenylate cyclase-related second messenger system. J Nucl Med 1993;34:1944–8. [cited 2015 Aug 25] Available from: http://www.ncbi.nlm.nih.gov/pubmed/8229239.

[203] Kiesewetter DO, Sassaman MB, Robbins J, Jagoda EM, Carson RE, Appel NM, et al. Synthesis and evaluation of an 18F analog of forskolin for imaging adenylyl cyclase. J Fluor Chem 2000;101:297–304.

[204] Jakobsen S, Kodahl GM, Olsen AK, Cumming P. Synthesis, radiolabeling and in vivo evaluation of [11C]RAL-01, a potential phosphodiesterase 5 radioligand. Nucl Med Biol 2006;33:593–7. [cited 2015 Aug 25] Available from: http://www.ncbi.nlm.nih.gov/pubmed/16843833.

[205] Vasdev N, LaRonde FJ, Woodgett JR, Garcia A, Rubie EA, Meyer JH, et al. Rationally designed PKA inhibitors for positron emission tomography: synthesis and cerebral biodistribution of *N*-(2-(4-bromocinnamylamino)ethyl)-*N*-[11C]methyl-isoquinoline-5-sulfonamide. Bioorg Med Chem 2008;16:5277–84. [cited 2015 Aug 25] Available from: http://www.ncbi.nlm.nih.gov/pubmed/18346896.

[206] Otani H, Kagaya Y, Imahori Y, Yasuda S, Fujii R, Chida M, et al. Myocardial 11C-diacylglycerol accumulation and left ventricular remodeling in patients after myocardial infarction. J Nucl Med 2005;46:553–9. [cited 2015 Aug 25] Available from: http://www.ncbi.nlm.nih.gov/pubmed/15809475.

[207] Imahori Y, Fujii R, Ueda S, Ido T, Nishino H, Moriyama Y, et al. No-carrier-added carbon-11-labeled sn-1,2- and sn-1,3-diacylglycerols by [11C]propyl ketene method.

J Nucl Med 1991;32:1622–6. [cited 2015 Aug 25] Available from: http://www.ncbi.nlm.nih.gov/pubmed/1869991.

[208] Langer O, Halldin C. PET and SPET tracers for mapping the cardiac nervous system. Eur J Nucl Med Mol Imaging 2002;29:416–34. [cited 2015 Aug 24] Available from: http://www.ncbi.nlm.nih.gov/pubmed/12002720.

[209] Strashun A. Adriamycin, congestive cardiomyopathy, and metaiodobenzylguanidine. J Nucl Med 1992;33:215–22. [cited 2015 Aug 25] Available from: http://www.ncbi.nlm.nih.gov/pubmed/1732443.

[210] Degrado TR, Zalutsky MR, Vaidyanathan G. Uptake mechanisms of meta-[123I]iodobenzylguanidine in isolated rat heart. Nucl Med Biol 1995;22:1–12. [cited 2015 Aug 26] Available from: http://www.ncbi.nlm.nih.gov/pubmed/7735158.

[211] Dae MW. Scintigraphy of myocardial innervation with metaiodobenzylguanidine (MIBG): is there a clinical application? J Nucl Cardiol 1995;2:151–4. [cited 2015 Aug 26] Available from: http://www.ncbi.nlm.nih.gov/pubmed/9420780.

[212] Dae MW, O'Connell JW, Botvinick EH, Chin MC. Acute and chronic effects of transient myocardial ischemia on sympathetic nerve activity, density, and norepinephrine content. Cardiovasc Res 1995;30:270–80. [cited 2015 Aug 26] Available from: http://www.ncbi.nlm.nih.gov/pubmed/7585815.

[213] Narula J, Sarkar K. A conceptual paradox of MIBG uptake in heart failure: retention with incontinence! J Nucl Cardiol 2003;10:700–4. [cited 2015 Aug 25] Available from: http://www.ncbi.nlm.nih.gov/pubmed/14668785.

[214] Matsuo S, Nakajima K, Yamashina S, Sakata K, Momose M, Hashimoto J, et al. Characterization of Japanese standards for myocardial sympathetic and metabolic imaging in comparison with perfusion imaging. Ann Nucl Med 2009;23:517–22. [cited 2015 Aug 25] Available from: http://www.ncbi.nlm.nih.gov/pubmed/19521747.

[215] Morozumi T, Kusuoka H, Fukuchi K, Tani A, Uehara T, Matsuda S, et al. Myocardial iodine-123-metaiodobenzylguanidine images and autonomic nerve activity in normal subjects. J Nucl Med 1997;38:49–52. [cited 2015 Aug 25] Available from: http://www.ncbi.nlm.nih.gov/pubmed/8998149.

[216] Geis WP, Kaye MP. Distribution of sympathetic fibers in the left ventricular epicardial plexus of the dog. Circ Res 1968;23:165–70. [cited 2015 Aug 25] Available from: http://www.ncbi.nlm.nih.gov/pubmed/5662572.

[217] Minisi AJ, Thames MD. Distribution of left ventricular sympathetic afferents demonstrated by reflex responses to transmural myocardial ischemia and to intracoronary and epicardial bradykinin. Circulation 1993;87:240–6. [cited 2015 Aug 25] Available from: http://www.ncbi.nlm.nih.gov/pubmed/8419013.

[218] Estorch M, Carrió I, Martínez-Duncker D, Berná L, Torres G, Alonso C, et al. Myocyte cell damage after administration of doxorubicin or mitoxantrone in breast cancer patients assessed by indium 111 antimyosin monoclonal antibody studies. J Clin Oncol 1993;11:1264–8. [cited 2015 Aug 24] Available from: http://www.ncbi.nlm.nih.gov/pubmed/8315423.

[219] Valdés Olmos RA, ten Bokkel Huinink WW, ten Hoeve RF, van Tinteren H, Bruning PF, van Vlies B, et al. Assessment of anthracycline-related myocardial adrenergic derangement by [123I]metaiodobenzylguanidine scintigraphy. Eur J Cancer 1995;31A:26–31. [cited 2015 Aug 24] Available from: http://www.ncbi.nlm.nih.gov/pubmed/7695974.

[220] Arimoto T, Takeishi Y, Niizeki T, Koyama Y, Okuyama H, Nozaki N, et al. Ongoing myocardial damage relates to cardiac sympathetic nervous disintegrity in patients with heart failure. Ann Nucl Med 2005;19:535–40. [cited 2015 Aug 25] Available from: http://www.ncbi.nlm.nih.gov/pubmed/16363617.

[221] Matsuo S, Nakamura Y, Tsutamoto T, Kinoshita M. Impairments of myocardial sympathetic activity may reflect the progression of myocardial damage or dysfunction in hypertrophic cardiomyopathy. J Nucl Cardiol 2002;9:407–12. [cited 2015 Aug 25] Available from: http://www.ncbi.nlm.nih.gov/pubmed/12161717.

[222] Ohshima S, Isobe S, Izawa H, Nanasato M, Ando A, Yamada A, et al. Cardiac sympathetic dysfunction correlates with abnormal myocardial contractile reserve in dilated cardiomyopathy patients. J Am Coll Cardiol 2005;46:2061–8. [cited 2015 Aug 25] Available from: http://www.ncbi.nlm.nih.gov/pubmed/16325043.

[223] Matsui T, Tsutamoto T, Maeda K, Kusukawa J, Kinoshita M. Prognostic value of repeated 123I-metaiodobenzylguanidine imaging in patients with dilated cardiomyopathy with congestive heart failure before and after optimized treatments—comparison with neurohumoral factors. Circ J 2002;66:537–43. [cited 2015 Aug 24] Available from: http://www.ncbi.nlm.nih.gov/pubmed/12074268.

[224] Fujimoto S, Inoue A, Hisatake S, Yamashina S, Yamashina H, Nakano H, et al. Usefulness of 123I-metaiodobenzylguanidine myocardial scintigraphy for predicting the effectiveness of beta-blockers in patients with dilated cardiomyopathy from the standpoint of long-term prognosis. Eur J Nucl Med Mol Imaging 2004; 31:1356–61. [cited 2015 Aug 24] Available from: http://www.ncbi.nlm.nih.gov/pubmed/15221293.

[225] Merlet P, Valette H, Dubois-Randé JL, Moyse D, Duboc D, Dove P, et al. Prognostic value of cardiac metaiodobenzylguanidine imaging in patients with heart failure. J Nucl Med 1992;33:471–7. [cited 2015 Aug 24] Available from: http://www.ncbi.nlm.nih.gov/pubmed/1552326.

[226] Nakata T, Miyamoto K, Doi A, Sasao H, Wakabayashi T, Kobayashi H, et al. Cardiac death prediction and impaired cardiac sympathetic innervation assessed by MIBG in patients with failing and nonfailing hearts. J Nucl Cardiol 1998;5:579–90. [cited 2015 Aug 24] Available from: http://www.ncbi.nlm.nih.gov/pubmed/9869480.

[227] Yamashina S, Yamazaki J. Neuronal imaging using SPECT. Eur J Nucl Med Mol Imaging 2007;34(Suppl. 1):S62–73. [cited 2015 Aug 24] Available from: http://www.ncbi.nlm.nih.gov/pubmed/17450357.

[228] Wakasugi S, Wada A, Hasegawa Y, Nakano S, Shibata N. Detection of abnormal cardiac adrenergic neuron activity in adriamycin-induced cardiomyopathy with iodine-125-metaiodobenzylguanidine. J Nucl Med 1992;33:208–14. [cited 2015 Aug 24] Available from: http://www.ncbi.nlm.nih.gov/pubmed/1732442.

[229] Wakasugi S, Fischman AJ, Babich JW, Aretz HT, Callahan RJ, Nakaki M, et al. Metaiodobenzylguanidine: evaluation of its potential as a tracer for monitoring doxorubicin cardiomyopathy. J Nucl Med 1993;34:1283–6. [cited 2015 Aug 24] Available from: http://www.ncbi.nlm.nih.gov/pubmed/8326385.

[230] Valdés Olmos RA, ten Bokkel Huinink WW, ten Hoeve RF, van Tinteren H, Bruning PF, van Vlies B, et al. Usefulness of indium-111 antimyosin scintigraphy in confirming myocardial injury in patients with anthracycline-associated left ventricular dysfunction. Ann Oncol 1994;5:617–22. [cited 2015 Aug 22] Available from: http://www.ncbi.nlm.nih.gov/pubmed/7993837.

[231] Panjrath GS, Jain D. Monitoring chemotherapy-induced cardiotoxicity: role of cardiac nuclear imaging. J Nucl Cardiol 2006;13:415–26. [cited 2015 Aug 24] Available from: http://www.ncbi.nlm.nih.gov/pubmed/16750786.

[232] Jeon TJ, Lee JD, Ha JW, Yang WI, Cho SH. Evaluation of cardiac adrenergic neuronal damage in rats with doxorubicin-induced cardiomyopathy using iodine-131 MIBG autoradiography and PGP 9.5 immunohistochemistry. Eur J Nucl Med 2000;27:686–93. [cited 2015 Aug 24] Available from: http://www.ncbi.nlm.nih.gov/pubmed/10901455.

[233] Meredith IT, Eisenhofer G, Lambert GW, Dewar EM, Jennings GL, Esler MD. Cardiac sympathetic nervous activity in congestive heart failure. Evidence for increased neuronal norepinephrine release and preserved neuronal uptake. Circulation 1993;88:136–45. [cited 2015 Aug 24] Available from: http://www.ncbi.nlm.nih.gov/pubmed/8391399.

[234] Takano H, Ozawa H, Kobayashi I, Hamaoka S, Nakajima J, Nakamura T, et al. Myocardial sympathetic dysinnervation in doxorubicin cardiomyopathy. J Cardiol 1996;27:49–55. [cited 2015 Aug 24] Available from: http://www.ncbi.nlm.nih.gov/pubmed/8919183.

[235] Pierpont GL, DeMaster EG, Reynolds S, Pederson J, Cohn JN. Ventricular myocardial catecholamines in primates. J Lab Clin Med 1985;106:205–10. [cited 2015 Aug 24] Available from: http://www.ncbi.nlm.nih.gov/pubmed/4020248.

[236] Stokkel MPM, de Wit-van der Veen LJ, Boekhout A. I-123-MIBG myocardial imaging in trastuzumab-based cardiotoxicity: the first experience. Nucl Med Commun 2013;34:19–24.

[237] Bengel FM. Clinical cardiovascular molecular imaging. J Nucl Med 2009;50:837–40. [cited 2015 Aug 25] Available from: http://www.ncbi.nlm.nih.gov/pubmed/19443581.

[238] Matsunari I, Aoki H, Nomura Y, Takeda N, Chen W-P, Taki J, et al. Iodine-123 metaiodobenzylguanidine imaging and carbon-11 hydroxyephedrine positron emission tomography compared in patients with left ventricular dysfunction. Circ Cardiovasc Imaging 2010;3:595–603. [cited 2015 Aug 26] Available from: http://www.ncbi.nlm.nih.gov/pubmed/20534790.

[239] Fallavollita JA, Luisi AJ, Michalek SM, Valverde AM, deKemp RA, Haka MS, et al. Prediction of arrhythmic events with positron emission tomography: PAREPET study design and methods. Contemp Clin Trials 2006;27:374–88. [cited 2015 Aug 26] Available from: http://www.ncbi.nlm.nih.gov/pubmed/16647885.

[240] Fallavollita JA, Heavey BM, Luisi AJ, Michalek SM, Baldwa S, Mashtare TL, et al. Regional myocardial sympathetic denervation predicts the risk of sudden cardiac arrest in ischemic cardiomyopathy. J Am Coll Cardiol 2014;63:141–9. [cited 2015 Aug 26] Available from: http://www.pubmedcentral.nih.gov/articlerender.fcgi?artid=3954563&tool=pmcentrez&rendertype=abstract.

[241] Merlet P, Delforge J, Syrota A, Angevin E, Mazière B, Crouzel C, et al. Positron emission tomography with 11C CGP-12177 to assess beta-adrenergic receptor concentration in idiopathic dilated cardiomyopathy. Circulation 1993;87:1169–78. [cited 2015 Aug 25] Available from: http://www.ncbi.nlm.nih.gov/pubmed/8096441.

[242] Choudhury L, Rosen SD, Lefroy DC, Nihoyannopoulos P, Oakley CM, Camici PG. Myocardial beta adrenoceptor density in primary and secondary left ventricular hypertrophy. Eur Heart J 1996;17:1703–9. [cited 2015 Aug 25] Available from: http://www.ncbi.nlm.nih.gov/pubmed/8922919.

[243] John AS, Mongillo M, Depre C, Khan MT, Rimoldi OE, Pepper JR, et al. Pre- and postsynaptic sympathetic function in human hibernating myocardium. Eur J Nucl Med Mol

Imaging 2007;34:1973–80. [cited 2015 Aug 26] Available from: http://www.ncbi.nlm.nih.gov/pubmed/17661029.

[244] Ohte N, Narita H, Iida A, Fukuta H, Iizuka N, Hayano J, et al. Cardiac β-adrenergic receptor density and myocardial systolic function in the remote noninfarcted region after prior myocardial infarction with left ventricular remodelling. Eur J Nucl Med Mol Imaging 2012;39:1246–53. [cited 2015 Aug 26] Available from: http://www.ncbi.nlm.nih.gov/pubmed/22588626.

[245] Kenk M, Thackeray JT, Thorn SL, Dhami K, Chow BJ, Ascah KJ, et al. Alterations of pre- and postsynaptic noradrenergic signaling in a rat model of adriamycin-induced cardiotoxicity. J Nucl Cardiol 2010;17:254–63. [cited 2015 Aug 25] Available from: http://www.ncbi.nlm.nih.gov/pubmed/20182926.

[246] Yu M, Bozek J, Lamoy M, Kagan M, Benites P, Onthank D, et al. LMI1195 PET imaging in evaluation of regional cardiac sympathetic denervation and its potential role in antiarrhythmic drug treatment. Eur J Nucl Med Mol Imaging 2012;39:1910–19. [cited 2015 Aug 25]Available from: http://www.ncbi.nlm.nih.gov/pubmed/22865199.

[247] Yu M, Bozek J, Lamoy M, Guaraldi M, Silva P, Kagan M, et al. Evaluation of LMI1195, a novel 18F-labeled cardiac neuronal PET imaging agent, in cells and animal models. Circ Cardiovasc Imaging 2011;4:435–43. [cited 2015 Aug 25] Available from: http://www.ncbi.nlm.nih.gov/pubmed/21555377.

[248] Ono M, Takahashi T. [123I-MIBG scintigraphy in cardiotoxicity related to antineoplastic agents]. Kaku Igaku 1994;31:451–8. [cited 2015 Aug 25] Available from: http://www.ncbi.nlm.nih.gov/pubmed/8028217.

[249] Nousiainen T, Vanninen E, Jantunen E, Remes J, Kuikka J, Hartikainen J. Anthracycline-induced cardiomyopathy: long-term effects on myocardial cell integrity, cardiac adrenergic innervation and fatty acid uptake. Clin Physiol 2001;21:123–8. [cited 2015 Aug 24] Available from: http://www.ncbi.nlm.nih.gov/pubmed/11168306.

[250] Kremer LC, Tiel-van Buul MM, Ubbink MC, Offringa M, Ottenkamp J, Olmos RV, et al. Indium-111-antimyosin scintigraphy in the early detection of heart damage after anthracycline therapy in children. J Clin Oncol 1999;17:1208. [cited 2015 Aug 22] Available from: http://www.ncbi.nlm.nih.gov/pubmed/10561180.

[251] Erselcan T, Kairemo KJ, Wiklund TA, Hernberg M, Blomqvist CP, Tenhunen M, et al. Subclinical cardiotoxicity following adjuvant dose-escalated FEC, high-dose chemotherapy, or CMF in breast cancer. Br J Cancer 2000;82:777–81. [cited 2015 Aug 25] Available from: http://www.pubmedcentral.nih.gov/articlerender.fcgi?artid=2374396&tool=pmcentrez&rendertype=abstract.

[252] Valdés Olmos RA, Carrió I, Hoefnagel CA, Estorch M, ten Bokkel Huinink WW, López-Pousa J, et al. High sensitivity of radiolabelled antimyosin scintigraphy in assessing anthracycline related early myocyte damage preceding cardiac dysfunction. Nucl Med Commun 2002;23:871–7. [cited 2015 Aug 25] Available from: http://www.ncbi.nlm.nih.gov/pubmed/12195092.

[253] Yu D, Hung MC. Overexpression of ErbB2 in cancer and ErbB2-targeting strategies. Oncogene 2000;19:6115–21. [cited 2015 Aug 24] Available from: http://www.ncbi.nlm.nih.gov/pubmed/11156524.

[254] Slamon DJ, Leyland-Jones B, Shak S, Fuchs H, Paton V, Bajamonde A, et al. Use of chemotherapy plus a monoclonal antibody against HER2 for metastatic breast cancer that overexpresses HER2. N Engl J Med 2001;344:783–92. [cited 2015 Jul 1] Available from: http://www.ncbi.nlm.nih.gov/pubmed/11248153.

[255] Molina MA, Codony-Servat J, Albanell J, Rojo F, Arribas J, Baselga J. Trastuzumab (herceptin), a humanized anti-Her2 receptor monoclonal antibody, inhibits basal and activated Her2 ectodomain cleavage in breast cancer cells. Cancer Res 2001; 61:4744–9. [cited 2015 Aug 24] Available from: http://www.ncbi.nlm.nih.gov/pubmed/11406546.

[256] Press MF, Pike MC, Chazin VR, Hung G, Udove JA, Markowicz M, et al. Her-2/neu expression in node-negative breast cancer: direct tissue quantitation by computerized image analysis and association of overexpression with increased risk of recurrent disease. Cancer Res 1993;53:4960–70. [cited 2015 Aug 24] Available from: http://www.ncbi.nlm.nih.gov/pubmed/8104689.

[257] Milenic DE, Wong KJ, Baidoo KE, Nayak TK, Regino CAS, Garmestani K, et al. Targeting HER2: a report on the in vitro and in vivo pre-clinical data supporting trastuzumab as a radioimmunoconjugate for clinical trials. MAbs 2010;2:550–64. [cited 2015 Aug 24] Available from: http://www.pubmedcentral.nih.gov/articlerender.fcgi?artid=2958576&tool=pmcentrez&rendertype=abstract.

[258] Ellis LM, Hicklin DJ. Resistance to targeted therapies: refining anticancer therapy in the era of molecular oncology. Clin Cancer Res 2009;15:7471–8. [cited 2015 Aug 24] Available from: http://www.ncbi.nlm.nih.gov/pubmed/20008847.

[259] Lub-de Hooge MN, Kosterink JGW, Perik PJ, Nijnuis H, Tran L, Bart J, et al. Preclinical characterisation of 111In-DTPA-trastuzumab. Br J Pharmacol 2004;143:99–106. [cited 2015 Aug 24] Available from: http://www.pubmedcentral.nih.gov/articlerender.fcgi?artid=1575276&tool=pmcentrez&rendertype=abstract.

[260] Robinson MK, Doss M, Shaller C, Narayanan D, Marks JD, Adler LP, et al. Quantitative immuno-positron emission tomography imaging of HER2-positive tumor xenografts with an iodine-124 labeled anti-HER2 diabody. Cancer Res 2005;65:1471–8. [cited 2015 Aug 24] Available from: http://www.ncbi.nlm.nih.gov/pubmed/15735035.

[261] Dijkers ECF, Kosterink JGW, Rademaker AP, Perk LR, van Dongen GAMS, Bart J, et al. Development and characterization of clinical-grade 89Zr-trastuzumab for HER2/neu immunoPET imaging. J Nucl Med 2009;50:974–81. [cited 2015 Aug 24] Available from: http://www.ncbi.nlm.nih.gov/pubmed/19443585.

[262] Goldstein R, Sosabowski J, Vigor K, Chester K, Meyer T. Developments in single photon emission computed tomography and PET-based HER2 molecular imaging for breast cancer. Expert Rev Anticancer Ther 2013;13:359–73. [cited 2015 Aug 24] Available from: http://www.ncbi.nlm.nih.gov/pubmed/23477521.

[263] Tamura K, Kurihara H, Yonemori K, Tsuda H, Suzuki J, Kono Y, et al. 64Cu-DOTA-trastuzumab PET imaging in patients with HER2-positive breast cancer. J Nucl Med 2013;54:1869–75. [cited 2015 May 27] Available from: http://www.ncbi.nlm.nih.gov/pubmed/24029656.

[264] Mortimer JE, Bading JR, Colcher DM, Conti PS, Frankel PH, Carroll MI, et al. Functional imaging of human epidermal growth factor receptor 2-positive metastatic breast cancer using (64)Cu-DOTA-trastuzumab PET. J Nucl Med 2014;55:23–9. [cited 2015 Jul 19] Available from: http://www.pubmedcentral.nih.gov/articlerender.fcgi?artid=4084518&tool=pmcentrez&rendertype=abstract.

[265] Beylergil V, Morris PG, Smith-Jones PM, Modi S, Solit D, Hudis CA, et al. Pilot study of 68Ga-DOTA-F(ab′)2-trastuzumab in patients with breast cancer. Nucl Med Commun 2013;34:1157–65. [cited 2015 Aug 24] Available from: http://www.pubmedcentral.nih.gov/articlerender.fcgi?artid=3815146&tool=pmcentrez&rendertype=abstract.

[266] Behr TM, Béhé M, Wörmann B. Trastuzumab and breast cancer. N Engl J Med 2001;345:995–6. [cited 2015 Aug 23] Available from: http://www.ncbi.nlm.nih.gov/pubmed/11575295.

[267] De Korte MA, de Vries EGE, Lub-de Hooge MN, Jager PL, Gietema JA, van der Graaf WTA, et al. 111Indium-trastuzumab visualises myocardial human epidermal growth factor receptor 2 expression shortly after anthracycline treatment but not during heart failure: a clue to uncover the mechanisms of trastuzumab-related cardiotoxicity. Eur J Cancer 2007;43:2046–51. [cited 2015 Aug 23] Available from: http://www.ncbi.nlm.nih.gov/pubmed/17719768.

[268] Perik PJ, Lub-De Hooge MN, Gietema JA, van der Graaf WTA, de Korte MA, Jonkman S, et al. Indium-111-labeled trastuzumab scintigraphy in patients with human epidermal growth factor receptor 2-positive metastatic breast cancer. J Clin Oncol 2006;24:2276–82. [cited 2015 Aug 24] Available from: http://www.ncbi.nlm.nih.gov/pubmed/16710024.

[269] Gavrieli Y, Sherman Y, Ben-Sasson SA. Identification of programmed cell death in situ via specific labeling of nuclear DNA fragmentation. J Cell Biol 1992;119:493–501. [cited 2015 Jul 25] Available from: http://www.pubmedcentral.nih.gov/articlerender.fcgi?artid=2289665&tool=pmcentrez&rendertype=abstract.

[270] Koopman G, Reutelingsperger CP, Kuijten GA, Keehnen RM, Pals ST, van Oers MH. Annexin V for flow cytometric detection of phosphatidylserine expression on B cells undergoing apoptosis. Blood 1994; 84:1415–20. [cited 2015 May 18] Available from: http://www.ncbi.nlm.nih.gov/pubmed/8068938.

[271] Chan A, Reiter R, Wiese S, Fertig G, Gold R. Plasma membrane phospholipid asymmetry precedes DNA fragmentation in different apoptotic cell models. Histochem Cell Biol 1998;110:553–8. [cited 2015 Aug 26] Available from: http://www.ncbi.nlm.nih.gov/pubmed/9860253.

[272] Boersma AW, Nooter K, Oostrum RG, Stoter G. Quantification of apoptotic cells with fluorescein isothiocyanate-labeled annexin V in chinese hamster ovary cell cultures treated with cisplatin. Cytometry 1996;24:123–30. [cited 2015 Aug 26] Available from: http://www.ncbi.nlm.nih.gov/pubmed/8725661.

[273] Orrenius S. Apoptosis: molecular mechanisms and implications for human disease. J Intern Med 1995;237:529–36. [cited 2015 Aug 26] Available from: http://www.ncbi.nlm.nih.gov/pubmed/7782723.

[274] Wu J. Apoptosis and angiogenesis: two promising tumor markers in breast cancer (review). Anticancer Res 1996;16:2233–9. [cited 2015 Aug 26] Available from: http://www.ncbi.nlm.nih.gov/pubmed/8694549.

[275] Olson M, Kornbluth S. Mitochondria in apoptosis and human disease. Curr Mol Med 2001;1:91–122. [cited 2015 Aug 26] Available from: http://www.ncbi.nlm.nih.gov/pubmed/11899246.

[276] Ameisen JC. On the origin, evolution, and nature of programmed cell death: a timeline of four billion years. Cell Death Differ 2002;9:367–93. [cited 2015 Aug 12] Available from: http://www.ncbi.nlm.nih.gov/pubmed/11965491.

[277] Martin SJ, Reutelingsperger CP, McGahon AJ, Rader JA, van Schie RC, LaFace DM, et al. Early redistribution of plasma membrane phosphatidylserine is a general feature of apoptosis regardless of the initiating stimulus: inhibition by overexpression of Bcl-2 and Abl. J Exp Med 1995;182:1545–56. [cited 2015 Aug 26] Available from: http://www.pubmedcentral.nih.gov/articlerender.fcgi?artid=2192182&tool=pmcentrez&rendertype=abstract.

[278] Evan GI, Vousden KH. Proliferation, cell cycle and apoptosis in cancer. Nature 2001;411:342–8. [cited 2015 Aug 1] Available from: http://www.ncbi.nlm.nih.gov/pubmed/11357141.

[279] Dive C, Hickman JA. Drug-target interactions: only the first step in the commitment to a programmed cell death? Br J Cancer 1991;64:192–6. [cited 2015 Aug 26] Available from: http://www.pubmedcentral.nih.gov/articlerender.fcgi?artid=1977304&tool=pmcentrez&rendertype=abstract.

[280] Blankenberg FG. In vivo detection of apoptosis. J Nucl Med 2008;49(Suppl. 2):81S–95S. [cited 2015 Aug 26] Available from: http://www.ncbi.nlm.nih.gov/pubmed/18523067.

[281] Martin SJ, Finucane DM, Amarante-Mendes GP, O'Brien GA, Green DR. Phosphatidylserine externalization during CD95-induced apoptosis of cells and cytoplasts requires ICE/CED-3 protease activity. J Biol Chem 1996;271:28753–6. [cited 2015 Aug 26] Available from: http://www.ncbi.nlm.nih.gov/pubmed/8910516.

[282] Van den Eijnde SM, Boshart L, Reutelingsperger CP, De Zeeuw CI, Vermeij-Keers C. Phosphatidylserine plasma membrane asymmetry in vivo: a pancellular phenomenon which alters during apoptosis. Cell Death Differ 1997;4:311–16. [cited 2015 Aug 26] Available from: http://www.ncbi.nlm.nih.gov/pubmed/16465246.

[283] Stace CL, Ktistakis NT. Phosphatidic acid- and phosphatidylserine-binding proteins. Biochim Biophys Acta 2006;1761:913–26. [cited 2015 Aug 26] Available from: http://www.ncbi.nlm.nih.gov/pubmed/16624617.

[284] Burtea C, Laurent S, Lancelot E, Ballet S, Murariu O, Rousseaux O, et al. Peptidic targeting of phosphatidylserine for the MRI detection of apoptosis in atherosclerotic plaques. Mol Pharm 2009;6:1903–19. [cited 2015 Jul 10] Available from: http://www.ncbi.nlm.nih.gov/pubmed/19743879.

[285] Igarashi K, Kaneda M, Yamaji A, Saido TC, Kikkawa U, Ono Y, et al. A novel phosphatidylserine-binding peptide motif defined by an anti-idiotypic monoclonal antibody. Localization of phosphatidylserine-specific binding sites on protein kinase C and phosphatidylserine decarboxylase. J Biol Chem 1995;270:29075–8. [cited 2015 Aug 1] Available from: http://www.ncbi.nlm.nih.gov/pubmed/7493929.

[286] Laumonier C, Segers J, Laurent S, Michel A, Coppée F, Belayew A, et al. A new peptidic vector for molecular imaging of apoptosis, identified by phage display technology. J Biomol Screen 2006;11:537–45. [cited 2015 Jul 10] Available from: http://www.ncbi.nlm.nih.gov/pubmed/16760366.

[287] Thapa N, Kim S, So I-S, Lee B-H, Kwon I-C, Choi K, et al. Discovery of a phosphatidylserine-recognizing peptide and its utility in molecular imaging of tumour apoptosis. J Cell Mol Med 2008;12:1649–60. [cited 2015 Jul 10] Available from: http://www.pubmedcentral.nih.gov/articlerender.fcgi?artid=3918081&tool=pmcentrez&rendertype=abstract.

[288] Hanshaw RG, Smith BD. New reagents for phosphatidylserine recognition and detection of apoptosis. Bioorg Med Chem 2005;13:5035–42. [cited 2015 Jun 21] Available from: http://www.ncbi.nlm.nih.gov/pubmed/15914007.

[289] Schutters K, Reutelingsperger C. Phosphatidylserine targeting for diagnosis and treatment of human diseases. Apoptosis 2010;15:1072–82. [cited 2015 Aug 26] Available from: http://www.pubmedcentral.nih.gov/articlerender.fcgi?artid=2929432&tool=pmcentrez&rendertype=abstract.

[290] Maurer-Fogy I, Reutelingsperger CP, Pieters J, Bodo G, Stratowa C, Hauptmann R. Cloning and expression of cDNA for human vascular anticoagulant, a Ca^{2+}-dependent

phospholipid-binding protein. Eur J Biochem 1988;174:585–92. [cited 2015 Aug 26] Available from: http://www.ncbi.nlm.nih.gov/pubmed/2455636.

[291] Boersma HH, Liem IH, Kemerink GJ, Thimister PWL, Hofstra L, Stolk LML, et al. Comparison between human pharmacokinetics and imaging properties of two conjugation methods for 99mTc-annexin A5. Br J Radiol 2003;76:553–60. [cited 2015 Aug 26] Available from: http://www.ncbi.nlm.nih.gov/pubmed/12893698.

[292] Kemerink GJ, Liu X, Kieffer D, Ceyssens S, Mortelmans L, Verbruggen AM, et al. Safety, biodistribution, and dosimetry of 99mTc-HYNIC-annexin V, a novel human recombinant annexin V for human application. J Nucl Med 2003;44:947–52. [cited 2015 Aug 26] Available from: http://www.ncbi.nlm.nih.gov/pubmed/12791824.

[293] Tait JF, Smith C, Levashova Z, Patel B, Blankenberg FG, Vanderheyden J-L. Improved detection of cell death in vivo with annexin V radiolabeled by site-specific methods. J Nucl Med 2006;47:1546–53. [cited 2015 Aug 26] Available from: http://www.ncbi.nlm.nih.gov/pubmed/16954565.

[294] Tait JF, Brown DS, Gibson DF, Blankenberg FG, Strauss HW. Development and characterization of annexin V mutants with endogenous chelation sites for (99m)Tc. Bioconjug Chem 2000;11:918–25. [cited 2015 Aug 26] Available from: http://www.ncbi.nlm.nih.gov/pubmed/11087342.

[295] Li X, Link JM, Stekhova S, Yagle KJ, Smith C, Krohn KA, et al. Site-specific labeling of annexin V with F-18 for apoptosis imaging. Bioconjug Chem 2008;19:1684–8. [cited 2015 Aug 26] Available from: http://www.pubmedcentral.nih.gov/articlerender.fcgi?artid=2646751&tool=pmcentrez&rendertype=abstract.

[296] Schellenberger E, Schnorr J, Reutelingsperger C, Ungethüm L, Meyer W, Taupitz M, et al. Linking proteins with anionic nanoparticles via protamine: ultrasmall protein-coupled probes for magnetic resonance imaging of apoptosis. Small 2008;4:225–30. [cited 2015 Aug 26] Available from: http://www.ncbi.nlm.nih.gov/pubmed/18203233.

[297] De Saint-Hubert M, Mottaghy FM, Vunckx K, Nuyts J, Fonge H, Prinsen K, et al. Site-specific labeling of "second generation" annexin V with 99mTc(CO)3 for improved imaging of apoptosis in vivo. Bioorg Med Chem 2010;18:1356–63. [cited 2015 Jul 30] Available from: http://www.ncbi.nlm.nih.gov/pubmed/20053567.

[298] Prinzen L, Miserus R-JJHM, Dirksen A, Hackeng TM, Deckers N, Bitsch NJ, et al. Optical and magnetic resonance imaging of cell death and platelet activation using annexin a5-functionalized quantum dots. Nano Lett 2007;7:93–100. [cited 2015 Aug 26] Available from: http://www.ncbi.nlm.nih.gov/pubmed/17212446.

[299] Van Tilborg GAF, Mulder WJM, Deckers N, Storm G, Reutelingsperger CPM, Strijkers GJ, et al. Annexin A5-functionalized bimodal lipid-based contrast agents for the detection of apoptosis. Bioconjug Chem 2006;17:741–9. [cited 2015 Aug 26] Available from: http://www.ncbi.nlm.nih.gov/pubmed/16704213.

[300] Garnier B, Bouter A, Gounou C, Petry KG, Brisson AR. Annexin A5-functionalized liposomes for targeting phosphatidylserine-exposing membranes. Bioconjug Chem 2009; 20:2114–22. [cited 2015 Aug 26] Available from: http://www.ncbi.nlm.nih.gov/pubmed/19835411.

[301] Murakami Y, Takamatsu H, Taki J, Tatsumi M, Noda A, Ichise R, et al. 18F-labelled annexin V: a PET tracer for apoptosis imaging. Eur J Nucl Med Mol Imaging 2004;31:469–74. [cited 2015 Aug 26] Available from: http://www.ncbi.nlm.nih.gov/pubmed/14666384.

[302] Lahorte CMM, van de Wiele C, Bacher K, van den Bossche B, Thierens H, van Belle S, et al. Biodistribution and dosimetry study of 123I-rh-annexin V in mice and humans. Nucl Med Commun 2003;24:871–80. [cited 2015 Aug 26] Available from: http://www.ncbi.nlm.nih.gov/pubmed/12869819.

[303] Keen HG, Dekker BA, Disley L, Hastings D, Lyons S, Reader AJ, et al. Imaging apoptosis in vivo using 124I-annexin V and PET. Nucl Med Biol 2005;32:395–402. [cited 2015 Jul 30] Available from: http://www.ncbi.nlm.nih.gov/pubmed/15878509.

[304] Cauchon N, Langlois R, Rousseau JA, Tessier G, Cadorette J, Lecomte R, et al. PET imaging of apoptosis with (64)Cu-labeled streptavidin following pretargeting of phosphatidylserine with biotinylated annexin-V. Eur J Nucl Med Mol Imaging 2007;34:247–58. [cited 2015 Aug 26] Available from: http://www.ncbi.nlm.nih.gov/pubmed/17021816.

[305] Rottey S, Loose D, Vakaet L, Lahorte C, Vermeersch H, Van Belle S, et al. 99mTc-HYNIC Annexin-V imaging of tumors and its relationship to response to radiotherapy and/or chemotherapy. Q J Nucl Med Mol Imaging Off Publ Ital Assoc Nucl Med [and] Int Assoc Radiopharmacol (IAR), [and] Sect Soc Radiopharm 2007;51:182–8. [cited 2015 Aug 26] Available from: http://www.ncbi.nlm.nih.gov/pubmed/17220821.

[306] Panjrath GS, Patel V, Valdiviezo CI, Narula N, Narula J, Jain D. Potentiation of Doxorubicin cardiotoxicity by iron loading in a rodent model. J Am Coll Cardiol 2007;49:2457–64. [cited 2015 Aug 7] Available from: http://www.ncbi.nlm.nih.gov/pubmed/17599610.

[307] Gabrielson KL, Mok GSP, Nimmagadda S, Bedja D, Pin S, Tsao A, et al. Detection of dose response in chronic doxorubicin-mediated cell death with cardiac technetium 99m annexin V single-photon emission computed tomography. Mol Imaging 2008;7:132–8. [cited 2015 Aug 25] Available from: http://www.ncbi.nlm.nih.gov/pubmed/19123983.

[308] Chatham JC, Cousins JP, Glickson JD. The relationship between cardiac function and metabolism in acute adriamycin-treated perfused rat hearts studied by 31P and 13C NMR spectroscopy. J Mol Cell Cardiol 1990;22:1187–97. [cited 2015 Aug 25] Available from: http://www.ncbi.nlm.nih.gov/pubmed/2095440.

[309] Ng TC, Daugherty JP, Evanochko WT, Digerness SB, Durant JR, Glickson JD. Detection of antineoplastic agent induced cardiotoxicity by 31P NMR of perfused rat hearts. Biochem Biophys Res Commun 1983;110:339–47. [cited 2015 Aug 25] Available from: http://www.ncbi.nlm.nih.gov/pubmed/6838522.

[310] Glickson JD, Forder JR, Chatham JC. Imaging of Cardiotoxicity. Mol Imaging 2008;7:115–17.

[311] Su H, Gorodny N, Gomez LF, Gangadharmath U, Mu F, Chen G, et al. Noninvasive molecular imaging of apoptosis in a mouse model of anthracycline-induced cardiotoxicity. Circ Cardiovasc Imaging 2015;8:1–18.

[312] Lopaschuk GD, Collins-Nakai RL, Itoi T. Developmental changes in energy substrate use by the heart. Cardiovasc Res 1992;26:1172–80. [cited 2015 Aug 25] Available from: http://www.ncbi.nlm.nih.gov/pubmed/1288863.

[313] Makinde AO, Kantor PF, Lopaschuk GD. Maturation of fatty acid and carbohydrate metabolism in the newborn heart. Mol Cell Biochem 1998;188:49–56. [cited 2015 Aug 25] Available from: http://www.ncbi.nlm.nih.gov/pubmed/9823010.

[314] Stanley WC, Lopaschuk GD, Hall JL, McCormack JG. Regulation of myocardial carbohydrate metabolism under normal and ischaemic conditions. Potential for pharmacological interventions. Cardiovasc Res 1997;33:243–57. [cited 2015 Aug 25] Available from: http://www.ncbi.nlm.nih.gov/pubmed/9074687.

[315] Liedtke AJ. Alterations of carbohydrate and lipid metabolism in the acutely ischemic heart. Prog Cardiovasc Dis 1981;23:321–36. [cited 2015 Aug 25] Available from: http://www.ncbi.nlm.nih.gov/pubmed/7012926.

[316] Mitra B, Panja M. Myocardial metabolism: pharmacological manipulation in myocardial ischaemia. J Assoc Physicians India 2005;53:552–60. [cited 2015 Aug 25] Available from: http://www.ncbi.nlm.nih.gov/pubmed/16121812.

[317] Bergmann SR. Imaging of myocardial fatty acid metabolism with PET. J Nucl Cardiol 2007;14:S118–24. [cited 2015 Aug 25] Available from: http://www.ncbi.nlm.nih.gov/pubmed/17556179.

[318] Takeishi Y, Sukekawa H, Sakurai T, Saito H, Nishimura S, Shibu T, et al. Noninvasive identification of anthracycline cardiotoxicity: comparison of 123I-MIBG and 123I-BMIPP imaging. Ann Nucl Med 1994;177–82. [cited 2015 Aug 25] Available from: http://www.ncbi.nlm.nih.gov/pubmed/7811559.

[319] Saito K, Takeda K, Okamoto S, Okamoto R, Makino K, Tameda Y, et al. Detection of doxorubicin cardiotoxicity by using iodine-123 BMIPP early dynamic SPECT: quantitative evaluation of early abnormality of fatty acid metabolism with the Rutland method. J Nucl Cardiol 2000;7:553–61. [cited 2015 Aug 22] Available from: http://www.ncbi.nlm.nih.gov/pubmed/11144469.

[320] Kitagawa K, Takeda K, Saito K, Okamoto S, Makino K, Maeda H, et al. Differences in fatty acid metabolic disorder between ischemic myocardium and doxorubicin-induced myocardial damage: assessment using BMIPP dynamic SPECT with analysis by the Rutland method. J Nucl Med 2002;43:1286–94. [cited 2015 Aug 22] Available from: http://www.ncbi.nlm.nih.gov/pubmed/12368365.

[321] Umezawa R, Takase K, Jingu K, Takanami K, Ota H, Kaneta T, et al. Evaluation of radiation-induced myocardial damage using iodine-123-methyl-iodophenyl pentadecanoic acid scintigraphy. J Radiat Res 2013;54:880–9. [cited 2015 Aug 25] Available from: http://www.pubmedcentral.nih.gov/articlerender.fcgi?artid=3766284&tool=pmcentrez&rendertype=abstract.

[322] Umezawa R, Takanami K, Kadoya N, Nakajima Y, Saito M, Ota H, et al. Assessment of myocardial metabolic disorder associated with mediastinal radiotherapy for esophageal cancer—a pilot study. Radiat Oncol 2015;10:96. [cited 2015 Aug 25] Available from: http://www.pubmedcentral.nih.gov/articlerender.fcgi?artid=4407329&tool=pmcentrez&rendertype=abstract.

[323] Peterson LR, Gropler RJ. Radionuclide imaging of myocardial metabolism. Circ Cardiovasc Imaging 2010;3:211–22. [cited 2015 Aug 25] Available from: http://www.pubmedcentral.nih.gov/articlerender.fcgi?artid=2892800&tool=pmcentrez&rendertype=abstract.

[324] Croteau E, Tremblay S, Gascon S, Dumulon-perreault V, Labbé SM, Rousseau JA, et al. [11 C]-Acetoacetate PET imaging: a potential early marker for cardiac heart failure. Nucl Med Biol 2014;41:863–70. Available from: http://dx.doi.org/10.1016/j.nucmedbio.2014.08.006.

[325] Ivanová M, Dovinová I, Okruhlicová L, Tribulová N, Simončíková P, Barte-ková M, et al. Chronic cardiotoxicity of doxorubicin involves activation of myocardial and circulating matrix metalloproteinases in rats. Acta Pharmacol Sin 2012;33:459–69. [cited 2015 Sep 1] Available from: http://www.pubmedcentral.nih.gov/articlerender.fcgi?artid=4003364&tool=pmcentrez&rendertype=abstract.

[326] Polegato BF, Minicucci MF, Azevedo PS, Carvalho RF, Chiuso-Minicucci F, Pereira EJ, et al. Acute doxorubicin-induced cardiotoxicity is associated with matrix metalloproteinase-

2 alterations in rats. Cell Physiol Biochem 2015;35:1924–33. [cited 2015 Sep 1] Available from: http://www.ncbi.nlm.nih.gov/pubmed/25871735.

[327] Meyersohn NNM, Pursnani A, Neilan TG. Detection of cardiac toxicity due to cancer treatment: role of cardiac MRI. Curr Treat Options Cardiovasc Med 2015;17:396. [cited 2015 Aug 23] Available from: http://www.ncbi.nlm.nih.gov/pubmed/26134969.

[328] Judenhofer MS, Wehrl HF, Newport DF, Catana C, Siegel SB, Becker M, et al. Simultaneous PET-MRI: a new approach for functional and morphological imaging. Nat Med 2008;14:459–65. [cited 2015 Aug 3] Available from: http://www.ncbi.nlm.nih.gov/pubmed/18376410.

[329] Majmudar MD, Nahrendorf M. Cardiovascular molecular imaging: the road ahead. J Nucl Med 2012;53:673–6. [cited 2015 Aug 17] Available from: http://www.pubmedcentral.nih.gov/articlerender.fcgi?artid=3744821&tool=pmcentrez&rendertype=abstract.

[330] Rischpler C, Nekolla SG, Kunze KP, Schwaiger M. PET/MRI of the heart. Semin Nucl Med 2015;45:234–47. [cited 2015 Aug 5] Available from: http://www.ncbi.nlm.nih.gov/pubmed/25841278.

Section V

Detection of Cardiac Dysfunction and Predictors of Cardiotoxicity

Chapter 23

Detection by Cardiac Imaging: LV Ejection Fraction, Diastolic Dysfunction, Tissue Doppler, and Speckle Tracking Echocardiography

J.C. Plana

Chapter Outline

LV EJECTION FRACTION

Historically the strategy for the detection of cardiac dysfunction has been based on the performance of serial echocardiograms aimed at recognizing an asymptomatic drop in left ventricular ejection fraction (LVEF). However, this approach has two important limitations. First, 2D echocardiography (2DE) is not well-suited for this task, as its temporal variability allows recognition of reductions of 10 points of ejection fraction or higher [1]. Second, the reduction in LVEF occurs at a late stage, at a point where LVEF recovery and cardiac event reduction may no longer be achievable despite aggressive heart failure therapy [2]. As a result, new imaging modalities have been evaluated for the early detection of cardiac dysfunction.

DIASTOLIC DYSFUNCTION

The recently published expert consensus for the multimodality imaging evaluation of the patient during and after cancer therapy recommends a comprehensive

Anticancer Treatments and Cardiotoxicity. DOI: http://dx.doi.org/10.1016/B978-0-12-802509-3.00023-6

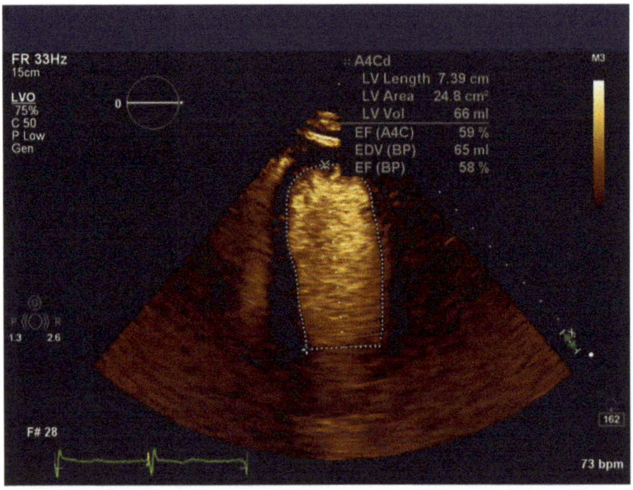

FIGURE 23.1 End-diastolic endocardial tracing obtained from the apical four-chamber view after the administration of contrast for the calculation of LVEF using the method of disks in a patient with inadequate 2D echocardiographical images. *From Plana JC, et al. Expert consensus for multimodality imaging evaluation of adult patients during and after cancer therapy: a report from the American Society of Echocardiography and the European Association of Cardiovascular Imaging. Eur Heart J Cardiovasc Imaging 2014;15(10):1063–1093.*

assessment of diastology including grading of diastolic function and providing an estimate of LV filling pressures (by using E/e′ ratios). Care should be exerted while using E/e′ ratio, as fluctuations of E and e′ velocities can be the result of changes in loading conditions and not the result of real change in left ventricular (LV) diastolic performance (Fig. 23.1).

Due to this limitation and to their inability to predict subsequent heart failure, they do not recommend the use of Doppler-derived diastolic indices in the early detection of cardiac dysfunction.

STRAIN IMAGING

Strain is a measurement of myocardial deformation. As the heart contracts, muscle shortens in the longitudinal and circumferential dimensions (negative strain), and thickens and lengthens in the radial direction (positive strain). Strain can be readily measured during routine echocardiography, providing an assessment of global and regional function. Strain imaging can be measured with the use of either tissue Doppler or two-dimensional-based methods.

Tissue Doppler-Based Strain

Tissue Doppler-based strain suffers from the same limitations as traditional Doppler echocardiography (i.e., angle dependency). That, along with the fact that the comparison of adjacent velocities is exquisitely sensitive to signal noise, makes its application for clinical purposes extremely challenging.

Two-Dimensional-Based Strain (Speckle Tracking Echocardiography)

The angle independency, signal noise ratio, and the ability to evaluate strain in two dimensions makes it attractive when compared to its tissue Doppler counterpart [3].

Two-dimensional speckle tracking echocardiography (STE) has evolved to be the imaging modality of choice for the detection of subclinical cardiac dysfunction. There are two recent studies describing normal global longitudinal strain values for the adult patient. Kocabay et al. reported a normal global longitudinal strain (GLS) (mean $\pm$ SD) of -20.7 ± 2 for males, and -22.1 ± 1.8 for females. Lower limits of normality (2 SD below the mean) are -16.7% in men, and -18.5% in women [4]. These values are almost identical to the ones previously reported by the JUSTICE study for the same vendor [5]. Cheng et al. recently evaluated the reproducibility of 2D STE in the Offspring Cohort of the Framingham Heart Study. The interobserver intraclass correlation coefficient was ≥ 0.84 for all global strain measurements, with an average coefficient of variation for GLS of $\leq 4\%$. The intraobserver intraclass correlation coefficient was ≥ 0.91 among time points spanning a total 8-month period, with an average of $\leq 6\%$ for GLS. The authors concluded that 2D-STE is reproducible when performed by trained operators [6]. However, there are no data as to the reproducibility of GLS in nonacademic centers or community hospitals. The presence of a learning curve makes dedicated training and monitoring of quality (i.e., intra-, interobserver and test retest variability) essential.

The most important limitation of 2D STE is the intervendor variability [5]. Different echo machines and software solutions may produce different strain results, making their comparison over time for a given patient challenging. Recognizing the critical need for standardization in strain imaging, the American Society of Echocardiography (ASE) and the European Association of Cardiovascular Imaging (EACVI) have recently completed an effort to reduce intervendor variability of strain measurement. Nevertheless, it is recommended to use the same vendor machine and software version for the serial evaluation of global longitudinal strain.

Strain imaging has been studied in two different settings in cardio-oncology:

1. Early detection of subclinical LV dysfunction.
   Studies performed in cardio-oncology patients receiving potentially cardiotoxic agents have shown that myocardial strain is more sensitive than LVEF in the detection of subclinical cardiac dysfunction.

A decrease of longitudinal and radial strain and strain rate was observed after the first anthracycline dose in children with leukemia, whereas LVEF remained unchanged until the second cycle had been completed [7]. This early decrease in deformation indices was confirmed by subsequent studies of adult patients treated with anthracyclines [8,9]. Similarly, myocardial strain decreased early after anthracyclines in breast cancer patients treated with anthracyclines followed by taxanes and trastuzumab [10–12].

2. Prognosis of cancer therapeutics-related cardiac dysfunction (CTRCD) using strain imaging.
   Strain imaging has been shown experimentally to predict subsequent CTRCD. In a mouse model of doxorubicin-induced cardiotoxicity, Neilan et al. demonstrated that radial strain rate predicted subsequent heart failure and death [13].
   A recent systematic review by Thavendiranathan et al. showed that as of 2014, 21 peer-reviewed studies evaluated the role of deformation indices (strain, strain rate, twist) in the detection of the subclinical left ventricular dysfunction in patients treated for cancer [14].
   The prognostic role of strain imaging has been evaluated clinically using two different strategies:
   a. Use of reduction of GLS below a cut-off.
      In the study by Sawaya et al. in 81 women with breast cancer treated with anthracyclines followed by taxanes and trastuzumab and evaluated every 3 months for a period of 15 months, a decrease in longitudinal strain below −19% after the initial anthracycline treatment predicted the occurrence of subsequent CTRCD with a sensitivity and specificity of 74% and 73%, respectively. The imaging strategy was superior to the biomarker one (ultrasensitive Tn I), where sensitivity and specificity were reported at 48 and 73% respectively. It is important to specify that the GLS was calculated as an average of the basal and midventricular peak systolic longitudinal strain measured in apical four- and two-chamber views [10].
   b. Use of a relative reduction of GLS.
      In a second study, Negishi et al. found that ΔGLS (percentage reduction in GLS when compared to baseline) was the strongest predictor of CTRCD. The optimal cutoff was a relative reduction in strain higher than 11% (95% confidence interval 8.3–14.6%), with sensitivity of 65% and specificity of 94%. It was concluded that a relative reduction of <8% was of no clinical significance, while a relative reduction of >15% was of definite clinical significance. In sequential models, the clinical model was improved with the addition of GLS. A net of 29% of patients without events were reclassified into lower categories, while a net of 48% of the patients reclassified into higher-risk categories [15] (Fig. 23.2).

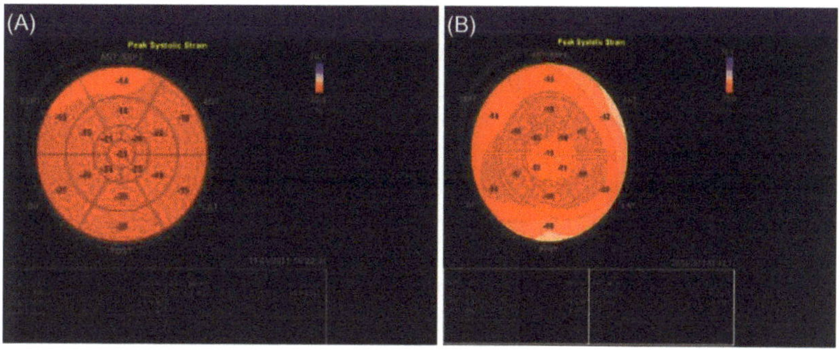

FIGURE 23.2 Bullseye plot showing GLS of patient with breast cancer treated with doxorubicin followed by trastuzumab. (A) GLS and regional longitudinal strain at baseline. (B) GLS and regional longitudinal strain 3 months during trastuzumab-based therapy after anthracyclines. GLS has decreased from −20.6% to −14.4% (30% decrease). The decrease is considered of clinical significance (>15% versus baseline). *From Plana JC et al. Expert consensus for multimodality imaging evaluation of adult patients during and after cancer therapy: a report from the American Society of Echocardiography and the European Association of Cardiovascular Imaging. Eur Heart J Cardiovasc Imaging 2014;15(10):1063–1093.*

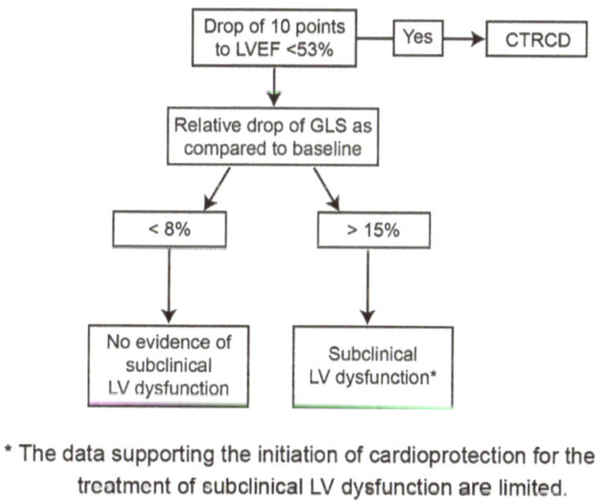

FIGURE 23.3 Early detection of subclinical cardiac dysfunction using GLS.

The ideal strategy for detection of subclinical cardiac dysfunction is to compare the measurements of GLS obtained during chemotherapy, with that obtained at baseline, allowing the patient to serve as her/his own control. A relative percentage reduction in GLS >15% is very likely to be abnormal and suggestive of subclinical LV dysfunction (Fig. 23.3). The abnormal GLS should be confirmed by a repeated study, performed 2–3 weeks following the initial abnormal one. When comparing GLS values, it is essential to keep in mind the load dependency of these measurements. The recently published ASE/EACVI expert consensus recommends reporting the timing of the echocardiogram with respect to the intravenous infusion of cancer therapeutics (number of days before or after treatment) as well as the vital signs measured during the test (BP and HR), recognizing that changes in loading conditions in the cancer patients are frequent, and may impact the GLS value (volume expansion due to the intravenous administration of chemotherapy or volume contraction due to vomiting or diarrhea) [16]. In the absence of a baseline GLS, the expert consensus refers the reader to the reference normal value table of the JUSTICE study, providing mean +/– SD for GLS. Subclinical LV dysfunction will be defined as a GLS 2 SD below the mean according to vendor, gender, and age.

CONCLUSIONS

Strain imaging appears to be a robust technique for the early identification of subclinical cardiac dysfunction and the prognostication of subsequent CTRCD. It is important to emphasize that the above-mentioned studies are small, and that larger studies with longer follow-up will be needed to independently validate these findings, and assess the value of deformation indices in the prediction of symptomatic heart failure and cardiac death.

REFERENCES

[1] Thavendiranathan P, et al. Reproducibility of echocardiographic techniques for sequential assessment of left ventricular ejection fraction and volumes: application to patients undergoing cancer chemotherapy. J Am Coll Cardiol 2013;61(1):77–84.

[2] Cardinale D, et al. Prevention of high-dose chemotherapy-induced cardiotoxicity in high-risk patients by angiotensin-converting enzyme inhibition. Circulation 2006;114(23):2474–81.

[3] Marwick TH. Measurement of strain and strain rate by echocardiography: ready for prime time? J Am Coll Cardiol 2006;47(7):1313–27.

[4] Kocabay G, et al. Normal left ventricular mechanics by two-dimensional speckle-tracking echocardiography. Reference values in healthy adults. Rev Esp Cardiol (Engl Ed) 2014;67(8):651–8.

[5] Takigiku K, et al. Normal range of left ventricular 2-dimensional strain: Japanese Ultrasound Speckle Tracking of the Left Ventricle (JUSTICE) study. Circ J 2012;76(11):2623–32.

[6] Cheng S, et al. Reproducibility of speckle-tracking-based strain measures of left ventricular function in a community-based study. J Am Soc Echocardiogr 2013;26(11):1258–66 e2.

[7] Ganame J, et al. Acute cardiac functional and morphological changes after Anthracycline infusions in children. Am J Cardiol 2007;99(7):974–7.

[8] Cadeddu C, et al. Protective effects of the angiotensin II receptor blocker telmisartan on epirubicin-induced inflammation, oxidative stress, and early ventricular impairment. Am Heart J 2010;160(3):487 e1–7.

[9] Jurcut R, et al. Strain rate imaging detects early cardiac effects of pegylated liposomal Doxorubicin as adjuvant therapy in elderly patients with breast cancer. J Am Soc Echocardiogr 2008;21(12):1283–9.

[10] Sawaya H, et al. Assessment of echocardiography and biomarkers for the extended prediction of cardiotoxicity in patients treated with anthracyclines, taxanes, and trastuzumab. Circ Cardiovasc Imaging 2012;5(5):596–603.

[11] Sawaya H, et al. Early detection and prediction of cardiotoxicity in chemotherapy-treated patients. Am J Cardiol 2011;107(9):1375–80.

[12] Fallah-Rad N, et al. The utility of cardiac biomarkers, tissue velocity and strain imaging, and cardiac magnetic resonance imaging in predicting early left ventricular dysfunction in patients with human epidermal growth factor receptor II-positive breast cancer treated with adjuvant trastuzumab therapy. J Am Coll Cardiol 2011;57(22):2263–70.

[13] Neilan TG, et al. Tissue Doppler imaging predicts left ventricular dysfunction and mortality in a murine model of cardiac injury. Eur Heart J 2006;27(15):1868–75.

[14] Thavendiranathan P, et al. Use of myocardial strain imaging by echocardiography for the early detection of cardiotoxicity in patients during and after cancer chemotherapy: a systematic review. J Am Coll Cardiol 2014;63(25 Pt A):2751–68.

[15] Negishi K, et al. Independent and incremental value of deformation indices for prediction of trastuzumab-induced cardiotoxicity. J Am Soc Echocardiogr 2013;26(5):493–8.

[16] Plana JC, et al. Expert consensus for multimodality imaging evaluation of adult patients during and after cancer therapy: a report from the American Society of Echocardiography and the European Association of Cardiovascular Imaging. Eur Heart J Cardiovasc Imaging 2014;15(10):1063–93.

Chapter 24

The Role of Biomarkers: Troponins, BNP, MPO, and Other Biomarkers

D. Cardinale and M. Scherrer-Crosbie

Chapter Outline

A novel strategy, based on the use of biochemical markers, in particular troponins, has emerged in the last 15 years, resulting in a diagnostic tool for early, real-time identification, assessment, and monitoring of cancer drug-induced cardiotoxicity. This approach seems to overcome most of the limitations of imaging techniques as it has proven to be more sensitive and more specific, cheaper, repeatable without damage to the patients, readily available even in small hospitals, and without interobserver variability [1,2].

TROPONINS

Troponins are considered the gold standard markers for myocardial injury from any cause [2]. In addition to the nearly absolute cardiac tissue specificity, troponins have a high-sensitivity (HS) for detecting small amounts of necrosis. In all clinical settings, they also allow for cardiac risk stratification, as their elevation correlates with the clinical severity of the disease and cardiac outcome [3]. As highlighted in a report by the Expert Working Group on Biomarkers of Drug-Induced Cardiac Toxicity of the Nonclinical Subcommittee of the Advisory Committee for Pharmaceutical Science, which is one of the expert panels of the Food and Drug Administration (FDA), one of the most important indications for using cardiac troponins in the evaluation of drug-induced cardiotoxicity is monitoring of therapy,

Anticancer Treatments and Cardiotoxicity. DOI: http://dx.doi.org/10.1016/B978-0-12-802509-3.00024-8

including potentially cardiotoxic anticancer drugs [4,5]. The role of cardiac troponins as indicators of early anthracycline-induced cardiotoxicity, and their ability to predict subsequent myocardial dysfunction, was first assessed in animal models [6,7]. In the clinical arena, their relevance is supported by data showing that troponin elevation during chemotherapy is associated with a significantly higher risk of left ventricular dysfunction (LVD). This association has been demonstrated in a number of children and adult populations, with evidence that troponin increments long precede changes on echocardiography (Table 24.1) [8–28]. Notably, assessment of troponins may provide useful information to clinicians: in addition to evaluate risk based solely on absolute troponin increase, monitoring and kinetics of troponins increase correlates with the degree of subsequent LVD, thus stratifying cardiac risk [29]. The largest study was performed in 703 patients with cancer, in whom Troponin I (TnI) was determined before chemotherapy, during the 3 days after the end of chemotherapy (early evaluation), and after 1 month (late evaluation) [13]. Three different troponin release patterns were identified. Troponin I was consistently within the normal range in 70% of cases, increased at only early evaluation in 21%, and increased at both early and late evaluations in 9% (Fig. 24.1). Patients without TnI elevation after chemotherapy showed no significant reduction in left ventricular ejection fraction (LVEF) and had a good prognosis, with a low incidence of cardiac events (1%) during the 3-year follow-up. Conversely, TnI-positive patients had a greater incidence of major adverse cardiac events. In particular, the persistence of the TnI elevation at late evaluation was associated with a greater cardiac impairment and a higher incidence of events, compared with patients showing only a transient increase in the marker (84% vs 37%; $P < 0.001$). Thanks to its high negative predictive value (99%), TnI allows identification of low-risk patients who will not require further cardiac monitoring. In contrast, TnI-positive patients require more stringent surveillance, particularly those showing a persistent TnI increase.

Troponins also may be used to identify early cardiac injury in patients undergoing treatment with newer targeted cancer drugs. The role of TnI also has been studied in 251 breast cancer patients treated with trastuzumab [18]. It was measured immediately before and immediately after each cycle, and it was shown to be increased in 14% of patients. LVD occurred in 62% of these, and in only 5% of patients with a normal TnI value ($P < 0.001$). Patients displaying an increase in TnI during trastuzumab treatment had a threefold lower chance of recovering from cardiac dysfunction, and an overall higher incidence of cardiac events, despite optimized heart failure treatment. Thus, troponin seems able to distinguish between reversible and irreversible cardiac injury.

More recently, Morris et al. [19] also demonstrated that TnI values increase in patients receiving both trastuzumab and the tyrosine kinase inhibitor lapatinib preceded by anthraycline-based chemotherapy. The timing of

TABLE 24.1 Paper Demonstrating Troponin as Predictor of Left Ventricular Dysfunction

Study (Year)	Patients (n.)	Cancer Type	Drug	Troponin	Cut Off	Timing of Assessment
Lipshultz et al. (1997) [8]	15[a]	All	AC	TnT	0.03 ng/mL	Before CT; 1–3 days after each dose
Cardinale et al. (2000) [9]	201	Various	HD CT	TnI	0.04 ng/mL	At 0-12-24-36-72 h after CT
Cardinale et al. (2002) [10]	232	Breast cancer	HD CT	TnI	0.04 ng/mL	At 0-12-24-36-72 h after CT
Auner et al. (2002) [11]	30	Hematological	HD Cycl	TnT	0.03 ng/mL	Before CT; 1–14 days after CT
Sandri et al. (2003) [12]	179	Various	HD CT	TnI	0.04 ng/mL	At 0-12-24-36-72-h after CT
Cardinale et al. (2004) [13]	703	Various	HD CT	TnI	0.04 ng/mL	At 0-12-24-36-72-h after CT
Specchia et al. (2005) [14]	79	Hematological	AC	TnI	0.15 ng/mL	Before CT; weekly × 4 times
Kilickap et al. (2005) [15]	41	Various	AC	TnT	0.10 ng/mL	Before CT; 3–5 days after first and last dose
Lee et al. (2008) [16]	86	Hematological	AC	TnI	0.20 ng/mL	Before each dose
Schmidinger et al. (2008) [17]	74	Renal carcinoma	sunitinib/sorafenib	TnI	0.03 ng/mL	Before CT; bimonthly during CT
Cardinale et al. (2010) [18]	251	Breast cancer	TRZ	TnI	0.04 ng/mL	Before and soon after each cycle
Morris et al. (2011) [19]	95	Breast cancer	AC + taxanes + TRZ/LAP	TnI	0.30 ng/mL	Every 2 weeks during chemotherapy

(*Continued*)

TABLE 24.1 (Continued)

Study (Year)	Patients (n.)	Cancer Type	Drug	Troponin	Cut Off	Timing of Assessment
Sawaya et al. (2011) [20]	43	Breast cancer	AC + taxanes + TRZ	HS-TnI	0.015 ng/mL	Before CT; after 3 and 6 months during CT
Lipshultz et al. (2012) [21]	205[a]	All	AC/ AC + dexrazoxane	TnI/TnT	any detectable amount	Before CT; 1–7 days after each dose;end CT
Sawaya et al. (2012) [22]	81	Breast cancer	AC + taxane + TRZ	HS-TnI	30 pg/mL	Before CT; after 3 and 6 months during CT
Geiger et al. (2012) [23]	50	Various	AC	TnT	n.a.	Before CT; after 6 h, 7 days, 3 months
Draft et al. (2013) [24]	53	Various	AC	TnI	0.06 ng/mL	Before CT; after 1, 3, 6 months
Mornos et al. (2013) [25]	74	Various	AC	HS-TnT	n.a.	Before CT; after 6, 12, 24, 52 weeks
Mavinkurve-Groothuis et al. (2013) [26]	60[a]	All	AC	HS-TnT	0.01 ng/mL	Before CT; after 3 and 12 months
Ky et al. (2014) [27]	78	Breast cancer	AC + taxanes + TRZ	HS-TnI	n.a.	Before CT; after 3 and 6 months during CT
Mornos et al. (2014) [28]	92	Various	AC	HS-TnT	n.a.	Before CT; after 12 and 36 weeks

AC, anthracycline-containing chemotherapy; ALL, acute lymphoblastic leukemia; CT, chemotherapy; HD, high-dose; Cycl, cyclophosphamide; LAP, lapatinib; TnI, troponin I; TnT, troponin T; TRZ, trastuzumab; US, ultra-sensitive.
[a]*Pediatric population.*

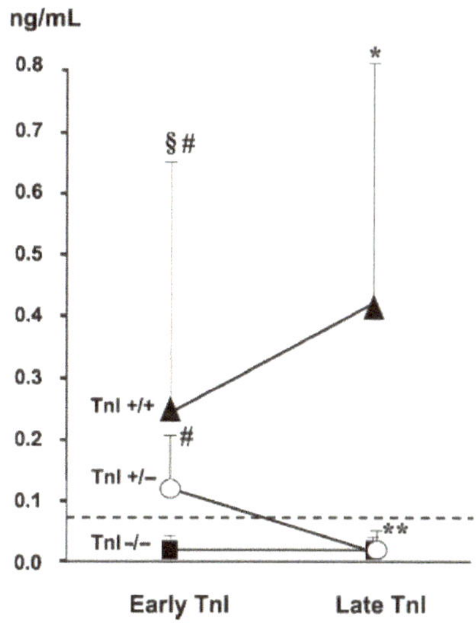

FIGURE 24.1 Early and late Troponin I (TnI) values in the three study groups. TnI +/+ ($n = 63$; 9%); TnI +/− ($n = 145$; 21%); TnI −/− ($n = 495$; 70%). * = $P < 0.05$ vs Early TnI; ** = $P < 0.001$ vs Early TnI; § = $P < 0.001$ vs TnI +/−; # = $P < 0.001$ vs TnI −/−. *Modified from Cardinale D, et al. Prognostic value of Troponin I in cardiac risk stratification of cancer patients undergoing high-dose chemotherapy. Circulation 2004;109:2749–54.*

maximum detectable TnI value preceded maximum decline in LVEF. In 86 patients with metastatic renal cancer treated with the tyrosine kinase inhibitor sunitinib or sorafenib, and monitored prospectively with serial TnT measurements, the increase in this marker was observed in 10% of patients [17]. 90% of these showed a later decrease in LVEF or regional contraction abnormalities. These data suggest that troponins may be useful for assessing cardiotoxicity in patients treated with both conventional and newer cancer therapies. Possibly, the release of troponin reflects a final common pathway for multiple cardiotoxic mechanisms. However, as repeated measurements of troponins are usually needed to detect positivity, the best timing at which the maximal sensitivity and specificity from a single sample of troponin could be obtained must still be clarified in further prospective studies.

HIGH-SENSITIVITY TROPONINS

Recent advances in assay technology have led to more sensitive and precise troponin assays. These new HS assays can now reliably measure small elevations that are undetectable using other troponin assays [30]. These tests could be of particular interest and offer some advantages in the field of cardiotoxicity, as we often deal with low concentrations of troponin, and it is of the utmost importance to use high-precision systems at low concentration levels.

The possible use of HS troponins in this setting was first presented by Sawaya et al. [22] in a recent multicenter study. The authors used HS troponins and echocardiographic parameters of myocardial deformation to detect LVD in patients receiving anthracyclines, taxanes, and trastuzumab. They evaluated global and regional myocardial function by using tissue Doppler and strain rate imaging, combined with HS TnI, at baseline and 3, 6, 9, 12, and 15 months during chemotherapy. Decreases in peak longitudinal strain and increases in HS TnI concentrations at the completion of the anthracycline-treatment were predictive of subsequent LVD. Conversely, changes in LVEF, diastolic function, and N-terminal pro-B-type natriuretic peptide (NT-proBNP), a hormone secreted by the ventricles in response to increased wall stretch [31], evaluated at the same time points were not predictive of later LVD.

More recently, Ky and coworkers [27] evaluated the association between multiple biomarker increases and the further development of cardiotoxicity in breast cancer patients treated with the same therapeutic schedule used in Sawaya's study. The levels of all these markers, with the exception of NT-proBNP and Galectin-3 increased from baseline. However, a greater risk of cardiotoxicity was only associated with HS TnI absolute values at the end of anthracyclines and with changes in TnI and myeloperoxidase, a marker of oxidative stress, even if for myeloperoxidase changes, the significance was less impressive. Further studies are needed to compare HS troponins with traditional troponin assays in identifying patients who will develop LVD in larger populations with longer follow-up.

OTHER BIOMARKERS

Brain-type natriuretic peptide (BNP) and NT-proBNP have been considered potentially important markers of cardiotoxicity and there is no doubt that they are elevated in marked LVD/symptomatic heart failure. As such, they are included, both by the American Heart Association (AHA) and the American College of Cardiology (ACC), [32] and by the common terminology criteria for adverse events used by oncologists [33], in the definition of early stages of cardiac insult. It has to be noted, however, that although BNP or NT-proBNP appear to increase after chemotherapy, in particular anthracycline therapy, the predictive value of these increases has not been consistently reported, and there are concerns about their variability and specificity in patients with cancer.

In patients treated with anthracyclines, the association of increased BNP levels with simultaneously decreased LVEF has been inconsistent; although most investigators have reported a correlation [34–36], some studies have not reproduced the findings [37,38]. Importantly, the predictive value of BNP or NT-proBNP in the detection of subsequent cardiotoxicity has not been demonstrated in most studies [22,34,39–42]. One explanation may be that in this population, multiple additional comorbidities such as anemia and even the presence of cancer may by themselves increase BNP or NT-proBNP levels [43].

Two studies, however, have reported encouraging results; in 71 patients with breast cancer, a persistent elevation in NT-proBNP (elevation detected after each of six anthracycline cycles) found in 30% of patients was associated with a decrease in LVEF at 12 months [44]. Moreover, the difference in baseline and peak NT-proBNP level also predicted an impairment of LV function at 12 months. Recently, Skovgaard et al. [45] prospectively measured BNP levels in 333 patients treated with cardiotoxic chemotherapy; 21 patients (6.3%) developed symptomatic heart failure over a mean follow-up of 3.7 years. A BNP concentration of >100 pg/mL predicted subsequent symptomatic heart failure with a sensitivity of 38% and a specificity of 92%. It is noteworthy, however, that the number of patients with this augmented BNP was not reported, the cardiovascular characteristics of the population and the timing of the sampling were not defined [45]. Therefore, the value of BNP or NT-proBNP in predicting cardiotoxicity is still unclear and the nonspecificity of an elevation in these biomarkers is a concern.

Myeloperoxidase, a marker of oxidative stress, may also be a marker of cardiotoxicity. In 78 women with breast cancer, an augmentation of myeloperoxidase levels after anthracycline therapy predicted subsequent cardiotoxicity [27]. In addition, measuring myeloperoxidase and troponin allowed to identify high-risk patients; patients in the 90th percentile of the elevation of both biomarkers had a 46.5% probability of developing subsequent cardiotoxicity over 12 months. Of note, the other biomarkers that were tested in this population (ST2 for cardiac remodeling, high-sensitivity (HS) C-reactive protein for inflammation, growth differentiation factor-15 for inflammation and oxidative stress, placental growth factor for angiogenesis, soluble fms-like tyrosine kinase receptor-1 for vascular remodeling, and galectin-3 for fibrosis) were nondiscriminatory.

REFERENCES

[1] Khouri MG, Douglas P, Mackey GR, et al. Cancer therapy–induced cardiac toxicity in early breast cancer. Addressing the unresolved issues. Circulation 2012;126:2749–63.

[2] O'Brien PJ. Cardiac troponin is the most effective translational safety biomarker for myocardial injury in cardiotoxicity. Toxicology 2008;245:206–18.

[3] Panteghini M. The new definition of myocardial infarction and the impact of troponin determination on clinical practice. Int J Cardiol 2006;106:298–306.

[4] Expert Working Group on Biomarkers of Drug-Induced Cardiac Toxicity report to the Nonclinical Studies Subcommittee of the Advisory Committee for Pharmaceutical Science, 2002. NICE website press release. <http://www.fda.gov/ohrms/dockets/ac/02/briefing/3891B101Troponin.Outline.pdf>.

[5] Adamcova M, Simunek T, Kaiserova H, Popelova O, Sterba M, Potacova A, et al. In vitro and in vivo examination of cardiac troponins as biochemical markers of drug-induced cardiotoxicity. Toxicology 2007;237:218–28.

[6] Seinyo Y, Tomita Y, Nagai Y, Kusama Y, Hayakawa H, Sasaki T, et al. Cardioprotective effects of ACE-inhibitor (Cilazapril) on adriamycin cardiotoxicity in spontaneously hypertensive rats. Circulation 1993;88:I-633.

[7] Herman EH, Zhang J, Lipshultz SE, Rifai N, Chadwick D, Takeda K, et al. Correlation between serum levels of cardiac troponin-T and the severity of the chronic cardiomyopathy induced by doxorubicin. J Clin Oncol 1999;17:2237–43.

[8] Lipshultz SE, Rifai N, Sallan SE, Lipsitz SR, Dalton V, Sacks DB. Predictive value of cardiac troponin T in pediatric patients at risk for myocardial injury. Circulation 1997;96:2641–8.

[9] Cardinale D, Sandri MT, Martinoni A, Tricca A, Civelli M, Lamantia G, et al. Left ventricular dysfunction predicted by early troponin I release after high-dose chemotherapy. J Am Coll Cardiol 2000;36:517–22.

[10] Cardinale D, Sandri MT, Martinoni A, Borghini E, Civelli M, Lamantia G. Myocardial injury revealed by plasma troponin I in breast cancer treatment with high dose chemotherapy. Ann Oncol 2002;13:710–15.

[11] Auner HW, Tinchon C, Linkesch W, Tiran A, Quehenberger F, Link H. Prolonged monitoring of troponin T for the detection of anthracycline cardiotoxicity in adults with hematological malignancies. Ann Hematol 2003;82:218–22.

[12] Sandri MT, Cardinale D, Zorzino L, Passerini R, Lentati P, Martinoni A. Minor increases in plasma troponin I predict decreased left ventricular ejection fraction after high-dose chemotherapy. Clin Chem 2003;49:248–52.

[13] Cardinale D, Sandri MT, Colombo A, Colombo N, Boeri M, Lamantia G. Prognostic value of Troponin I in cardiac risk stratification of cancer patients undergoing high-dose chemotherapy. Circulation 2004;109:2749–54.

[14] Specchia G, Buquicchio C, Pansini N, Di Serio F, Liso V, Pastore D. Monitoring of cardiac function on the basis of serum troponin I levels in patients with acute leukemia treated with anthracyclines. J Lab Clin Med 2005;145:212–20.

[15] Kilickap S, Barista I, Akgul E, Aytemir K, Aksoyek S, Aksoy S. cTnT can be a useful marker for early detection of anthracycline cardiotoxicity. Ann Oncol 2005;16:798–804.

[16] Lee HS, Son CB, Shin SH, Kim YS. Clinical correlation between brain natriutetic peptide and anthracyclin-induced cardiac toxicity. Cancer Res Treat 2008;40(3):121–6.

[17] Schmidinger M, Zielinski CC, Vogl UM, Bojic A, Bojic M, Schukro C. Cardiac toxicity of sunitinib and sorafenib in patients with metastatic renal cell carcinoma. J Clin Oncol 2008;26:5204–12.

[18] Cardinale D, Colombo A, Torrisi R, Sandri MT, Civelli M, Salvatici M. Trastuzumab-induced cardiotoxicity: clinical and prognostic implications of troponin I evaluation. J Clin Oncol 2010;28:3910–16.

[19] Morris PG, Chen C, Steingart RM, Fleisher M, Lin N, Moy B. Troponin I and C-reactive protein are commonly detected in patients with breast cancer treated with dose-dense chemotherapy incorporating trastuzumab and lapatinib. Clin Cancer Res 2011;17:3490–9.

[20] Sawaya H, Sebag IA, Plana JC, Januzzi JL, Ky B, Cohen V, et al. Early detection and predictor of cardiotoxicity in chemotherapy-treated patients. Am J Cardiol 2011;107:1375–80.

[21] Lipshultz SE, Miller TL, Scully RE, Lipsitz SR, Rifai N, Silverman LB, et al. Changes in cardiac biomarkers during doxorubicin treatment of pediatric patients with high-risk acute lymphoblastic leukemia: associations with long-term echocardiographic outcomes. J Clin Oncol 2012;30(10):1042–9.

[22] Sawaya H, Sebag IA, Plana JC, Januzzi JL, Ky B, Tan TC, et al. Assessment of echocardiography and biomarkers for the extended prediction of cardiotoxicity in patients treated with anthracyclines, taxanes and trastuzumab. Circ Cardiovasc Imaging 2012;5:596–603.

[23] Geiger S, Stemmler HJ, Suhl P, Stieber P, Lange V, Baur D, et al. Anthracycline-induced cardiotoxicity: cardiac monitoring by continuous wave-Doppler ultrasound cardiac output monitoring and correlation to echocardiography. Onkologie 2012;35(5):241–6.

[24] Drafts BC, Twomley KM, D'Agostino Jr R, Lawrence J, Avis N, et al. Low to moderate dose anthracycline-based chemotherapy is associated with early noninvasive imaging evidence of subclinical cardiovascular disease. JACC Cardiovasc Imaging 2013;6(8):877–85.

[25] Mornoş C, Petrescu L. Early detection of anthracycline-mediated cardiotoxicity: the value of considering both global longitudinal left ventricular strain and twist. Can J Physiol Pharmacol 2013;91(8):601–7.

[26] Mavinkurve-Groothuis AM, Marcus KA, Pourier M, Loonen J, Feuth T, Hoogerbrugge PM, et al. Myocardial 2D strain echocardiography and cardiac biomarkers in children during and shortly after anthracycline therapy for acute lymphoblastic leukaemia (ALL): a prospective study. Eur Heart J Cardiovasc Imaging 2013;14(6):562–9.

[27] Ky B, Putt M, Sawaya H, French B, Januzzi JL, Sebag IA, et al. Early increases in multiple biomarkers predict subsequent cardiotoxicity in patients with breast cancer treated with doxorubicin, taxanes, and trastuzumab. J Am Coll Cardiol 2014;63 (8):809–16.

[28] Mornoş C, Manolis AJ, Cozma D, Kouremenos N, Zacharopoulou I, Ionac A. The value of left ventricular global longitudinal strain assessed by three-dimensional strain imaging in the early detection of anthracyclinemediated cardiotoxicity. Hellenic J Cardiol 2014;55 (3):235–44.

[29] Christenson ES, James T, Agrawal V, Park BH. Use of biomarkers for the assessment of chemotherapy-induced cardiac toxicity. Clin Biochem 2015;48(4–5):223–35.

[30] Reichlin T, Hochholzer W, Bassett S, Steuer S, Stelzig C, Hartwiger S, et al. Early diagnosis of myocardial infarction with sensitive cardiac troponin assays. N Engl J Med 2009;361:858–67.

[31] De Lemos JA, MacGuire DK, Drazner MH. B-type natriuretic peptide in cardiovascular disease. Lancet 2003;362:316–22.

[32] Yancy CW, Jessup M, Bozkurt B, Butler J, Casey DE, Drazner MH, et al. American College of Cardiology Foundation/American Heart Association Task Force on Practice Guidelines. 2013 ACCF/AHA guideline for the management of heart failure: a report of the American College of Cardiology Foundation/American Heart Association Task Force on practice guidelines. 2013. p. e240–327.

[33] Common Terminology Criteria for Adverse Events v4.03 (CTCAE). 2010 [cited 2015 Mar 22]; Available from: http://evs.nci.nih.gov/ftp1/CTCAE.

[34] Daugaard G, Lassen U, Bie P, Pedersen EB, Jensen KT, Abildgaard U, et al. Natriuretic peptides in the monitoring of anthracycline induced reduction in left ventricular ejection fraction. Eur J Heart Fail 2005;7:87–93.

[35] Vogelsang TW, Jensen RJ, Hesse B, Kjaer A. BNP cannot replace gated equilibrium radionuclide ventriculography in monitoring of anthracycline-induced cardiotoxity. Inter J Cardiol 2008;124:193–7.

[36] Okumura H, Iuchi K, Yoshida T, Nakamura S, Takeshima M, Takamatsu H, et al. Brain natriuretic peptide is a predictor of anthracycline-induced cardiotoxicity. Acta Haematol 2000;104:158–63.

[37] Nousiainen T, Jantunen E, Vanninen E, Remes J, Vuolteenaho O, Hartikainen J. Natriuretic peptides as markers of cardiotoxicity during doxorubicin treatment for non-Hodgkin's lymphoma. Eur J Haematol 1999;62:135–41.

[38] Meinardi MT, van Veldhuisen DJ, Gietema JA, Dolsma WV, Boomsma F, van den Berg MP, et al. Prospective evaluation of early cardiac damage induced by epirubicin-containing adjuvant chemotherapy and locoregional radiotherapy in breast cancer patients. J Clin Oncol 2001;19:2746–53.

[39] Dodos F, Halbsguth T, Erdmann E, Hoppe UC. Usefulness of myocardial performance index and biochemical markers for early detection of anthracycline-induced cardiotoxicity in adults. Clin Res Cardiol 2008;97:318–26.

[40] Horacek JM, Pudil R, Jebavy L, Tichy M, Zak P, Maly J. Assessment of anthracycline-induced cardiotoxicity with biochemical markers. Exp Oncol 2007;29:309–13.

[41] Knobloch K, Tepe J, Rossner D, Lichtinghagen R, Luck HJ, Busch KH, et al. Combined NT-pro-BNP and CW-Doppler ultrasound cardiac output monitoring (USCOM) in epirubicin and liposomal doxorubicin therapy. Int J Cardiol 2008;128:316–25.

[42] Knobloch K, Tepe J, Lichtinghagen R, Luck HJ, Vogt PM. Monitoring of cardiotoxicity during immunotherapy with Herceptin using simultaneous continuous wave Doppler depending on N-terminal pro-brain natriuretic peptide. Clin Med 2007;7:88–9.

[43] Burjonroppa SC, Tong AT, Xiao L-C, Johnson MM, Yusuf SW, Lenihan DJ. Cancer patients with markedly elevated B-type natriuretic peptide may not have volume overload. Am J Clin Oncol 2007;30:287–93.

[44] Romano S, Fratini S, Ricevuto E, Procaccini V, Stifano G, Mancini M, et al. Serial measurements of NT-proBNP are predictive of not-high-dose anthracycline cardiotoxicity in breast cancer patients. Br J Cancer 2011;105:1663–8.

[45] Skovgaard D, Hasbak P, Kjaer A. BNP predicts chemotherapy-related cardiotoxicity and death: comparison with gated equilibrium radionuclide ventriculography. PLoS One 2014;9:e96736.

Chapter 25

Screening and Comprehensive Follow-Up Evaluation

R. Hinojar and J.L. Zamorano Gómez

Chapter Outline

AN INTEGRATED APPROACH OF MARKERS AND CARDIAC IMAGING

Increasing evidence is rapidly accumulating and supports the use of conventional and novel echocardiographic indices and biomarkers for the detection of early cardiac injury [1–5]. Decreases in myocardial strain and strain rate have been described after anthracycline-based chemotherapies, and speckle-tracking echocardiography (STE) has been proposed as the imaging technique of choice for detection of subclinical left ventricular (LV) dysfunction. Troponin I variations over time have been shown to be predictive of subsequent cardiotoxicity [6–7], with high positive and negative predictive value. Moreover, different biomarkers such as myeloperoxidase in combination with TnI can provide additional value to predict cardiovascular (CV) risk.

Based on this evidence, an integrated approach combining echocardiographic and biomarker information may provide incremental value in predicting subsequent cardiac dysfunction. This additional benefit was suggested by the results of Sawaya and collaborators in 81 breast cancer patients treated with anthracycline and trastuzumab, in which ultrasensitive troponin levels (usTnI) were obtained at the same time as STE-derived strain imaging after anthracycline exposure [8]. Although longitudinal strain (<19%) was identified as the only independent

Anticancer Treatments and Cardiotoxicity. DOI: http://dx.doi.org/10.1016/B978-0-12-802509-3.00025-X

predictor of cardiotoxicity, the specificity to predict cardiotoxicity improved to 93% compared to 73% when an elevated usTnI concentration ($\geq$30 pg/mL) was used in combination. Furthermore, if just one or the other parameter was present the sensitivity increased to 87% and negative predictive value to 91%.

Some centers have already adopted an integrated approach with the use of echocardiography and biomarker assessment at preselected intervals. Whether this approach may have an impact on clinical management and prognosis has to be validated in further studies.

IMPLICATIONS OF EARLY DETECTION ON THERAPEUTIC APPROACH

Current efforts are directed to prevent or identify cardiac toxicity at the subclinical stage given the modest effects to therapy when it is diagnosed late in its course. Small studies have suggested that a variety of agents such as dexrazoxane, β-blockers, angiotensin-receptor blockers, and statins may be helpful in the prevention or early treatment of cardiac injury; however, no definitive recommendations can be set with the current available data, even in patients with cardiac risk factors or underlying cardiac disease [9]. Furthermore, for the time being, the effectiveness of screening techniques for detecting subclinical CV injury in asymptomatic survivors of cancer is not established. Accordingly, there are no evidence-based guidelines that support the application of the newer methodologies (biomarkers, advanced imaging with echocardiography, or CV magnetic resonance) for CV monitoring during therapy. Most of the management algorithms have focused on the primary use of noninvasive imaging to assess left ventricular ejection fraction (LVEF). In fact, the definition of cardiotoxicity is usually established in the presence of symptomatic LVEF reduction of 5% or an asymptomatic fall of >10% both to an LVEF of <55% [10]. Despite its unquestionable value, LVEF is not sensitive enough to detect minor changes in LV status and major changes in LVEF may reflect an advanced stage of cardiac dysfunction. Subsequently, LVEF may not reflect the underlying subclinical CV disease that could predict the development of CV events in patients actively treated for or those that survive cancer.

Novel cardiac imaging parameters and biomarkers have the potential to predict CV injury in a subclinical stage, providing a scope for changes on therapeutic management algorithms and improvement on cardiac outcomes.

One of the most promising techniques to identify cardiac injury is the assessment of global longitudinal strain (GLS) by STE. Longitudinal LV mechanics have been shown to constitute the most sensible and highly reproducible component of LV mechanics that can be assessed with well-performed transthoracic echocardiography [11–13]. A significant number of studies have established the potential role of GLS to predict the development of cardiotoxicity. Reductions of more than 10% of GLS and radial strain have been observed after 1 week of anthracycline treatment [14]. In addition,

Sawaya and collaborators [15] showed that a reduction of >10% of GLS after 3 months of cancer treatment with an anthracycline and trastuzumab predicted the later development of a reduction of LVEF 6 months after initiation of these therapies with high negative predictive value. In this same study, LVEF did not help to predict cardiotoxicity. A recent systematic review confirmed the value of the assessment of myocardial mechanics for the early detection of myocardial changes and prediction of cardiotoxicity in patients receiving cancer therapy [16]. An early reduction of 10–15% in GLS by STE during therapy appeared to be the most useful parameter for the prediction of cardiotoxicity, defined as a drop in LVEF or heart failure.

Whether the detection of early left ventricular dysfunction will allow a more individualized use of prophylactic pharmacological interventions (dexrazoxane, β-blocker, statin, or angiotensin antagonists) and reduce the frequency and the magnitude of cardiotoxic responses still needs to be tested in future clinical studies [17].

PRACTICAL USE OF IMAGING FOR FOLLOW-UP EVALUATION

When applying imaging to detect cardiac injury in patients actively or previously treated for cancer it is essential to consider that the timing of LV dysfunction can vary among different agents and therefore they cannot be viewed as a single class of drugs. While in patients under anthracyclines, the damage occurs immediately after the exposure, for others the timing appears to be more variable, even years or decades after receiving the cardiotoxic treatment.

To date, very few established guidelines exist regarding the implementation of noninvasive imaging techniques for monitoring patients receiving treatment for cancer. However, several suggested management algorithms have been published over the last decade, particularly focused on the assessment of patients receiving radiation, anthracyclines, or trastuzumab [18–23]. Recently, the American Society of Echocardiography and the European Association of Cardiovascular Imaging published an expert consensus providing follow-up recommendations, which for the first time address the use of newer methodologies available (biomarkers, advanced imaging with 3D echocardiography, or speckle-tracking techniques) that may provide evidence of early injury before a decline in LVEF [24].

Regarding the evaluation of those patients receiving *radiation therapy*, the European Association of Cardiovascular Imaging and the American Society of Echocardiography published an expert consensus statement for multimodality imaging evaluation of CV complications of radiotherapy in adults [18]. Although the radiation-induced cardiac injury may develop acutely, most often they become clinically apparent several years after irradiation. Importantly, the risk of LV dysfunction, valvular abnormality, and coronary artery disease (CAD) has been documented in those patients treated in the 1980s with chest irradiation. The current risk with modern radiotherapy techniques has not been fully defined, although follow-up evaluations are still desirable. Fig. 25.1 summarizes a proposed algorithm for patients after chest radiotherapy. Briefly, a pretreatment CV screening for risk factors, careful clinical examination and baseline echocardiographic evaluation should be performed in all patients. During follow-up, a yearly anamnesis and physical examination with close attention to symptoms and signs of CV disease is essential; the development of any CV sign or symptom should prompt transthoracic echocardiography examination. In otherwise asymptomatic patients screening echocardiography should be performed 10 years after treatment or after 5 years in high-risk patients and later every 5 years. Given the increased risk for CAD, noninvasive stress imaging should be performed every 5 years. Because of its higher specificity stress echocardiography or stress cardiovascular magnetic resonance (CMR) may be preferred to exercise ECG.

In regard to receipt of *anthracycline-based chemotherapy*, the European Society for Medical Oncology provided recommendations to help clinicians

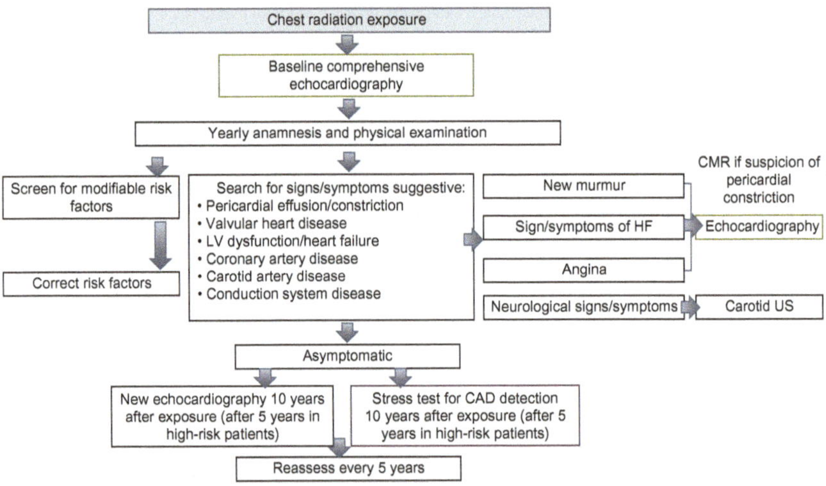

FIGURE 25.1 Algorithm for patient management after chest radiotherapy. *LV*, left ventricle; *US*, ultrasound. High-risk patients: anterior or left-side chest irradiation with ≥1 risk factor for radiation-induced heart disease (RIHD) (risk factors for RIHD: high cumulative dose of radiation (>30 Gy); younger patients (<50 years); high dose of radiation fractions (>2 Gy/day); presence and extent of tumor in or next to the heart; lack of shielding; concomitant chemotherapy (the anthracyclines considerably increase the risk); cardiovascular risk factors (i.e., diabetes mellitus, smoking, overweight, ≥moderate hypertension, hypercholesterolemia); preexisting cardiovascular disease). *Adapted from Lancellotti P, et al. Expert consensus for multi-modality imaging evaluation of cardiovascular complications of radiotherapy in adults: a report from the European Association of Cardiovascular Imaging and the American Society of Echocardiography. Eur Heart J Cardiovasc Imaging 2013;14(8):721–40.*

to identify patients at higher risk, which have been recently updated, by the recommendations of the European Association of Cardiovascular Imaging and the American Society of Echocardiography [19,24]. The anthracycline-associated abnormalities and their related cardiac insult represent an irreversible form of chemotherapy or type I-related cardiac dysfunction in which the best predictor of cardiotoxicity is the total cumulative dose of anthracycline [25,26]. Additional risk factors include ageing, preexisting cardiac dysfunction, longstanding hypertension, intercurrent cardiotoxic therapies, and prior irradiation therapy, particularly when anthracyclines are given in high cumulative doses with bolus administration.

Before the start of the therapy, clinicians should screen patients to identify patient- and treatment-related CV risk factors and plan proactive treatment of those modifiable risk factors. For instance, hypertensive patients should receive medication such as ACE inhibitors and other lifestyle advice to reduce blood pressure before and during anthracycline treatment. A baseline evaluation including electrocardiography and measurements of LVEF, preferably by 3D-echocardiography or contrast 2D-echocardiography, GLS, and troponin is recommended (Fig. 25.2). If any are abnormal, a cardiology consultation is recommended. Follow-up is recommended at the completion of therapy and 6 months later for doses <240 mg/m^2 or its equivalent. Once

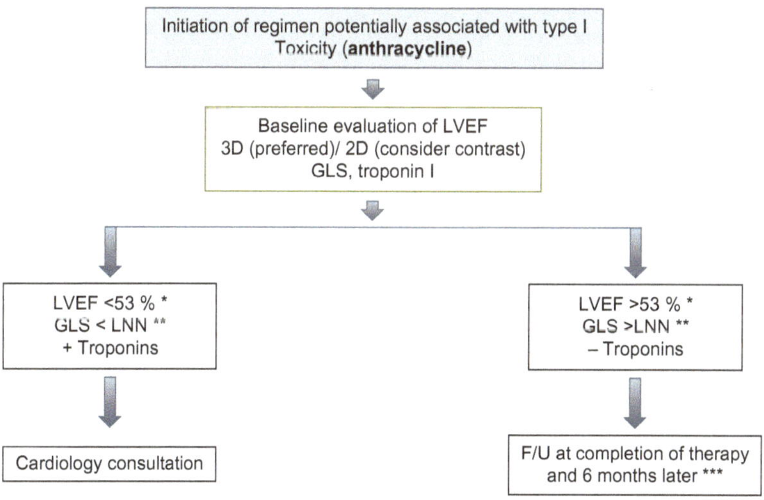

FIGURE 25.2 Initiation of a regimen potentially associated with type I toxicity. * Consider confirmation with CMR; ** *LLN*, lower limit of normal; *** If the dose is higher than 240 mg/m^2 (or its equivalent) recommend measurement of LVEF, GLS, and troponin prior to each additional 50 mg/m^2. *Adapted from Plana JC et al. Expert consensus for multimodality imaging evaluation of adult patients during and after cancer therapy: a report from the American Society of Echocardiography and the European Association of Cardiovascular Imaging. J Am Soc Echocardiogr 2014 Sep;27(9):911–39.*

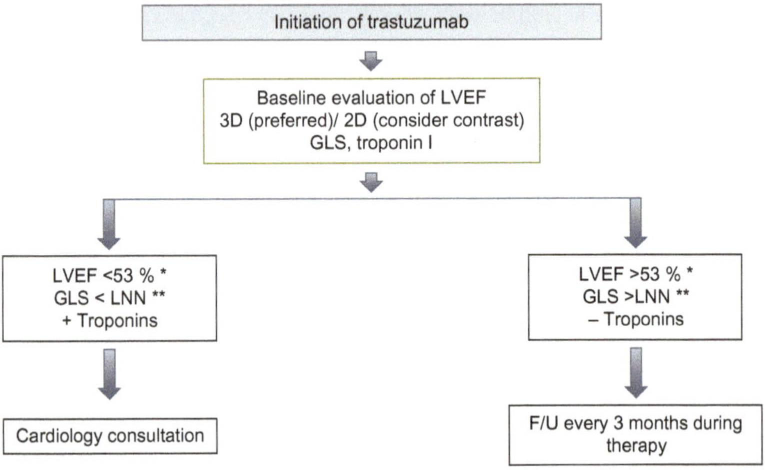

FIGURE 25.3 Initiation of trastuzumab. * Consider confirmation with CMR; ** *LLN*, lower limit of normal. *Adapted from Plana JC, et al. Expert consensus for multimodality imaging evaluation of adult patients during and after cancer therapy: a report from the American Society of Echocardiography and the European Association of Cardiovascular Imaging. J Am Soc Echocardiogr 2014 Sep;27(9):911–39.*

this dose is exceeded, measurements of LVEF, GLS, and troponin are recommended before each additional 50 mg/m^2.

Lastly, *trastuzumab toxicity* constitutes a type II-related cardiac dysfunction, which is not dose-related, does not occur in all patients, and is not associated with any significant structural abnormalities. Furthermore, this type of toxicity appears to be reversible, with a high likelihood of recovery. Fig. 25.3 summarizes practical follow-ups for patients starting trastuzumab [24]. A baseline evaluation, including measurements of LVEF, GLS, and troponin is recommended. If any are abnormal, a cardiology consultation is recommended. Measurements of LVEF, GLS, and troponin are recommended every 3 months during therapy. A similar approach is recommended when trastuzumab is started after a regimen associated with type I toxicity, but an additional screening with LVEF, GLS, and troponin after 6 months of the treatment is also recommended.

FOCUS ON THE PATIENT WITH KNOWN CARDIAC DISEASE

Several targeted drugs used in oncology have a detrimental impact on CV physiology through on-target or off-target effects. The type and duration of cancer treatment plays an important role in determining CV injury or toxicity; moreover, the same drug may be associated with different cardiotoxicities. CV toxicity can be caused by direct injury to or death of cardiac myocytes; by stimulation of myocardial fibrosis; by provocation of stress-induced myocardial ischemia via endothelial dysfunction; by vascular injury; by myocardial and/or pericardial inflammation; by arrhythmogenic or conduction abnormalities; by autonomic dysfunction; by valvular disease; or by exacerbation of known CV risk factors.

During screenings and follow-ups of patients, recognition of previous cardiac disease and the recognition of modifiable and nonmodifiable risk factors such as hypertension, diabetes, and obesity are essential as they may predispose individuals to develop cardiac injury. Primary prevention of known modifiable risk factors represents an important step in the baseline management.

For instance, Hequet and collaborators investigated the potential role of conventional CV risk factors to predispose to cardiac dysfunction in 141 patients who previously received doxorubicin-based chemotherapy for lymphoma [27]. In a multivariate analysis, male gender, older age, and being overweight were identified as independent risk factors for the development of cardiomyopathy. Similarly, the contribution of conventional CV risk factors was explored in 476 patients with aggressive nonHodgkin lymphoma treated with at least six cycles of doxorubicin-based chemotherapy [28]. The age at the start of chemotherapy, preexisting hypertension, and smoking increased the risk of heart failure. In a large registry of 43,338 anthracycline-treated women with breast cancer, baseline characteristics such as aging, hypertension, diabetes, black race, and previous history of CAD were predictors of congestive heart failure. Similar results were found by Hershman et al. [29]; their study confirmed that CV risk factors (hypertension, diabetes) and previous history of CAD increased the risk of heart failure in 9438 patients who received doxorubicin-based chemotherapy. Only hypertension was found to have a synergistic with doxorubicin for the development of heart failure.

REFERENCES

[1] Thavendiranathan P, Poulin F, Lim KD, Plana JC, Woo A, Marwick TH. Use of myocardial strain imaging by echocardiography for the early detection of cardiotoxicity in patients during and after cancer chemotherapy: a systematic review. J Am Coll Cardiol 2014;63:2751–68.

[2] Neilan TG, Jassal DS, Perez-Sanz TM, Raher MJ, Pradhan AD, Buys ES, et al. Tissue Doppler imaging predicts left ventricular dysfunction and mortality in a murine model of cardiac injury. Eur Heart J 2006;27:1868–75.

[3] Ganame J, Claus P, Eyskens B, Uyttebroeck A, Renard M, D'hooge J, et al. Acute cardiac functional and morphological changes after Anthracycline infusions in children. Am J Cardiol 2007;99:974–7.

[4] Jurcut R, Wildiers H, Ganame J, D'hooge J, De Backer J, Denys H, et al. Strain rate imaging detects early cardiac effects of pegylated liposomal Doxorubicin as adjuvant therapy in elderly patients with breast cancer. J Am Soc Echocardiogr 2008;21:1283–9.

[5] Hare JL, Brown JK, Leano R, Jenkins C, Woodward N, Marwick TH. Use of myocardial deformation imaging to detect preclinical myocardial dysfunction before conventional measures in patients undergoing breast cancer treatment with trastuzumab. Am Heart J 2009;158:294–301.

[6] Cardinale D, Sandri MT, Colombo A, et al. Prognostic value of troponin I in cardiac risk stratification of cancer patients undergoing high-dose chemotherapy. Circulation 2004; 109:2749–54.

[7] Ky B, Putt M, Sawaya H, French B, Januzzi Jr JL, Sebag IA, et al. Early increases in multiple biomarkers predict subsequent cardiotoxicity in patients with breast cancer treated with doxorubicin, taxanes, and trastuzumab. J Am Coll Cardiol 2014;63(8):809–16.

[8] Sawaya H, Sebag IA, Plana JC, Januzzi JL, Ky B, Tan TC, et al. Assessment of echocardiography and biomarkers for the extended prediction of cardiotoxicity in patients treated with anthracyclines, taxanes, and trastuzumab. Circ Cardiovasc Imaging 2012;5: 596–603.

[9] Hensley ML, Hagerty KL, Kewalramani T, Green DM, Meropol NJ, Wasserman TH, et al. American Society of Clinical Oncology 2008 clinical practice guideline update: use of chemotherapy and radiation therapy protectants. J Clin Oncol 2009;27(1):127–45.

[10] Yeh ET, Bickford CL. Cardiovascular complications of cancer therapy: incidence, pathogenesis, diagnosis, and management. J Am Coll Cardiol 2009;53:2231–47.

[11] Biswas M, Sudhakar S, Nanda NC, et al. Two and three-dimensional speckle tracking echocardiography: clinical applications and future directions. Echocardiography 2013;30: 88–105.

[12] Dorosz JL, Lezotte DC, Weitzenkamp DA, Allen LA, Salcedo EE. Performance of 3-dimensional echocardiography in measuring left ventricular volumes and ejection fraction: a systematic review and meta-analysis. J Am Coll Cardiol 2012;59:1799–808.

[13] Geyer H, Caracciolo G, Abe H, et al. Assessment of myocardial mechanics using speckle tracking echocardiography: fundamentals and clinical applications. J Am Soc Echocardiogr 2010;23(4):351–69.

[14] Stoodley PW, Richards DA, Hui R, et al. Two dimensional myocardial strain imaging detects changes in left ventricular systolic function immediately after anthracycline chemotherapy. Eur J Echocardiogr 2011;12:945–52.

[15] Sawaya H, Sebag IA, Plana JC, et al. Early detection and prediction of cardiotoxicity in chemotherapy-treated patients. Am J Cardiol 2011;107:1375–80.

[16] Thavendiranathan P, Poulin F, Lim K, Plana JC, Woo A, Marwick TH. Use of myocardial strain imaging by echocardiography for the early detection of cardiotoxicity in patients during and after cancer chemotherapy–a systematic review. J Am Coll Cardiol 2014;63:2751–68.

[17] Kalam K, Marwick TH. Role of cardioprotective therapy for prevention of cardiotoxicity with chemotherapy: a systematic review and metaanalysis. Eur J Cancer 2013;49:2900–9.

[18] Lancellotti P, Nkomo VT, Badano LP, et al. Expert consensus for multi-modality imaging evaluation of cardiovascular complications of radiotherapy in adults: a report from the European Association of Cardiovascular Imaging and the American Society of Echocardiography. Eur Heart J Cardiovasc Imaging 2013;14:721–40.

[19] Barrett-Lee PJ, Dixon JM, Farrell C, et al. Expert opinion of the use of anthracyclines in patients with advanced breast cancer at cardiac risk. Ann Oncol 2009;20:816–27.

[20] Schwartz RG, McKenzie WB, Alexander J, et al. Congestive heart failure and left ventricular dysfunction complicating doxorubicin therapy. Seven-year experience using serial radionuclide angiocardiography. Am J Med 1987;82:1109–18.

[21] Steinherz LJ, Graham T, Hurwitz R, et al. Guidelines for cardiac monitoring of children during and after anthracycline therapy: report of the Cardiology Committee. Pediatrics 1992;89(5 Pt 1):942–9.

[22] Raschi E, De Ponti F. Cardiovascular toxicity of anticancer-targeted therapy: emerging issues in the era of cardio-oncology. Intern Emerg Med 2012;7:113–31.

[23] Keefe DL. Trastuzumab-associated cardiotoxicity. Cancer 2002;95:1592–600.

[24] Plana JC, Galderisi M, Barac A, Ewer MS, Ky B, Scherrer-Crosbie M, et al. Expert consensus for multimodality imaging evaluation of adult patients during and after cancer therapy: a report from the American Society of Echocardiography and the European Association of Cardiovascular Imaging. J Am Soc Echocardiogr 2014;27(9):911–39.

[25] Swain SM, Whaley FS, Ewer MS. Congestive heart failure in patients treated with doxorubicin: a retrospective analysis of three trials. Cancer 2003;97:2869–79.

[26] Lipshultz SE, Adams MJ, Colan SD. Longterm cardiovascular toxicity in children, adolescents, and young adults who receive cancer therapy: pathophysiology, course, monitoring, management, prevention, and research directions: a scientific statement for the American Heart Association. Circulation 2013;128:1927–95.

[27] Hequet O, Le QH, Moullet I, Pauli E, Salles G, Espinouse D, et al. Subclinical late cardiomyopathy after doxorubicin therapy for lymphoma in adults. J Clin Oncol 2004;22 (10):1864–71.

[28] Moser EC, Noordijk EM, van Leeuwen FE, le Cessie S, Baars JW, Thomas J, et al. Long-term risk of cardiovascular disease after treatment for aggressive non-Hodgkin lymphoma. Blood 2006;107(7):2912–19.

[29] Hershman DL, McBride RB, Eisenberger A, Tsai WY, Grann VR, Jacobson JS. Doxorubicin, cardiac risk factors, and cardiac toxicity in elderly patients with diffuse B-cell non-Hodgkin's lymphoma. J Clin Oncol 2008;26(19):3159–65.

Chapter 26

Preoperative Assessment for Noncardiac Surgery

V. Sánchez

Chapter Outline

Over the past few decades, there has been an increasing incidence of cancer diagnoses. Survival has improved due to earlier detection and the development of more efficient cancer-specific treatment regimens. Consequently, there will be an increasing number of patients with a history of cancer requiring possible surgical treatment.

RISK CALCULATION OF PERIOPERATIVE CARDIAC MORBIDITY

Cardiac risk evaluation is initially based on clinical characteristics and type of surgery. Several risk indices have been developed during the past 30 years and represent the relationship between clinical characteristics and perioperative cardiac mortality and morbidity.

The Lee index or "revised cardiac risk" index [1] was designed to predict postoperative myocardial infarction, pulmonary edema, ventricular fibrillation or cardiac arrest, and complete heart block. This risk index comprises six variables: high-risk type of surgery, history of ischemic heart disease, history of congestive heart failure (HF), history of cerebrovascular disease, preoperative treatment with insulin, and preoperative creatinine >2 mg/dL.

Anticancer Treatments and Cardiotoxicity. DOI: http://dx.doi.org/10.1016/B978-0-12-802509-3.00026-1

A new predictive model was recently developed to assess the risk of intraoperative/postoperative myocardial infarction or cardiac arrest, using the American College of Surgeons National Surgical Quality Improvement Program (NSQIP) database [2]. The NSQIP model provides a model-based estimate of the probability of myocardial infarction/cardiac arrest for an individual patient. This model includes the variable "disseminated cancer," defined as the patient who has a primary cancer that has metastasized to a major organ and meets at least one of the following: active treatment for the cancer within 1 year of the surgery date and the surgical procedure is the treatment for the metastatic cancer, the patient has elected not to receive treatment for the metastatic disease or the patient's metastatic cancer has been deemed untreatable. The following cancers are considered as disseminated cancer: acute lymphocytic leukemia (ALL), acute myelogenous leukemia (AML), and stage IV lymphoma. The following are not considered as disseminated cancer: chronic lymphocytic leukemia (CLL), chronic myelogenous leukemia (CML), stages I through III lymphomas or multiple myeloma. This risk calculator may offer the best estimation of surgery-specific risk of a major adverse cardiac event (MACE) and death.

The NSQIP and Lee risk index models provide complementary prognostic perspectives and can help the clinician in the decision-making process. Risk models do not dictate management decisions but should be of help to complete the evaluation with the information at the physician's disposal.

The last recommendations in the ACC/AHA Guideline on Perioperative Cardiovascular Evaluation and Management of Patients Undergoing Noncardiac Surgery [3] include that a validated risk-prediction tool can be useful in predicting the risk of perioperative MACE in patients undergoing noncardiac surgery (level of evidence: B). For patients with a low risk of perioperative MACE, further testing is not recommended before the planned operation.

However, the majority of risk calculator models do not include cancer or previous chemotherapy as variables. In oncology patients the timing of left ventricular (LV) dysfunction can vary among agents so, in the evaluation of preoperative cardiac risk in these patients it is important to identify the risk of cardiotoxicity and the need of further tests to rule out it. The greatest risk factor for anthracycline-induced cardiotoxicity is the cumulative dose. In addition, other risk factors have been identified that increase the risk of anthracycline-induced cardiotoxicity, including young or old age, female gender, underlying cardiovascular disease, history of prior irradiation, hypertension [4], and concomitant treatment with cyclophosphamide, trastuzumab, or paclitaxel. In the case of anthracyclines, the damage occurs immediately after the exposure; for others, the timeframe between drug administration and detectable cardiac dysfunction appears to be more variable. Thus, cardiac damage may not become apparent until years or even decades after receiving the cardiotoxic treatment. This is of particular importance in asymptomatic patients who are evaluated for an elective surgical procedure.

Echocardiography is the cornerstone in the cardiac imaging evaluation of patients treated with anticancer drugs. Evaluation of left ventricle ejection fraction has emerged as the most widely used strategy for monitoring the changes in cardiac function after the administration of potentially cardiotoxic cancer treatment.

It should be noted that the 2011 appropriate use criteria for echocardiography state that it is "inappropriate" to assess ventricular function in patients without signs or symptoms of cardiovascular disease in the preoperative setting [5]. Although there are few data on the preoperative evaluation in oncology patients, evaluation of LV function seems to be reasonable in preoperative assessment, especially in patients treated with anthracycline and high risk of development of cardiotoxicity.

Also, there is little information on the preoperative evaluation of patients with specific nonischemic cardiomyopathies before noncardiac surgery. This group of patients includes oncology patients with or at risk of cardiotoxicity. Preoperative recommendations must be based on a thorough understanding of the pathophysiology of the cardiomyopathy, assessment, and management of the underlying process, and overall management of the HF.

In patients exposured to cancer therapeutics, left ventricular ejection fraction (LVEF) decrease may be categorized as symptomatic or asymptomatic [4]. According to this classification, the preoperative risk for noncardiac surgery will be different.

ASYMPTOMATIC PATIENTS WITH NORMAL LV FUNCTION

For patients with a low risk of perioperative MACE and normal LV function in echocardiogram, further testing is not recommended before the planned operation.

HEART FAILURE

Patients with clinical HF or a history of HF are at significant risk for perioperative complications, and widely used indices of cardiac risk include HF as an independent prognostic variable [1,2].

HF is defined by a combination of signs and symptoms, such as history of HF, pulmonary edema, or paroxysmal nocturnal dyspnea; physical examination showing bilateral rales or third heart sound gallop; and chest X-ray showing pulmonary vascular redistribution. Despite the changes in treatment strategies, and advances in the perioperative area, different studies have demonstrated that HF remains a significant risk for perioperative morbidity and mortality. In fact, patients with active HF have a significantly higher risk of postoperative death than patients with coronary artery disease.

SYMPTOMATIC LV DYSFUNCTION

Although signs and/or symptoms of decompensated HF give the highest risk, severe LV dysfunction (<30%) itself is an independent contributor to perioperative outcome and a long-term risk factor for death in patients with HF undergoing intermediate- or high-risk noncardiac surgery and with high mortality in the longer term [6].

ASYMPTOMATIC PATIENTS WITH LV DYSFUNCTION

The effect of asymptomatic LV dysfunction on perioperative outcomes is unknown. One study that includes 1005 consecutive patients demonstrated that asymptomatic LV dysfunction is a predictor of cardiovascular outcome in open vascular surgery patients [7]. These data suggest that preoperative risk stratification should not solely include symptomatic HF but also routine preoperative echocardiography to risk-stratify open vascular surgery patients. No data are available in patients treated with anticancer drugs and asymptomatic LV dysfunction.

NATRIURETIC PEPTIDES IN PERIOPERATIVE RISK OF HF

Preoperative natriuretic peptide levels independently predict cardiovascular events in the first 30 days after vascular surgery. Measurement of biomarkers, especially natriuretic peptides, may be helpful in assessing patients with HF. In oncology patients persistent increases in cardiac troponin I or B-type natriuretic peptide concentrations seem to identify patients at risk of cardiotoxicity (except in the presence of the syndrome of inappropriate ADH secretion for the latter). A useful approach could be performing baseline assessment of biomarker concentrations especially in patients with LV dysfunction. Further prospective randomized studies are needed to assess the utility of such a strategy.

In summary, there is little information on the preoperative evaluation of patients treated with anticancer drugs. Risk index models provide complementary prognostic perspectives and can help the clinician in the decision-making process, but the majority of risk calculator models do not include cancer or previous chemotherapy as a variable. Preoperative recommendations in oncology patients with or at risk of cardiotoxicity must be based on a thorough understanding of the pathophysiology of the cardiomyopathy, assessment, and management of the underlying process, and overall management of the HF. Evaluation of LV function should be considered in preoperative evaluation, especially in patients treated with anthracycline and high risk of development of cardiotoxicity. Determination of preoperative natriuretic peptide levels at baseline could be a useful approach, especially in patients with LV dysfunction.

REFERENCES

[1] Lee TH, Marcantonio ER, Mangione CM, et al. Derivation and prospective validation of a simple index for prediction of cardiac risk of major noncardiac surgery. Circulation 1999;100:1043–9.

[2] Gupta PK, Gupta H, Sundaram A, et al. Development and validation of a risk calculator for prediction of cardiac risk after surgery. Circulation 2011;124:381–7.

[3] Fleisher LA, Fleischmann KE, Auerbach AD, et al. 2014 ACC/AHA guideline on perioperative cardiovascular evaluation and management of patients undergoing noncardiac surgery: a report of the American College of Cardiology/American Heart Association Task Force on Practice Guidelines. J Am Coll Cardiol 2014;64:e77–e137.

[4] Bovelli D, Plataniotis G, Roila F, Group ObotEGW. Cardiotoxicity of chemotherapeutic agents and radiotherapy-related heart disease: ESMO Clinical Practice Guidelines. Ann Oncol 2010;21:v277–82.

[5] Douglas PS, Garcia MJ, Haines DE, et al. ACCF/ASE/AHA/ASNC/HFSA/HRS/SCAI/SCCM/SCCT/SCMR 2011 Appropriate Use Criteria for Echocardiography: A Report of the American College of Cardiology Foundation Appropriate Use Criteria Task Force, American Society of Echocardiography, American Heart Association, American Society of Nuclear Cardiology, Heart Failure Society of America, Heart Rhythm Society, Society for Cardiovascular Angiography and Interventions, Society of Critical Care Medicine, Society of Cardiovascular Computed Tomography, and Society for Cardiovascular Magnetic Resonance Endorsed by the American College of Chest Physicians. J Am Coll Cardiol 2011;57:1126–66.

[6] Healy KO, Waksmonski CA, Altman RK, Stetson PD, Reyentovich A, Maurer MS. Perioperative outcome and long-term mortality for heart failure patients undergoing intermediate- and high-risk noncardiac surgery: impact of left ventricular ejection fraction. Congest Heart Fail 2010;16:45–9.

[7] Flu MDW J, van Kuijk MDJ-P, Hoeks PDSE, et al. Prognostic implications of asymptomatic left ventricular dysfunction in patients undergoing vascular surgery. J Am Soc Anesthesiol 2010;112:1316–24.

Section VI

Cardiotoxicity in Childhood

Chapter 27

Cardiotoxicity of Childhood Cancer Treatments

J.L. Zamorano Gómez, J. Ramos, G. Alcidi and M. Galderisi

Chapter Outline

CHILDHOOD CANCER SURVIVAL: PREAMBLE

Despite the fact that cancer is not a frequent pathology among children, it represents the second commonest cause of mortality among them in developed countries [1].

The incidence rate of cancer in children under 14 varies with age, sex, or ethnicity [2,3], and generally, it is higher in industrialized countries [4,5]. It is in the first year of life where the highest incidence rates are found, with malignant tumors during the first 5 years being almost twice as frequent as among the 5–14-year-old group. Males have a 20% increased risk when compared to females [6]. Fig. 27.1 shows age- and sex-adjusted incidence rates for childhood malignancies.

The variety of cancer types described in children is wider than in adults. During childhood leukemia (especially acute lymphoblastic leukemia), solid tumors of the central nervous system, neuroblastomas, and lymphomas represent the four most common types of malignancies in Europe, while carcinomas

Anticancer Treatments and Cardiotoxicity. DOI: http://dx.doi.org/10.1016/B978-0-12-802509-3.00027-3

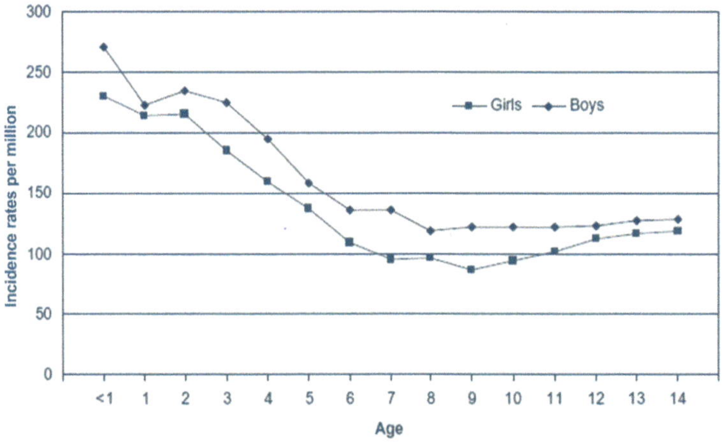

FIGURE 27.1 Age- and sex-specific incidence rates per million children for childhood cancer (age 0–14). *From German Childhood Cancer Registry. Annual Report 2008; available at http://www.unimedizin-mainz.de/index.php?id=22653.*

are a rare diagnosis in this age-group [6]. Similar patterns of incidence are found in the United States [7].

Incidence rates have experienced an average yearly increase of 1.1% [8] during recent decades for reasons that are largely unknown. Improvement of diagnostic methods, better access to medical care, or environmental changes may contribute to this rising rate.

Survival after childhood cancer is now generally good and better than for adults. Statistics [9,10] have shown an improvement of survival rates for childhood cancer with a continuous dropping of death risk among these patients.

Early diagnosis methods, continuous advances in treatment, enhanced supportive care including intensive care, blood banking, or better management of concomitant infectious diseases have led to this better and longer survival of cancer patients.

Most recent data for European trends in terms of survival come from the EUROCARE-5 study [11]. For all types of cancer combined for children diagnosed in 2000–07, 1-year survival was 90.6%, 3-year survival was 81.0%, and 5-year survival was 77.9%. American statistics show similar 5-year survival rates [7].

Naturally, survivorship varies with the type of cancer. In general, the best diagnosis-related survival rates are seen for retinoblastoma and Hodgkin lymphoma (over 95%) and the worst are found in acute myeloid leukemia and CNS tumors (around 60%) [11]. Table 27.1 summarizes the 5-year survival rates for different International Classification of Childhood Cancer diagnostic groups.

However, increasing survival comes at a price; depending on the type of pathology and received therapy, survivors of cancer during childhood may

TABLE 27.1 Five-Year Survival Rates by ICCC (International Classification of Childhood Cancer) Groups for Patients Diagnosed 2000–07 [11]

ICCC Diagnostic Group	
All cancers	77.9
Ia: acute lymphoid leukemia	86.3
Ib: acute myeloid leukemia	62.7
IIa: Hodgkin's lymphoma	95.4
IIb: nonHodgkin's lymphoma (excepts Burkitt's lymphoma)	84
IIc: Burkitt's lymphoma	90.2
III: CNS and miscellaneous intracranial and intraspinal neoplasms	57.5
IVa: neuroblastoma and ganglioneuroblastoma	70.6
V: retinoblastoma	96.4
VIa: nephroblastoma and other nonepithelial renal tumors	89.4
VIIIa: osteosarcoma	69.3
VIIIc: Ewing's sarcoma and related sarcomas of bone	67.9
IXa: rhabdomyosarcomas	67.7

remain at risk of developing subsequent malignancies, chronic disease, and functional impairments [12].

Globally, these patients have an eightfold risk of developing severe, disabling, life-threatening, or fatal conditions for several chronic diseases when compared to a sibling comparison group [13].

With regards to geographical distribution, EUROCARE-5 shows that the 5-year survival for all cancers combined is increasing in Europe. The most notable improvements occurred in Eastern Europe, where 5-year survivorship rose from 65% (1999–2001) to 70% (2000–07).

Despite these improvements, in most eastern European countries there is still a low rate of survival among children after cancer diagnosis in comparison with the rest of Europe.

Many factors contribute to worse results in eastern countries, e.g., a lower gross domestic product [14], which may led to less sensitive diagnostic methods with subsequent retard in diagnosis [15], lack of drugs and other cancer therapies [16], no availability of multidisciplinary teams [17], or worse outcomes in management of secondary effects of treatments [16].

The current panorama brings a challenging situation, especially in order to solve international inequalities and to ensure multidisciplinary follow-up for correct monitoring of childhood cancer survivors.

CHRONIC CARDIOTOXICITY AND LONG-TERM EFFECT OF RADIOTHERAPY IN CHILDHOOD

Epidemiology

A steadily growing number of childhood cancer survivors have to face life-long side effects of anticancer therapies, some of them affecting the cardiovascular system.

Irradiation of the heart as a consequence of chest radiation can cause functional and anatomic cardiac disease in children.

Radiation-related heart damage encompasses a wide range of pathologies such as pericarditis [18] which rarely evolves to cardiac tamponade, myocardial fibrosis [19], coronary artery disease, valvular alterations, conduction abnormalities, and vascular disease [20–22]. Table 27.2 lists the wide spectrum of radiotherapy-induced cardiac abnormalities.

Cardiovascular pathology is often asymptomatic for a long period of time. However, the course may be severe with acute coronary syndrome or sudden death as the initial manifestation [23].

There is evidence of the high long-term risk of cardiac death in cancer survivors having received radiotherapy. The standardized hazard ratio for

TABLE 27.2 Effects of Radiotherapy on Heart Function

Radiation-Related Cardiac Diseases

Structural
• Valve disease
  • Mitral regurgitation/stenosis
  • Aortic regurgitation/stenosis
• Pericardial disease
  • Acute pericarditis
  • Pericardial effusions
  • Constrictive pericarditis

Vascular • Microvascular dysfunction • Coronary artery disease
Myocardial • Restrictive cardiomyopathy • Systolic dysfunction • Diastolic dysfunction
Electrical and conduction abnormalities • Bundle branch blocks • Ectopy • QT prolongation • Sick sinus syndrome

cardiac death is around 6 when compared with the general population. The relative risk for death is proportional to the radiation dose (RR 3 for <4.9 Gy to RR 25 with >15 Gy) [24].

A recent large follow-up trial [25] found cardiovascular complications in 8.1% of more than 32,000 children who survived cancer. The highest rates were described for heart failure, valvular dysfunction, and cerebrovascular disease, varying considerably with age (an almost 20-fold increase in young people compared to 1.3 for those beyond the age of 60). This study also showed that hospitalization risk was increased twofold, and first hospitalization occurred, on average, 7 years earlier in cancer survivors than in control group.

Pathophysiology

Ionizing radiation damages both cancer and healthy cells by producing reactive oxygen molecules which cause disruption in DNA strands. In addition, irradiation triggers vasodilatation of small vessels, increasing their permeability. These lead to the activation of an inflammatory cascade [26] which disturbs the normal structure of the endothelium.

This results in thickening of the vessel wall due to collagen deposition and fibrosis [27].

Similarly to atheromatosis, but differing in its microvascular location, this leads to a progressive reduction of irrigation with increasing ischemia and cell death [28].

Pericardial Disease

Acute pericarditis might be one of the earliest complications of radiotherapy, appearing typically a few weeks after treatment. Its incidence, proportional to dose and volume of irradiation [29] has remarkably decreased from 20% to 2.5% [30,31] with modern methods, low doses, and shielding technics.

Acute pericarditis is usually self-limited, but in 10–20% of cases it can evolve to chronic pericarditis after 5–10 years of treatment. When chronic pericarditis appears with pericardial effusions it is referred as to effusive-constrictive pericarditis, a well-described pathology in radiation-treated cancer survivors [32,33].

Myocardial Dysfunction and Heart Failure

The absence of myocyte division makes myocardium relatively resistant to irradiation. Nevertheless, marked interstitial fibrosis is common in radiotherapy-induced cardiotoxicity, with lesions of variable volumes and distribution.

The result is an alteration of diastolic function with restrictive cardiomyopathy pattern [34].

Systolic dysfunction is generally observed after concomitant use of anthracyclines and radiotherapy.

Diastolic abnormalities are seven times more common in individuals treated with thoracic radiotherapy [35], whereas systolic dysfunction has a relative risk of 5.2 compared with control groups [25].

Valve Disease

Radiation may directly affect cardiac valves and surrounding myocardium, producing a progressive thickening of the valve leaflets, valvular retraction, and late calcification.

Survivors of Hodgkin's lymphoma treated with mediastinal radiotherapy are at a high risk of developing progressive valvular deterioration and subsequent aortic stenosis 20–30 years after treatment [36]. Valvular regurgitation is reported to be the most frequent valve disease during the first decade after irradiation, affecting about 30% [36] of survivors, meanwhile it might take valves up to 20 years to became significantly thickened, calcified, and stenotic [36].

Symptoms of valvular heart disease are the same in cancer survivors as in the general population. However, the relative risk of needing valve surgery can rise up to 8 [21] compared to general population.

Coronary Artery Disease

Survivors treated with thoracic radiotherapy are at increased risk of radiation-associated coronary artery disease, which is an established cause of early mortality [37].

Radiation injury to the coronaries is caused by endothelial damage with a subsequent acceleration of atherosclerosis [38]. Ostial lesions are frequent and life-threatening complications.

The evolution might be quick and severe with acute coronary syndrome or even sudden death, but is more likely to develop a silent coronary disease for a long time before symptoms. The risk of myocardial infarction in patients radiated for Hodgkin's lymphoma is 2–7-fold higher than in the general population with a cumulative incidence of 13% after 30 years of chest irradiation [39].

Arrhythmias

Abnormalities along the entire conduction system have been described in childhood cancer survivors treated with radiotherapy. These include varying degrees of atrioventricular block, sick sinus syndrome, prolonged QT, and supraventricular and ventricular tachycardia [40].

Ventricular ectopy might occur in up to 50% [41] of children treated with radiation. The most common conduction abnormality seems to be right bundle branch block, possibly due to its anterior location [42].

CARDIOTOXICITY RISK FACTORS IN THE PEDIATRIC AGE

Since survival rates with childhood cancer are steadily improving, there is a greater responsibility to monitor these survivors for late adverse health outcomes related to cancer treatment. Development of secondary malignancies and major cardiac events are the most common effects of all the late toxicities tracked in childhood cancer survivors [43].

Chemotherapeutic cardiotoxicity can be characterized as either type I or type II cardiotoxicity based on the effect of the agent on cardiomyocytes. Type I cardiotoxicity is caused by cardiomyocyte death, either through necrosis or apoptosis, and as a result is not reversible. Type II cardiotoxicity is caused by cardiomyocyte dysfunction rather than cell death and therefore may be reversible.

An established direct relationship between radiotherapy dose and major cardiac events has been described. Anthracycline exposure $>250\ mg/m^2$ is also an independent risk factor for heart failure, pericardial disease, and valvular abnormalities [44].

Furthermore, the combined effect of chest radiation and anthracyclines is stronger than either exposure alone, developing cardiac disease in a shorter period of time [45].

In terms of exposure to these cardiotoxic treatments, anthracyclines are used in over 50% [46] of childhood cancer treatments, whereas chest irradiation is used in almost 25% of children surviving cancer [47].

Anthracycline

Anthracycline cardiotoxicity has three different types (acute, early onset, and late onset) depending on the time between administration and development of signs and symptoms of cardiac disease. Table 27.3 includes the main characteristics of the different types of anthracycline-induced cardiotoxicity.

Acute abnormalities within the first week of treatment may be transient. The long-term cardiotoxicity caused by the anthracyclines includes cardiomyocyte death and therefore represents a type I toxicity which is irreversible.

These acute changes during anthracycline therapy range from minor abnormalities to fatal heart failure. Ecocardiography can reveal systolic dysfunction and it is not rare to see electrocardiographic alterations, most often asymptomatic until late in the disease process.

Many more survivors experience late-onset cardiotoxicity. Total accumulative dose of anthracyclines is the most important risk factor for permanent cardiac dysfunction [48] which appears as long as two decades after therapy,

TABLE 27.3 Characteristics of the Different Types of Anthracycline Cardiotoxicity

Characteristic	Acute Cardiotoxicity	Early-Onset Progressive Cardiotoxicity	Late-Onset Progressive Cardiotoxicity
Onset	Within the first week of anthracycline treatment	<1 year after completion of anthracycline treatment	≥1 year after completion of anthracycline treatment
Risk factor dependence	Unknown	Yes[a]	Yes[a]
Clinical features in children	Transient depression of myocardial contractility	Restrictive cardiomyopathy and/or dilated cardiomyopathy	Dilated cardiomyopathy
Course	Usually reversible on discontinuation of anthracycline	Can be progressive	Can be progressive

[a]*Risk factors for early-onset and late-onset cardiotoxicity are shown in Table 27.4.*

but it is unclear if there is a time limit. This is due to dose-related toxicity, with myocyte loss and damage, leading to a progressive left ventricle dilatation, wall thinning, and decreased contractility [49]. Table 27.4 includes risk factors for developing cardiotoxicity in children under anthracycline therapy.

Radiation

Children having received heart radiation are at risk of developing radiation-induced cardiac disease. Modern techniques using lower total doses, hyperfractionation, and cardiac shielding are less likely to cause damage.

Whether the heart sustains injury after radiation treatment depends on several factors including: [52]

- Host factors
  - Young age at irradiation. High risk if younger than 5 years
  - Ethnicity (high risk if African descent)
  - Medical conditions (hypertension, obesity, dyslipidemia, coronary artery disease, diabetes mellitus, febrile illness)
  - Behavioral factors (smoking, isometric exercise, drug use)
- Treatment factors
  - Radiation dose ≥20 Gy to chest
  - Total body irradiation

TABLE 27.4 Risk Factors for Anthracycline-Induced Cardiotoxicity [48]

Risk Factors	Features
Total cumulative dose	Most significant predictor of abnormal cardiac function
Age	For comparable cumulative doses, younger age predisposes to greater cardiotoxicity (especially <5 years of age)
Length of follow-up	Longer follow-up results in higher prevalence of myocardial impairment
Sex	Females more vulnerable for comparable doses
Genetics	CBR3 genotype [50]
	C282Y genotype [51]
Concomitant mantle radiation	Evidence of enhanced cardiotoxicity; not clear whether additive or synergistic
Others	Concomitant exposure to cyclophosphamide, bleomycin, vincristine, amsacrine, or mitoxantrone may predispose to cardiotoxicity; trisomy 21 and black race have been associated with higher risk of early clinical cardiotoxicity
Rate of anthracycline administration	Higher rate was thought to predispose to greater toxicity, but current trials do not support this

  - Combined with radiomimetic chemotherapy (e.g., doxorubicin, dactinomicyn)
  - Combined with other cardiotoxic chemotherapy (anthracyclines, cyclophosphamide, amsacrine)
- Treatment highest-risk factors
  - Anteriorly weighted radiation fields
  - Lack of subcarinal shielding
  - Doses ≥ 30 Gy having received anthracyclines
  - Doses ≥ 40 Gy not having received anthracyclines
  - Longer time since treatment.

Additional Risk Factors

There is substantial evidence suggesting that anthracyclines and chest radiation place survivors of childhood cancer at increased risk for late-onset cardiotoxicity. However, as the lifespan of these patients is rising, traditional, modifiable cardiovascular factors should be considered in developing late cardiac outcomes.

This population, even if not treated with either anthracyclines or radiotherapy, has a higher proportion of certain cardiovascular risk factors

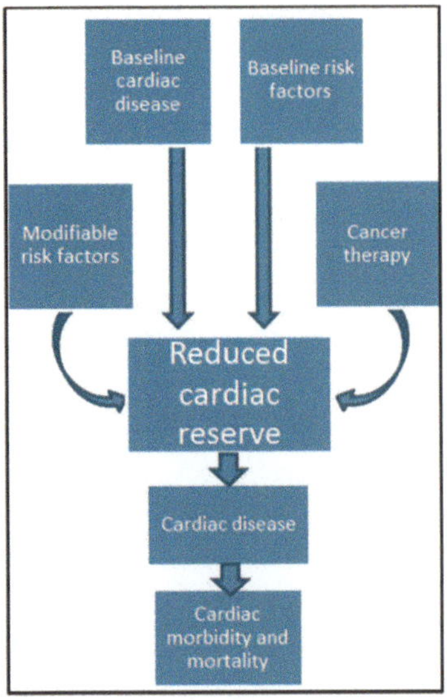

FIGURE 27.2 The multiple-hit hypothesis of cancer therapy-related cardiotoxicity.

(e.g., elevated body mass index, insulin level, a nonhigh-density lipoprotein cholesterol), compared to a sibling population [53].

The multiple-hit hypothesis (Fig. 27.2) integrates cardiac disease and risk factors that in combination with cancer therapy contribute to increase the burden of cardiac disease among cancer survivors.

DETECTION AND MONITORING OF CARDIOTOXICITY IN CHILDREN

Monitoring and screening of childhood cancer survivors is absolutely needed in order to detect early signs of cardiotoxicity in higher-risk patients. A baseline cardiac evaluation including medical history and physical exam is recommended before beginning chemotherapy [54–56].

Theoretically, *endomyocardial biopsy* should be the best means to provide in-treatment histological information but the performance of serial biopsies is not suggested in the clinical practice because they are highly invasive and expensive.

As in adults, *serum cardiac biomarkers* as cardiac troponin T, N-terminal probrain-natriutetic-peptide (NT-proBNP) and high-sensitivity C-reactive protein appear to be very promising for serial evaluations. They may identify childhood populations experiencing cardiotoxicity and those more prone to subsequent cardiotoxicity. In children with acute lymphoblastic leukemia treated with doxorubicin, elevated troponin T levels in the first 90 days of therapy were associated with reduced left ventricular (LV) mass 4 years after therapy,

NT-proBNP concentrations were elevated in 89% of patients before treatment and in 48% of posttreatment patients, whereas the levels of C-reactive proteins remained in the normal range [57]. Of note, an increase in troponin T concentrations is associated with high probability of major cardiac events within the first year of follow-up, whereas patients with persistently normal troponin levels would not develop cardiotoxicity, with a negative predictive value of 99% [58]. Increased hs-cTnT levels are detectable also in a substantial proportion of adult survivors of childhood acute leukemias, these being related to higher cumulative anthracycline dose received and cardiac irradiation [59]. High-sensitivity cTnI assay could also be more effective in identifying cardiac injury. In another study, however, cardiac TnT did not contribute to identify late-onset anthracycline-induced cardiotoxicity while abnormal levels of NT-pro-BNP were detected in 13% of 122 asymptomatic, long-term survivors of childhood cancer [60]. The International Late Effects of Childhood Cancer Guideline Harmonization Group has dealt recently with the issue of monitoring late cardiotoxic effects in survivors of childhood anthracycline-induced cardiotoxicity [61].

Echocardiography is highly recommended in primary and periodic evaluation of children exposed to the cardiotoxic effects of chemotherapeutics. It has to be taken into account that subjects undergoing anthracycline therapy in the pediatric age group are subjected to an LV remodeling induced by a thinning of LV walls. Therefore, LV mass index can often be reduced, since the increase of LV internal diameters occurs only in the advanced stages, it being accompanied by a depression of LV chamber function. The assessment of LV systolic function in this setting of patients is commonly performed by estimation of ejection fraction (EF) but endocardial fractional shortening obtained by LV linear measurements at end-diastole and end-systole has been also used in some studies [9]. As in adults, anthracycline treatment should be discontinued if EF or fractional shortening drop by 10% or more below the normal EF (50%). Even in cases of inadequate ultrasound windows, MUGA assessment of EF should be discouraged and eventually favored the performance of magnetic resonance imaging (MRI) in children.

In general, also in childhood, LVEF appears to have a limited role for identifying early, subclinical cardiotoxicity and should therefore be combined with assessment of additional echocardiographic measurements of cardiac function. Asymptomatic pediatric cancer survivors at high risk for anthracycline cardiotoxicity have some evidence of LV diastolic abnormalities, including prolongation of E velocity deceleration time [62] and of isovolumic relaxation [62,63], abnormal pulmonary venous flow pattern [63], reduction of pulsed tissue Doppler-derived e′ velocity of the mitral annulus and increase of E/e′ ratio [64]. A recent study demonstrated the superiority of global longitudinal strain (GLS) in detecting early, subclinical cardiotoxicity in children [62,65,66] as it occurs in adults. Reduced GLS in childhood cancer survivors can be attributed to the loss of myocites and increased collagen deposit resulting in myocardial fibrosis.

TABLE 27.5 List of Cardiac Imaging Parameters to Detect Cardiotoxicity of Cancer Treatments in Childhood

Echocardiography	Left ventricular mass index
	Ejection fraction
	Deceleration time of E′ velocity and IVRT
	E′ velocity and E/e′ ratio
	Global longitudinal strain
Cardiac MRI	Ejection fraction
	LGE
	T1 mapping

Cardiac MRI can be more than a simple alternative to echocardiography in childhood cancer survivors [67]. It may be significantly more accurate in estimating EF. However, recent findings support the use of cardiac MRI for the evaluation of the left atrial volume, as an early marker of diastolic dysfunction, and myocardial delayed enhancement, as a marker of myocardial fibrosis and scarring in this clinical setting [68]. Moreover, myocardial T1 and extracellular volume have been found to be early tissue markers of LV remodeling, they being expressions of diffuse fibrosis in children with normal EF postanthracycline therapy, and being related to cumulative dose, exercise capacity, and myocardial wall thinning [69]. Table 27.5 summarizes the main parameters for detecting and monitoring cardiac function and structure in childhood cancer survivors by different cardiac imaging modalities.

PREVENTION OF CARDIOTOXICITY IN CHILDREN

The prevention of anthracycline-induced cardiotoxicity is very important in children who can be expected to survive for decades after being cured of their malignancy. Attempts to reduce anthracycline cardiotoxicity have been directed towards:

1. Decreasing myocardial concentrations of anthracyclines and their metabolites by dose limitation, schedule modification and route of administration;
2. Developing and using less cardiotoxic analogs;
3. Administering cardioprotective agents to attenuate the effects of anthracyclines on the heart [70].

As regards schedule modification, avoidance of anthracycline peak levels may reduce the pathologic and clinical cardiotoxicity, although this has not always been observed. Reduced cumulative anthracycline dose is one of the most commonly accepted heart damage prevention methods. Accordingly, the recommended highest doxorubicin dose should fall within the range of 400–550 mg/m^2 and not exceed 240 mg/m^2 in children and adolescents. Another possibility is represented by the route of administration [71]. It is likely that heart injury does not depend on the cumulative dose only but also on peak serum anthracycline levels. Despite controversial results in different studies, it could be postulated that a continuous anthracycline infusion could have a cardioprotective effect by decreasing the maximum serum drug concentration. Based on this assumption, several pediatric treatment schemes recommend continuous infusion, although long-term observation does not sustain its efficacy [71].

The analogs of doxorubicin, such as epirubicin, have similar cardiotoxicity to that of doxorubicin when given in amounts of equivalent myelotoxicity. Liposomal (third-generation) anthracyclines are a new class of agent that may allow more specific organ targeting, thereby producing less cardiac toxicity. This technology made it possible to transport doxorubicin on a liposomal carrier and to prolong the time it remains within the circulation, just like the continuous infusion. Liposomes are capable of transporting active substances selectively to the neoplastic tissue [72]. However, liposomal anthracycline forms are very expensive, which limits their use, however more studies are required to assess the effective advantages, if any, of these preparations over classical anthracyclines.

The cardioprotective agent, dexrazoxane, an iron chelator, is highly effective and provides short-term cardioprotection to most patients receiving even the most intensive doxorubicin-containing regimens. Preliminary results have shown cardioprotective effects of dexrazoxane in pediatric cancer patients at early stages of treatment. Its long-term benefits remain to be determined. In addition, it has been observed that it could reduce the efficacy of cancer therapies [73]. The use of β-blockers and ACE inhibitors has been also proposed, similarly to adult cancer patients but dosages remain to be well established in children. In children developing heart failure, therapy with ACE inhibitors induces improvement in LV structure and function, but this improvement appears to be transient.

Subtle, subclinical abnormalities, related to anthracycline treatment in childhood, can develop into cardiomyopathy, which may progress toward heart failure during time. In the presence of heart failure, the use of digitalis and diuretic therapy can be suggested. In children who have refractory hemodynamic decompensation, heart transplantation is indicated.

REFERENCES

[1] Howlader N, Noone AM, Krapcho M, et al., editors. SEER cancer statistics review, 1975–2010. Bethesda, MD: National Cancer Institute; 2013.

[2] Bhatia S. Disparities in cancer outcomes: lessons learned from children with cancer. Pediatr Blood Cancer 2011;56:994–1002.

[3] Pui CH, Pei D, Pappo AS, et al. Treatment out comes in black and white children with cancer: results from the SEER database and St Jude Children's Research Hospital, 1992 through 2007. J Clin Oncol 2012;30:2005–12.

[4] Bunin GR. Nongenetic causes of childhood cancers: evidence from international variation, time trends, and risk factor studies. Toxicol Appl Pharmacol 2004;199:91–103.

[5] Stiller CA, Parkin DM. Geographic and ethnic variations in the incidence of childhood cancer. Br Med Bull 1996;52:682–703.

[6] German Childhood Cancer Registry. Annual report 2008, <http://www.kinderkrebsregister.de/english/content08.html>; 2009.

[7] Ward E, De Santis C, Robbins A, Kohler B, Jemal A. Childhood and adolescent cancer statistics, 2014. CA Cancer J Clin 2014;64:83–103.

[8] Kaatsch P, Steliarova-Foucher E, Crocetti E, Magnani C, Spix C, Zambon P. Time trends of cancer incidence in European children (1978–1997): report from the automated childhood cancer information system project. Eur J Cancer 2006;42:1961–71.

[9] Gatta G, Zigon G, Capocaccia R, et al. The Eurocare Working Group Survival of European children and young adults with cancer diagnosed 1995–2002. Eur J Cancer 2009;45:992–1005.

[10] Gatta G, Capocaccia R, Stiller C, Kaatsch P, Berrino F, Terenziani M, et al. Childhood cancer survival trends in Europe: a Eurocare Working Group study. J Clin Oncol 2005;23:3742–51.

[11] Gatta G, et al. Childhood cancer survival in Europe 1999–2007: results of Eurocare-5—a population-based study. Lancet Oncol 2014;15:35–47.

[12] Armstrong GT, Liu Q, Yasui Y, et al. Late mortality among 5-year survivors of childhood cancer: a summary from the Childhood Cancer Survivor Study. J Clin Oncol 2009;27:2328–38.

[13] Diller L, Chow EJ, Gurney JG, Hudson MM, Kadin-Lottick NS, Kawashima TI, et al. Chronic disease in the Childhood Cancer Survivor Study cohort: a review of published findings. J Clin Oncol 2009;27:2339–55.

[14] GDP per capita, <http://data.worldbank.org/indicator/NY.GDP.PCAP.CD/countries> [accessed 19.08.13].

[15] SIOPE. Standards of Care for Children with Cancer, <http://www.siope.eu/european-research-and-standards/standards-of-care-inpaediatric-oncology/> [accessed 19.08.13].

[16] Sullivan R, Kowalczyk JR, Agarwal B, et al. New policies to address the global burden of childhood cancers. Lancet Oncol 2013;14:e125–35.

[17] Pritchard-Jones K, Pieters R, Reaman GH, et al. Sustaining innovation and improvement in the treatment of childhood cancer: lessons from high-income countries. Lancet Oncol 2013;14:e95–103.

[18] Stewart JR, Fajardo LF, Gillette SM, Constine LS. Radiation injury to the heart. Int J Radiat Oncol Biol Phys 1995;31:1205–11.

[19] Lipshultz SE, Sallan SE. Cardiovascular abnormalities in long-term survivors of childhood malignancy. J Clin Oncol 1993;11:1199–203.

[20] Adams MJ, Lipshultz SE, Schwartz C, et al. Radiation-associated cardiovascular disease: manifestations and management. Semin Radiat Oncol 2003;13:346–56.

[21] Hull MC, Morris CG, Pepine CJ, Mendenhall NP. Valvular dysfunction and carotid, subclavian, and coronary artery disease in survivors of Hodgkin lymphoma treated with radiation therapy. JAMA 2003;290:2831–7.

[22] Green DM, Grigoriev YA, Nan B, et al. Congestive heart failure after treatment for Wilms' tumor: a report from the National Wilms' Tumor Study group. J Clin Oncol 2001;19:1926–34.

[23] Totterman K, Pesonene E, Siltanen P. Radiation related chronic heart disease. Chest 1983;6:875–8.

[24] Tukenova M, Guibout C, Oberlin O, Doyon F, Mousannif A, Haddy N, et al. Role of cancer treatment in long-term overall and cardiovascular mortality after childhood cancer. J Clin Oncol 2010;28:1308–15.

[25] Gudmundsdottir T, Winther JF, de Fine Licht S, Bonnesen TG, Asdahl PH, Tryggvadottir L, et al. Cardiovascular disease in adult life after childhood cancer in Scandinavia: a population-based cohort study of 32,308 one-year survivors. Int J Cancer 2015;121 (5):800. Available from: http://dx.doi.org/10.1002/ijc.29468.

[26] Hatoum OA, Otterson MF, Kopelman D, et al. Radiation induces endothelial dysfunction in murine intestinal arterioles via enhanced production of reactive oxygen species. Arterioscler Thromb Vasc Biol 2006;26:287–94.

[27] Gaya AM, Ashford RF. Cardiac complications of radiation therapy. Clin Oncol (R Coll Radiol) 2005;17:153–9.

[28] Ng AK, Abramson JS, Digumarthy SR, Reingold JS, Stone JR. Case records of the Massachusetts General Hospital. Case 24–2010. A 56-year-old woman with a history of Hodgkin's lymphoma and sudden onset of dyspnea and shock. N Engl J Med 2010;363:664–75.

[29] van Rijswijk S, Huijbregts MA, Lust E, Strack van Schijndel RJ. Minire view on cardiac complications after mediastinal irradiation for Hodgkin lymphoma. Neth J Med 2008;66:234–7.

[30] Carmel RJ, Kaplan HS. Mantle irradiation in Hodgkin's disease. An analysis of technique, tumor eradication, and complications. Cancer 1976;37:2813–25.

[31] Mauch PM, Weinstein H, Botnick L, Belli J, Cassady JR. An evaluation of long-term survival and treatment complications in children with Hodgkin's disease. Cancer 1983;51:925–32.

[32] Hancock EW. Subacute effusive-constrictive pericarditis. Circulation 1971;43:183–92.

[33] Sagrista-Sauleda J, Angel J, Sanchez A, Permanyer-Miralda G, SolerSoler J. Effusive-constrictive pericarditis. N Engl J Med 2004;350:469–75.

[34] Chello M, Mastroroberto P, Romano R, Zofrea S, Bevacqua I, Marchese AR. Changes in the proportion of types I and III collagen in the left ventricular wall of patients with post-irradiative pericarditis. Cardiovasc Surg 1996;4:222–6.

[35] Heidenreich PA, Hancock SL, Vagelos RH, Lee BK, Schnittger I. Diastolic dysfunction after mediastinal irradiation. Am Heart J 2005;150:977–82.

[36] Wethal T, Lund MB, Edvardsen T. Valvular dysfunction and left ventricular changes in Hodgkin's lymphoma survivors. A longitudinal study. Br J Cancer 2009;101:575–81.

[37] Hancock SL, Donaldson SS, Hoppe RT. Cardiac disease following treatment of Hodgkin's disease in children and adolescents. J Clin Oncol 1993;11:1208–15.

[38] Adams MJ, Lipshultz SE. Pathophysiology of anthracycline- and radiation-associated cardiomyopathies: implications for screening and prevention. Pediatr Blood Cancer 2005;44:600–6.

[39] van Leeuwen-Segarceanu EM, Bos WJ, Dorresteijn LD, Rensing BJ, der Heyden JA, Vogels OJ, et al. Screening Hodgkin lymphoma survivors for radiotherapy induced cardiovascular disease. Cancer Treat Rev 2011;37:391–403.

[40] Orzan F, Brusca A, Gaita F, et al. Associated cardiac lesions in patients with radiation-induced complete heart block. Int J Cardiol 1993;39:151–6.

[41] Larsen RL, Jakacki RI, Vetter VL, Meadows AT, Silber JH, Barber G. Electrocardiographic changes and arrhythmias after cancer therapy in children and young adults. Am J Cardiol 1992;70:73–7.

[42] Adams MJ, Lipsitz SR, Colan SD, et al. Cardiovascular status in long-term survivors of Hodgkin's disease treated with chest radiotherapy. J Clin Oncol 2004;22:3139–48.

[43] Armstrong GT, Kawashima T, Leisenring W, et al. Aging and risk of severe, disabling, life-threatening, and fatal events in the childhood cancer survivor study. J Clin Oncol 2014;32:1218–27.

[44] Mulrooney DA, Yeazel MW, Kawashima T, et al. Cardiac outcomes in a cohort of adult survivors of childhood and adolescent cancer: retrospective analysis of the Childhood Cancer Survivor Study cohort. BMJ 2009;339:b4606.

[45] Van Der Pal HJ, Van Dalen EC, Van Delden E, et al. High risk of symptomatic cardiac events in childhood cancer survivors. J Clin Oncol 2012;30:1429–37.

[46] Albini A, Pennesi G, Donatelli F, Cammarota R, De Flora S, Noonan DM. Cardiotoxicity of anticancer drugs: the need for cardio-oncology and cardio-oncological prevention. J Natl Cancer Inst 2010;102:14–25.

[47] Armstrong GT, Oeffinger KC, Chen Y, et al. Modifiable risk factors and major cardiac events among adult survivors of childhood cancer. J Clin Oncol 2013;31:3673–80.

[48] Lipshultz SE, Adams MJ, Colan SD, et al. Long-term cardiovascular toxicity in children, adolescents, and young adults who receive cancer therapy: pathophysiology, course, monitoring, management, prevention, and research directions: a scientific statement from the American Heart Association. Circulation 2013;128:1927–95.

[49] Kim DH, Landry 3rd AB, Lee YS, Katz AM. Doxorubicin-induced calcium release from cardiac sarcoplasmic reticulum vesicles. J Mol Cell Cardiol 1989;21:433–6.

[50] Lipshultz SE, Lipsitz SR, Kutok JL, Miller TL, Colan SD, Neuberg DS, et al. Impact of hemochromatosis gene mutations on cardiac status in doxorubicin-treated survivors of childhood high-risk leukemia. Cancer 2013;119:3555–62.

[51] Blanco JG, Sun CL, Landier W, Chen L, Esparza-Duran D, Leisenring W, et al. Anthracycline-related cardiomyopathy after childhood cancer: role of polymorphisms in carbonyl reductase genes-a report from the Children's Oncology Group. J Clin Oncol 2012;30:1415–21.

[52] Children's Oncology Group. Long-term follow-up guidelines for survivors of childhood, adolescent and young adult cancers. Version 4.0. Monrovia, CA: Children's Oncology Group, <www.survivorshipguidelines.org>; 2013.

[53] Lipshultz SE, Landy DC, Lopez-Mitnik G, et al. Cardiovascular status of childhood cancer survivors exposed and unexposed to cardiotoxic therapy. J Clin Oncol 2012;30:1050–7.

[54] Bovelli D, Plataniotis G, Roila F. Cardiotoxicity of chemotherapeutic agents and radiotherapy-related heart disease: ESMO Clinical Practice Guidelines. Ann Oncol 2010;21(Suppl. 5):v277–82.

[55] Trachtenberg BH, Landy DC, Franco VI, Henkel JM, Pearson EJ, Miller TL, et al. Anthracycline-associated cardiotoxicity in survivors of childhood cancer. Pediatr Cardiol 2011;32:342–53.

[56] Gottsauner-Wolf M, Schedlmayer-Duit J, Porenta G, Gwechenberger M, Huber K, et al. Assessment of left ventricular function: comparison between radionuclide angiography and semiquantitative two-dimensional echocardiographic analysis. Eur J Nucl Med 1996;23:1613–18.

[57] Lipshultz SE, Miller TL, Scully RE, Lipsitz SR, Rifai N, Silverman LB, et al. Changes in cardiac biomarkers during doxorubicin treatment of pediatric patients with high-risk acute lymphoblastic leukemia: associations with long-term echocardiographic outcomes. J Clin Oncol 2012;30:1042–9.

[58] Dolci A, Dominici R, Cardinale D, Sandri MT, Panteghine M. Biochemical markers for prediction of chemotherapy-induced cardiotoxicity: systematic review of the literature and recommendations for use. Am J Clin Pathol 2009;130:688–95.

[59] Cheung YF, Yu W, Cheuk DK, Cheng FW, Yang JY, Yau JP, et al. Plasma high sensitivity troponin T levels in adult survivors of childhood leukaemias: determinants and associations with cardiac function. PLoS One 2013;8:e77063.

[60] Mavinkurve-Groothuis AM, Groot-Loonen J, Bellersen L, Pourier MS, Feuth T, Bökkerink JP, et al. Abnormal NT-pro-BNP levels in asymptomatic long-term survivors of childhood cancer treated with anthracyclines. Pediatr Blood Cancer 2009;52:631–6.

[61] Armenian SH, Hudson MM, Mulder RL, Chen MH, Constine LS, Dwyer M, et al. Recommendations for cardiomyopathy surveillance for survivors of childhood cancer: a report from the International Late Effects of Childhood Cancer Guideline Harmonization Group. Lancet Oncol 2015;16:e123–36.

[62] Iarussi D, Galderisi M, Ratti G, Tedesco MA, Indolfi P, Casale F, et al. Left ventricular systolic and diastolic function after anthracycline chemotherapy in childhood. Clin Cardiol 2001;24:663–9.

[63] Ganame J, Claus P, Uyttebroeck A, Renard M, D'hooge J, Bijnens B, et al. Myocardial dysfunction late after low-dose anthracycline treatment in asymptomatic pediatric patients. J Am Soc Echocardiogr 2007;20:1351–8.

[64] Karakurt C, Koçak G, Ozgen U. Evaluation of the left ventricular function with tissue tracking and tissue Doppler echocardiography in pediatric malignancy survivors after anthracycline therapy. Echocardiography 2008;25:880–7.

[65] Toro-Salazar OH, Gillan E, O'Loughlin MT, Burke GS, Ferranti J, Stainsby J, et al. Occult cardiotoxicity in childhood cancer survivors exposed to anthracycline therapy. Circ Cardiovasc Imaging 2013;6:873–80.

[66] Mavinkurve-Groothuis AM, Marcus KA, Pourier M, Loonen J, Feuth T, Hoogerbrugge PM, et al. Myocardial 2D strain echocardiography and cardiac biomarkers in children during and shortly after anthracycline therapy for acute lymphoblastic leukaemia (ALL): a prospective study. Eur Heart J Cardiovasc Imaging 2013;14:562–9

[67] Basar EZ, Corapcioglu F, Babaoglu K, Anik Y, GorurDaglioz G, Dedeoglu R. Are cardiac magnetic resonance imaging and radionuclide ventriculography good options against echocardiography for evaluation of anthracycline induced chronic cardiotoxicity in childhood cancer survivors? Pediatr Hematol Oncol 2014;31:237–52.

[68] de Ville de Goyet M, Brichard B, Robert A, Renard L, Veyckemans F, Vanhoutte L, et al. Prospective cardiac MRI for the analysis of biventricular function in children undergoing cancer treatments. Pediatr Blood Cancer 2015;62:867–74.

[69] Tham EB, Haykowsky MJ, Chow K, Spavor M, Kaneko S, Khoo NS, et al. Diffuse myocardial fibrosis by T1-mapping in children with subclinical anthracycline cardiotoxicity: relationship to exercise capacity, cumulative dose and remodeling. J Cardiovasc Magn Reson 2013;15:48.

[70] Iarussi D, Indolfi P, Casale F, Martino V, Di Tullio MT, Calabrò R. Anthracycline-induced cardiotoxicity in children with cancer: strategies for prevention and management. Paediatr Drugs 2005;7:67–76.

[71] Franco VI, Henkel JM, Miller TL, Lipshultz SE. Cardiovascular effects in childhood cancer survivors treated with anthracyclines. Cardiol Res Pract 2011;11:346–79.

[72] Sieswerda E, Kremer L, Caron H, van Dalen E. The use of liposomal anthracycline analogues for childhood malignancies: a systematic review. Eur J Cancer 2011;47:2000–8.

[73] Tebbi CK, London WB, Friedman D, Villaluna D, De Alarcon PA, Constine LS, et al. Dexrazoxane-associated risk for acute myeloid leukemia/myelodysplastic syndrome and other secondary malignancies in pediatric Hodgkin's disease. J Clin Oncol 2007;25(5):493–500.

Section VII

Management of Anticancer Drugs Related Cardiotoxicity

Chapter 28

Nonpharmacologic Therapy

G.L. Alonso Salinas and J.L. Zamorano Gómez

Chapter Outline

One important item needs to be addressed clinically: only a subgroup of patients who are treated with certain chemotherapy, targeted therapy, or chemoprevention regimens will develop cardiovascular complications, the risk being individual.

The best treatment for chemotherapy-induced cardiotoxicity is prevention. The first step in this process should be a careful selection of candidates for chemotherapy. Before starting chemotherapeutic interventions, a complete medical history and physical examination should be obtained to appropriately risk-stratify patients and optimize cardiac surveillance. Preexisting cardiac disease is often underestimated, but that is also manageable if the patients have careful cardiovascular monitoring and cardiac adjusted treatment.

RISK FACTORS

An accurate family and personal history will lead to identifying high-risk patients. Environmental and genetic factors determine susceptibility to develop cardiotoxicity of any kind. The genetic component is polygenic and different genes cooperate in an epistatic manner. Epigenetic factors also contribute to the genetic susceptibility to cardiotoxicity.

Moreover, familial risk of coronary artery disease or cardiac heart failure has been associated with an additional risk of developing these conditions in the treated population. Age, sex, and other characteristics or events related to personal history, including previous or concurrent therapies, should be included.

Anticancer Treatments and Cardiotoxicity. DOI: http://dx.doi.org/10.1016/B978-0-12-802509-3.00028-5

Cardiotoxity increases with age, although it can appear in all ages. Toxicity can also develop months after the last chemotherapy dose, and late reactions can be seen years later when they present as new-onset cardiomyopathy [1].

Also, men and women have differences in risk of cardiotoxicity. As in the noncancer population, premenopausal women are less likely than men of the same age to develop atherosclerosis. However, after the menopause the rate of atherosclerosis rapidly increases. Thus, gender is important to take into account in risk stratification in these patients [2].

Early stratification of high-risk patients should be a primary goal for oncologists in the development of personalized antineoplastic therapeutic strategies or interventions. The improvement of diagnostic tools in cardiology and in oncology has led to an increased number of patients who have been treated for cancer and diagnosed with cardiovascular disease. It may sometimes be necessary for oncology patients to undergo cardiothoracic surgery to survive heart problems, when their risk from cardiovascular disease outweighs their risk from cancer. Therefore, risk versus benefit or risk versus risk evaluations should de performed by a cardio-oncology interdisciplinary unit.

Baseline cardiovascular examination with careful cardiovascular management could not only prevent adverse events from antineoplastic drugs but could also be used to exclude their use in potentially high-risk individuals and thereby enable assessment of the effectiveness of these therapeutic or prevention agents in low- and moderate-risk individuals. One simple approach to monitor the cardiotoxicity of chemotherapy is arterial pressure measurement to identify hypertension.

Hypertension is a relatively common and dose-related side effect of several antiangiogenic drugs [3,4], mainly due to inhibition of vascular endothelial growth factor, which decreases nitrous oxide in the wall of arterioles. It can occur at any time during therapy, and preexisting hypertension is an important risk factor for cardiovascular complications. Aggressive hypertensive monitoring and intervention are needed before and during therapy. Heart failure agents, such as β-blockers and angiotensin inhibitors are preferred, since chemotherapy can cause left ventricular dysfunction.

Lipid profile is another target to control in high-risk oncology patients. Lipid-lowering agents have been described and indicated as protective agents against anthracycline-mediated cardiotoxicity; in particular statins seem to have a chemotherapy cardiotoxicity preventive and direct antitumor effect [5].

Active smoking has been shown to be a predictor of myocardial infarction or coronary artery disease in breast cancer, requiring intervention prior to chemotherapy [6].

Another mandatory approach is performing electrocardiography before chemotherapy. QRS voltage reduction in ECG limbs leads and prolonged

QTc interval have been identified as early markers of left ventricular dysfunction after chronic anthracycline-based treatment. However, oncology patients can have multiple risk factors for QTc prolongation at baseline due to preexisting cardiac disease, kidney or liver disorders, and concomitant medications, which make this parameter even less reliable in the risk assessment.

The most frequently used and effective approach to monitor cardiac function is by echocardiography. Left ventricular ejection fraction (LVEF) and its decrease are an indicator of cardiovascular risk and heart failure during and after chemotherapy [7]. However, decrease of LVEF does not identify early subclinical myocardial dysfunction. In contrast, it seems that early identification of left ventricular diastolic impairment can be crucial in patients who may develop left ventricular systolic dysfunction and overt heart failure. Two parameters that reveal signs of early cardiac dysfunction are tissue Doppler imaging and myocardial deformation imaging (strain and strain rate). Alterations in these two modalities can predict LVEF decrease in an early phase.

Other imaging techniques are also available and can help us in prechemotherapy stratification. Nuclear imaging can provide an evaluation of cardiac function independent from geometrical assumptions of ventricular shape, although its use might be limited because of high cost and radiation exposure. Cardiovascular magnetic resonance (CMR) imaging can characterize cardiac tissue with a prognostic value in patients treated with cardiotoxic drugs. It is proved that an increase of relative myocardial contrast enhancement predicts a significant decline in LVEF at 28 days [8].

EXERCISE

It has been proposed that aerobic exercise as a nonpharmacologic therapy may mitigate the deleterious effects of heart failure. It has been shown that exercise encourages nitric oxide formation and improves cardiac and skeletal muscle energy metabolism and function, despite improving diastolic filling and increasing stroke volume. All of these changes improve both systolic and diastolic functions, cardiac output and increase oxygen uptake, resulting in better exercise tolerance and decreasing fatigability [9].

Moreover, some studies have shown that there is an inverse relation of physical exercise practice and cancer appearance. It is described that physical activity may decrease renal cancer risk [10].

The aerobic capacity in women treated with doxorubicin is approximately 30% below that of age-matched sedentary untreated women, despite normal left ventricle ejection fraction [11]. These data suggest that doxorubicin-induced injury affects not only the myocardium but also other oxygen-transport organs, such as the lungs. Several studies in animals have investigated the effects of aerobic exercise training before and during doxorubicin therapy, but nowadays there is no evidence from human studies.

Aerobic exercise might be particularly effective for preventing the functional decrease that chemotherapy can cause. It can simultaneously increase the reserve capacity of multiple oxygen-transport organs, thereby leading to improvements in aerobic capacity.

NUTRITION AND DIET

Correct nutrition is one of the pillars of any cardiovascular risk-reduction strategy. A complete and polyunsaturated fat-free diet, with a correct balance between proteins, lipids, and carbohydrates, and with the correct quantity of fiber, vitamins, and other essential nutritive complements, has been shown to be primordial in primary and secondary prevention. One example of a healthy diet is the so-called Mediterranean diet.

The Mediterranean diet is the most evidence-based diet to prevent not only cardiovascular disease but also other chronic diseases, as it becomes the standard for health eating and a dietary template of particular value. Diet and its components have been found to reduce cardiovascular risk by mechanisms including reductions of blood pressure, lipids, endothelial dysfunction, glucose, body mass index, and waist circumference as well as by providing increased nitric oxygen bioavailability, antioxidant properties, and antiinflammatory effects [12,13].

Many of these mentioned mechanisms are also implied in chemotherapy-induced cardiotoxicity as has been previously shown in this chapter. A good prevention strategy should consider a complete and equilibrated diet, such as the Mediterranean diet, although prospective human evidence studies are needed to enforce this recommendation.

SERUM MARKERS

Cardiac biomarkers are a valid diagnostic tool for identification and monitoring of cardiotoxicity in early stages. A biomarker strategy would lead the physician to early intervention with cardioprotective medication or alteration of the chemotherapy regimen to prevent cardiac dysfunction. Some markers have been studied including troponin, natriuretic peptide, or C-reactive protein.

Classic troponin I is a sensitive and specific marker for myocardial injury, not only in acute coronary syndromes but also in any kind of myocardial damage. It has been proved that in populations treated with high-dose chemotherapy, patients with a positive troponin level had a more marked reduction in LVEF that persists after treatment [14]. Moreover, patients without troponin I elevation after treatment had a good prognosis, with no significant reduction in LVEF and a very low incidence of cardiac events.

More sensitive troponin assays have been recently developed which allow earlier detection of myocyte stress. It has been studied for predicting cardiotoxicity among breast cancer patients, and it showed that a rise of its levels above 30 pg/mL was associated with a subsequent decline in LVEF and symptomatic cardiac heart failure [15].

Natriuretic peptides have been extensively studied for diagnostic and prognostic roles in cardiotoxicity. Unlike troponin, there are insufficient data to recommend the routine measurement of these peptides in cardiotoxicity in clinical practice.

C-reactive protein has been recently demonstrated to have high sensitivity (92.9%) and negative predictive value (94.1%) for predicting trastuzumab-induced cardiotoxicity [16]. However, additional studies are needed to validate the utility before application in clinical practice.

REFERENCES

[1] Albini A, Pennesi G, Donatelli F, et al. Cardiotoxicity of anticancer drugs: the need for cardio-oncology and cardio-oncological prevention. J Natl Cancer Inst 2010;102:14–25.

[2] Mancia G, Fagard R, Narkiewitcz K, et al. ESH/ESC Guidelines for the management of arterial hypertension. Eur Heart J 2013;34:2159–219.

[3] Todaro M, Oreto L, Qamar R, et al. Cardioncology: state of the heart. In J Cardiol 2013;168:680–7.

[4] Milan A, Puglisi E, Ferrrari L, et al. Arterial hypertension and cancer. Int J Cancer 2014;134:2269–77.

[5] Kuoppala J, Lamminpaa A, Pukkala E. Statins and cancer: a systematic review and meta-analysis. Eur J Cancer 2008;44(5):2122–32.

[6] Steingart R, Yadav N, Manrique C, et al. Cancer survivorship: cardiotoxic therapy in the adult cancer patient; cardiac outcomes with recommendarions for patient management. Semin Oncol 2013;40:690–708.

[7] Carver J, Shapiro C, Ng A, et al. American society of clinical oncology clinical evidence review on the ongoing care of adult cancer survivors: cardiac and pulmonary late effects. J Clin Oncol 2007;25:3991–4008.

[8] Wassmuth R, Lentzsch S, Erdbruegger U, et al. Subclinical cardiotoxic effects of anthracyclines as assessed by magnetic resonance imaging—a pilot study. Am Heart J 2001;141:1007–13.

[9] Yu AF, Steingart RM, Fuster V. Cardiomyopathy associated with cancer therapy. J Card Fail 2014;20(11):841–52.

[10] Behrens G, Leitzmann MF. The association between physical activity and renal cancer: systematic review and meta-analysis. Br J Cancer 2013;108:798–811.

[11] Khakoo AY, Lui PP, Force T, et al. Cardiotoxicity due to cancer therapy. Tex Heart Inst J 2011;38(3):253–6.

[12] Widmer RJ, Flammer AJ, Lerman LO, et al. The mediterranean diet, its components, and cardiovascular disease. Am J Med 2015;128(3):229–38. Available from: http://dx.doi.org/10.1016/j.amjmed.2014.10.014.

[13] Martínez-González MA, García-López M, Bes-Rastrollo M, et al. Mediterranean diet and the incidence of cardiovascular disease: a Spanish cohort. Nutr Metab Cardiovas Dis 2011;21:237–44.

[14] Cardinale D, Sandri MT. Role of biomarkers in chemotherapy-induced cardiotoxicity. Prog Cardiovasc Dis 2010;53:121–9.

[15] Sawaya H, Sebag IA, Plana JC, et al. Assessment of echocardiography and biomarkers for the extended prediction of cardiotoxicity in patients treated with anthracyclines, taxanes and trastuzumab. Circ Cardiovascu Imaging 2012;5:596–603.

[16] Onitilo AA, Engel JM, Stankowski RV, et al. High-sensivity C-reactive protein (hs-CRP) as a biomarker for trastuzumab-induced cardiotoxicity in HER2-positive early-stage breast cancer: a pilot study. Breast Cancer Res 2012;134:291–8.

Chapter 29

Beta-Blockers

G.L. Alonso Salinas and J.L. Zamorano Gómez

Chapter Outline

On one hand, intensive treatment of malignancies is a success history in modern medicine. However, intensive treatment creates a risk for developing heart failure. Thus, treating a high-mortality disease with a medication that can induce another life-threatening disease is problematic.

On the other hand, beta-blockers (β-blockers) are one of the most commonly used and most studied heart failure medications. They have been long known to improve survival with congestive heart failure, cardiac hypertrophy, and reperfusion abnormalities. They have also been studied in chemotherapy-induced cardiotoxicity, although there is no prolific evidence in this field.

PHYSIOLOGY OF β-BLOCKERS IN CARDIOTOXICITY

The exact mechanisms of cardioprotection with β-blockers remain unclear, but there are a number of key effects that can mitigate anthracycline cardiotoxicity. Certain β-blockers, such as carvedilol, nebivolol, or alprenolol inhibit β-adrenergic receptor-mediated G protein-coupled receptor signaling while preserving β-adrenergic receptor recruitment of β-arrestin. β-Arrestin has been shown to be cardioprotective under long-term catecholamine stimulation, with an attenuation of anthracycline-induced cardiotoxicity [1]. Carvedilol, nebivolol, and alprenolol also activate the ErB-mediated prosurvival mitogen-activated protein kinase/ERK1/2 pathway via recruitment of β-arrestin.

Anticancer Treatments and Cardiotoxicity. DOI: http://dx.doi.org/10.1016/B978-0-12-802509-3.00029-7

EVIDENCE-BASED DATA

Carvedilol has been shown in animal models to mitigate myocardial oxidative stress. It also prevents doxorubicin-induced mitochondrial respiration alterations and changes in mitochondrial calcium-loading capacity [2].

Limited data support the recommendation of β-blocker use at chemotherapy initiation. In a small, randomized placebo-controlled study, patients treated with carvedilol at anthracycline regimen initiation showed attenuation of the decline of the left ventricular ejection fraction (LVEF) and diastolic function compared with patients treated with placebo at 6 months [3]. Furthermore, in a retrospective study of patients treated with trastuzumab, dual therapy with angiotensin-converting enzyme inhibitors and carvedilol was effective for the recovery of LVEF at 12 months [4].

Recently the OVERCOME trial (preventiOn of left Ventricular dysfunction with Enalapril and caRvedilol in patients submitted to intensive ChemOtherapy for the treatment of Malignant hEmopathies) has been published. The primary endpoint was to measure the change from baseline in global LVEF. Echocardiographic LVEF was similar in the intervention and control groups at baseline. At 6 months no serial changes were observed in the enalapril- and carvedilol-treated group while patients in the control group had a decrease that resulted in a global absolute intergroup difference of 3.11 points. It concluded that combined treatment with enalapril and carvedilol may prevent left ventricular systolic dysfunction in patients with malignant hemopathies treated with intensive chemotherapy [5].

Besides the protection against LVEF decrease, the OVERCOME trial also found significant differences in the combined event of death or heart failure, and of death, heart failure, or a final LVEF under 45%.

CLINICAL PRACTICE

As seen, limited data support the idea that some β-blockers may be effective for cardiac dysfunction prevention. It has been described that some β-blockers may have improved benefit in comparison with others of the same family. The most commonly studied being carvedilol.

Carvedilol has shown a potential benefit in animal trials, in retrospective trials, and in addition to enalapril for preventing cardiotoxicity due to aggressive chemotherapy in malignant hemopathies. Alprenolol and nebivolol may have the same molecular advantages as carvedilol; however there are no human-based studies with these two β-blockers.

To conclude, it seems that it is too early to recommend carvedilol or another β-blocker due to the limited evidence available. However, the potential lines that are being developed suggest that this therapy may change the natural course of cardiotoxicity in future years.

REFERENCES

[1] Shalkey Hahn V, Lenihan DJ, Ky B. Cancer therapy-induced cardiotoxicity: basic mechanisms and potential cardioprotective therapies. J Am Heart Assoc 2014;3(2):e000665. Available from: http://dx.doi.org/10.1161/JAHA.113.000665.

[2] Santos DL, Moreno AJ, Leino RL, et al. Carvedilol protects against doxorubicin-induced mitochondrial cardiomyopathy. Toxicol Appl Pharmacol 2002;185:218–27.

[3] Kalay N, Basar E, Ozdogru I, et al. Protective effects of carvedilol angainst anthraciclyne-induced cardiomyopathy. J Am Coll Cardiol 2006;48:2258–62.

[4] Oliva S, Cioffi G, Frattini S, et al. Administration of angiotensin-converting enzyme inhibitors and bet-blockers during adjuvant trastuzumab chemotherapy for nonmetastatic breast cancer: marker risk of cardioprotection in the world? Oncologist 2012;17:917–24.

[5] Bosch X, Rovira M, Sitges M, et al. Enalapril and carvedilol for preventing chemotherapy-induced left ventricular systolic dysfunction in patients with malignant hemopathies. The OVERCOME trial (preventiOn of left Ventricular dysfunction with Enalapril and caRvedilol in patients submitted to intensive ChemOtherapy for the treatment of Malignant hEmopathies). J Am Coll Cardiol 2013;61(23):2355–62.

Chapter 30

Angiotensin-Converting Enzyme Inhibition

G.L. Alonso Salinas and J.L. Zamorano Gómez

Chapter Outline

Angiotensin-converting enzyme inhibitors have been shown to slow the progression of left ventricular dysfunction in several clinical settings. They block cardiac-associated renin–angiotensin system activity, reduce left ventricle remodeling, and decrease oxidative stress.

Cancer therapy produces myocardial dysfunction and injury. Angiotensin-converting enzyme inhibitors may prevent this damage and could be an important support for avoiding cardiotoxicity during chemotherapy.

PHYSIOLOGY

It has been suggested that angiotensin-converting enzyme inhibitors may reduce interstitial fibrosis, attenuate oxidative stress, improve intracellular calcium handling, and modify gene expression, affecting cardiomyocyte metabolism and mitochondrial function.

Angiotensin-converting enzyme inhibitors protect against anthracycline cardiotoxicity and may repair its damage, possibly because it is a potent downregulator of the actions of the NRG-1/ErbB system, an important target of anthracyclines that may produce cardiac damage [1]. Whether angiotensin receptor blockers also have a beneficial effect in preventing trastuzumab cardiotoxicity remains unknown.

Anticancer Treatments and Cardiotoxicity. DOI: http://dx.doi.org/10.1016/B978-0-12-802509-3.00030-3

EVIDENCE-BASED DATA

The role of angiotensin-converting enzyme inhibitors for the prevention of cardiotoxicity has been investigated by multiple animal and human studies.

In a randomized-controlled trial of 473 patients with elevated troponin I after a high dose of chemotherapy, comparing enalapril with a no-intervention group, it seemed to prevent the development of late cardiotoxicity [2]. In this trial, 20 mg enalapril daily, started 1 month after chemotherapy and continued for 1 year, prevented a decrease of >10% and <50% decrease in left ventricular ejection fraction (LVEF).

In addition to this trial, the OVERCOME trial, as shown in Chapter 29, Beta-Blockers, compared enalapril and carvedilol treatment versus placebo for prevention of malignant hemopathy chemotherapy cardiotoxicity. At 6 months it concluded that combined treatment with enalapril and carvedilol may prevent left ventricular systolic dysfunction in patients with malignant hemopathies treated with intensive chemotherapy [3].

CLINICAL PRACTICE

Angiotensin-converting enzyme inhibitors seem to be effective in cardiac dysfunction inhibition during high-dose chemotherapy. Enalapril is the most-studied, but currently other angiotensin-converting enzyme inhibitors are being investigated, such as perindopril [4].

In conclusion, evidence-based data confirm the potential cardioprotective effect of angiotensin-converting enzyme inhibitors, especially enalapril. However, these data need to be confirmed in larger randomized-controlled human trials.

ANGIOTENSIN II RECEPTOR BLOCKERS

Angiotensin II receptor blockers are an important first-line treatment in hypertension, especially if there is any kind of intolerance to angiotensin-converting enzyme inhibitors. The mechanism of action of inhibiting angiotensin, similar to angiotensing-converting enzyme inhibitors, turns them into a possible target in cardiotoxicity prevention. However, evidence about the role of angiotensin II receptor blockers in chemotherapy cardiotoxicity is still limited.

Some animal studies suggest the potential effect of this treatment. It has been shown in rats that olmesartan and aliskiren have protective effects against tacrolimus-induced cardiotoxicity [5].

Human data have shown some findings in that way. A small randomized-controlled 40-patient trial proved that valsartan may prevent left ventricle dilatation, QT interval increasing and brain natriuretic peptide rising during cyclophosphamide, doxorubicin, vincristine, and prednisolone chemotherapy regimen [6].

Another recent study, a 100-patient single-blind placebo trial, investigated telmisartan effect and its duration on epirubicin chemotherapy cardiotoxicity, assessed by serial strain rate. It concluded that it has a protective long-lasting effect, probably by ensuring a permanent defense against chronic or late-onset types of anthracycline-induced cardiotoxicity [7].

In conclusion, angiotensin II receptor blockers have limited evidence in chemotherapy cardiac harm protection. There are some studies that suggest a protective effect, but this has to be confirmed in future trials.

REFERENCES

[1] Shalkey Hahn V, Lenihan DJ, Ky B. Cancer therapy-induced cardiotoxicity: basic mechanisms and potential cardioprotective therapies. J Am Heart Assoc 2014. Available from: http://dx.doi.org/10.1161/JAHA.113.000665.

[2] Cardinale D, Colombo A, Sandri MT, et al. Prevention of high-dose chemotherapy-induced cardiotoxicity in high-risk patients by angiotensin-converting enzyme inhibitors. Circulation 2006;114:2474–81.

[3] Bosch X, Rovira M, Sitges M, et al. Enalapril and carvedilol for preventing chemotherapy-induced left ventricular systolic dysfunction in patients with malignant hemopathies. The OVERCOME Trial (preventiOn of left Ventricular dysfunction with Enalapril and caRvedilol in patients submitted to intensive ChemOtherapy for the treatment of Malignant hEmopathies). J Am Coll Cardiol 2013;61(23):2355–62.

[4] Pituskin E, Haykowsky M, Mackey JR, et al. Rationale and design of the Multidisciplinary Approach to Novel Therapies in Cardiology Oncology Research Trial (MANTICORE 101-Breast): a randomized, placebo-controlled trial to determine if conventional heart failure pharmacotherapy can prevent trastuzumab-mediated left ventricular remodeling among patients with HER2+ early breast cancer using MRI. BMC Cancer 2011;11:318.

[5] Al-Harbi N, Imam F, Nadeem A, et al. Protection against tacrolimus-induced cardiotoxicity in rats by olmesartan and aliskiren. Toxicol Mech Method 2011;21(9):697–702.

[6] Nakamae H, Tsumura K, Terada Y, et al. Notalbe effects of angiotensin II receptor blocker, valsartan, on acute cardiotoxic changes after standard chemotherapy with cyclophosphamide, doxorubicin, vincristine, and prednisolone. Cancer 2005;104(11):2492–8.

[7] Dessi M, Madeddu C, Piras A, et al. Long-term, up to 18 months, protective effects of tha angiotensin II receptor blocker telmisartan on Epirubin-induced inflammation and oxidative stress assessed by serial strain rate. Springerplus 2013;2:198.

Chapter 31

Diuretics

D. Rodríguez Muñoz

Chapter Outline

Traditionally, diuretics have played a dual role in heart failure: on one side, they are the cornerstone of symptomatic treatment; on the other side, aldosterone antagonists have been shown to reduce morbidity and mortality in patients with severe heart failure and previous myocardial infarction through their effect on cardiac fibrosis and remodeling [1–3]. Similarly, the role of this group of drugs in heart failure secondary to the cardiotoxic effects of cancer treatment can be divided into cardioprotective and symptomatic treatment.

CARDIOPROTECTIVE TREATMENT

Spironolactone is an aldosterone antagonist that blocks the final steps of the renin–angiotensin–aldosterone system. A dose of 25 mg/day of spironolactone has proved to be an effective cardioprotective strategy, preserving left ventricular systolic function against the cardiotoxic effect of anthracyclines [4]. It has also been shown to prevent adverse cardiac remodeling, preserving systolic and diastolic diameters and diastolic function. Additionally, markers of oxidative stress were also reduced in patients under spironolactone treatment who underwent chemotherapy with anthracyclines [4]. A cardioprotective effect has also been suggested for spironolactone in patients under treatment with trastuzumab through the inhibition of aldosterone transactivated epidermal growth factor receptors upregulation, but this hypothesis has not yet been tested in the clinical field [5].

SYMPTOMATIC TREATMENT

Diuretics and, especially, loop diuretics such as furosemide, are the cornerstone of symptomatic treatment in acute and chronic heart failure [6]. Its use

Anticancer Treatments and Cardiotoxicity. DOI: http://dx.doi.org/10.1016/B978-0-12-802509-3.00031-5

is key in heart failure both in reduced and preserved ejection fraction. The aim of diuretic treatment in cardiotoxicity is to restore and maintain the patient's euvolemia. Combination of different diuretics may be necessary and can be of use to reduce the side effects of one drug or to increase the effect, especially in patients with severe symptoms and respiratory compromise or in those with suspected or confirmed loop diuretic resistance [7].

REFERENCES

[1] Solomon SD, Pfeffer MA. Aldosterone antagonism and myocardial infarction: from animals to man and back. J Am Coll Cardiol 2003;42:1674–6.

[2] Pitt B, Zannad F, Remme WJ, Cody R, Castaigne A, Perez A, et al. The effect of spironolactone on morbidity and mortality in patients with severe heart failure. Randomized aldactone evaluation study investigators. N Engl J Med 1999;341:709–17.

[3] Pitt B, Remme W, Zannad F, Neaton J, Martinez F, Roniker B, et al. Eplerenone post-acute myocardial infarction heart failure efficacy and survival study investigators. Eplerenone, a selective aldosterone blocker, in patients with left ventricular dysfunction after myocardial infarction. N Engl J Med 2003;348:1309–21.

[4] Akpek M, Ozdogru I, Sahin O, Inanc M, Dogan A, Yazici C, et al. Protective effects of spironolactone against anthracycline-induced cardiomyopathy. Eur J Heart Fail 2015;17:81–9.

[5] Yavas G, Elsurer R, Yavas C, Elsurer C, Ata O. Does spironolactone ameliorate trastuzumab-induced cardiac toxicity? Med Hypotheses 2013;81:231–4.

[6] McMurray JJ, Adamopoulos S, Anker SD, Auricchio A, Böhm M, Dickstein K, et al. ESC Committee for Practice Guidelines. ESC Guidelines for the diagnosis and treatment of acute and chronic heart failure 2012: the task force for the diagnosis and treatment of acute and chronic heart failure 2012 of the European Society of Cardiology. Developed in collaboration with the Heart Failure Association (HFA) of the ESC. Eur Heart J 2012;33:1787–847.

[7] Cox ZL, Lenihan DJ. Loop diuretic resistance in heart failure: resistance etiology-based strategies to restoring diuretic efficacy. J Card Fail 2014;20:611–22.

Chapter 32

Antiarrhythmic Drugs

D. Rodríguez Muñoz

Chapter Outline

The development of arrhythmias is a common complication in treated cancer patients, with some series reporting an incidence of more than 30% of patients [1]. Management depends on the mechanism and type of arrhythmia, and is primarily aimed at correcting the potential causative factors. Choice of antiarrhythmic drug will also depend on these factors.

SUPRAVENTRICULAR ARRHYTHMIAS

Supraventricular arrhythmias may appear during or after anticancer treatment, both related to chemo- and radiotherapy. The most common is atrial fibrillation, which can be related both to patient comorbidities and to the toxic effect of the oncologic treatment [2].

- Beta-blockers and nondihydropyridine calcium channel blockers are good options for rate control and have an additional effect in reducing supraventricular tachycardias. These drugs must, however, be used with caution in patients with previous systolic dysfunction or who are under treatment with anticancer regimens with known risk for cardiotoxicity, given its negative inotropic effects. Its use must be avoided in patients with severe heart failure or hemodynamic instability. In these patients, digoxin is a good alternative for rate control and an initial dose of 500–1000 μg can be administered intravenously in 4–8 h if necessary and depending on the patient's response. If adequate rate control is not achieved with this treatment regimen, amiodarone may be used in patients with severely depressed ejection fraction or in a situation of severe heart failure [3].

Anticancer Treatments and Cardiotoxicity. DOI: http://dx.doi.org/10.1016/B978-0-12-802509-3.00032-7

- The decision to adopt a rhythm control strategy during cancer treatment should be based on a careful assessment of the patient's symptomatic situation and cardiac function and structure. Class IC antiarrhythmic drugs may not be adequate in patients undergoing potentially cardiotoxic treatment, who are at risk for development of left ventricular (LV) dilatation, fibrosis, and ventricular arrhythmias. Amiodarone can be used safely in these scenarios, but the risk of adverse events and drug interactions must be taken into consideration when considering it as a maintenance treatment. Sotalol may be an adequate option, but its antiarrhythmic power is lower than the previously mentioned options. QT prolongation is common with amiodarone and sotalol, and therefore should be avoided in patients under treatment with drugs with known or potential risk for prolonging QT-interval.
- Anticoagulation for stroke prevention in atrial flutter or atrial fibrillation requires an individual approach based on a careful evaluation of thrombotic and bleeding risk, both of which are increased in cancer patients through different mechanisms [2]. The use of CHA_2DS_2-VASc and HAS-BLED scores can guide decision-making in the initiation of antithrombotic treatment, but the presence and type of cancer are not rated as part of them, and therefore this must be incorporated into the global assessment (see chapter 33: Anticoagulation in Cancer Patients).

VENTRICULAR ARRHYTHMIAS

Ventricular arrhythmias can be linked to QT interval prolongation or to direct effects of chemo- and radiotherapy. LV dilatation, dysfunction, fibrosis, and ischemia are all factors that predispose to the development of ventricular arrhythmias. QT duration should be monitored before and during treatment. Common screening and early cardiotoxicity diagnosis strategies involve periodic echocardiographic exams, which serve as a diagnostic tool for the aforementioned structural changes that can lead to ventricular arrhythmias.

Correction of the underlying causes is essential in patients with polymorphic ventricular tachycardia, Torsade de Pointes or ventricular fibrillation that can be linked to correctable causes common in cancer patients such as nausea, emesis, diarrhea, use of loop diuretics, electrolyte imbalance or concurrent use of QT-prolonging drugs (Table 32.1).

Choice of antiarrhythmic drug should be based on the mechanism and patient's situation and concomitant medications. The decision to implant a cardioverter-defibrillator must consider life expectancy and quality of life.

TABLE 32.1 Cardiac Arrhythmias Induced by Chemotherapeutic Regimens

Type of Arrhythmia	Causative Drug
Bradycardia, AV block, and other conduction disturbances	Arsenic trioxide, anthracyclines, bortezomib, cladribine, cisplatin, cyclophosphamide, cytarabine, 5-FU, ifosfamide, imatinib, interferons, IL-2, methotrexate, mitoxantrone, paclitaxel, pentostatin, rituximab, taxanes, thalidomide
Tachycardia	Anthracyclines, carmustine
Atrial fibrillation and other supraventricular tachycardias	Alkylating agents, amsacrine, anthracyclines, antimetabolites, bortezomib, doxorubicin, IL-2, interferons, paclitaxel, rituximab, romidepsin, TKIs, toposiomerase II inhibitors, taxanes, vinca alkaloids
Ventricular tachycardia/ fibrillation	Alkylating agents (cisplatin, cyclophosphamide, ifosfamide), amsacrine, antimetabolites (capecitabine, 5-FU, gemcitabine), arsenic trioxide, doxorubicin, interferons, IL-2, metothrexate, paclitaxel, proteasome inhibitors (bortezomib, carfilzomib), rituximab, romidepsin
Sudden cardiac death	Anthracyclines, arsenic trioxide, 5-FU, interferons, nilotinib, romidepsin

BRADYCARDIA, SINUS NODE DYSFUNCTION AND CONDUCTION DEFECTS

Both chemo- and radiotherapy can cause bradycardia and alterations in heartbeat generation and conduction. Correction of underlying factors, whenever possible, is the priority in the initial approach to management of these patients. However, a careful risk/benefit analysis of each patient must be performed, considering the impact on cancer prognosis that any switch in anticancer treatment may have. Asymptomatic bradycardia may require periodic evaluation and follow-up. Evaluation of symptoms attributable to bradycardia can be challenging in cancer patients in whom syncope, fatigue, and loss of strength and physical capacity can be related to several other factors including their disease and side effects of anticancer treatment.

Treatment options for ambulatory patients are limited. Hospitalized patients should be assessed based on two main aspects: possibility to correct the causative mechanism of the bradyarrhythmia and risk of evolving toward complete heart block or cardiac arrest. The result of this evaluation should guide the use of transient measures (pharmacologic, with continuous infusion of isoprenaline in patients with low risk of cardiac arrest, or temporary pacing, in those with high-degree block) or definitive ones (permanent pacemaker implant).

REFERENCES

[1] Yeh ET, Bickford CL. Cardiovascular complications of cancer therapy: incidence, pathogenesis, diagnosis, and management. J Am Coll Cardiol 2009;53(24):2231–47.

[2] Farmakis D, Parissis J, Filippatos G. Insights into onco-cardiology: atrial fibrillation in cancer. J Am Coll Cardiol 2014;63(10):945–53.

[3] Camm AJ, Lip GY, De Caterina R, Savelieva I, Atar D, Hohnloser SH, et al. 2012 Focused update of the ESC Guidelines for the management of atrial fibrillation: an update of the 2010 ESC Guidelines for the management of atrial fibrillation. Developed with the special contribution of the European Heart Rhythm Association. Eur Heart J 2012;33:2719–47.

Chapter 33

Anticoagulation in Cancer Patients

D. Rodríguez Muñoz

Chapter Outline

Thrombotic risk is increased in cancer patients due to different mechanisms. Procoagulant status, alteration in fibrinolytic pathways, and proaggregating activity contribute to this situation, together with proinflamatory and proangiogenic cytokines and increased adhesion between the endothelium and blood cells [1]. Additionally, anticancer therapies increase this risk [2].

Anticoagulation in cancer patients may be indicated as part of a therapeutic regimen or preventive strategy.

THERAPEUTIC ANTICOAGULATION

Venous thromboemolism (VTE) occurs frequently in cancer patients, with up to 20% of hospitalized patients suffering at least one episode [3]. Chemotherapy increases the risk of VTE sixfold, and the risk of VTE recurrence twofold [4]. This is partly due to the effect of the drugs used, but can also be related to implications of cancer treatment such as the placement of central venous catheters. Detection of thrombotic events is based on clinical suspicion, since systematic screening has shown no benefit.

- Symptomatic thrombosis: following clinical suspicion for VTE and a positive diagnosis, the most effective treatment regimen consists of the administration of low-molecular-weight heparin (LMWH) over a period of 3–6 months. Clinical trials have shown a superior reduction of VTE events with LMWH compared to vitamin K antagonists (VKA), with no increase in bleeding risk, although VKA seem a reasonable alternative with the advantage of oral administration [5]. Available data on the effect

Anticancer Treatments and Cardiotoxicity. DOI: http://dx.doi.org/10.1016/B978-0-12-802509-3.00033-9

of non-VKA oral anticoagulants (NOACs) suggest efficacy and bleeding risk are similar to that of VKA on cancer patients, although these data come from subgroup analysis from large trials [6,7]. Comparison between NOACs and LMWH has not yet been performed. When considering the use of NOACs, it is important to pay careful attention to potential renal or hepatic failure that may contraindicate its use or require dose adjustment [7].

A decision on anticoagulation should also be based on the patient's bleeding risk profile and life expectancy. Bleeding risk under anticoagulation is increased sixfold in cancer patients [8]. In patients considered at high bleeding risk, placement of a vena cava filter can be considered.

Thrombolysis may be considered in hemodynamically unstable patients suffering pulmonary embolism (PE) due to high early mortality risk, but data on the benefits of this approach are inconclusive [5]. Surgical embolectomy may be considered as an alternative option, but it also entails substantial bleeding risk due to the need for intensive anticoagulation [5].

- Silent thrombosis: an incidental finding of venous thrombosis or PE is not uncommon in diagnostic tests frequently performed during cancer diagnosis, stratification, and follow-up. Although the management of these cases is still not clearly defined, most centers treat the patient with the same anticoagulation regimens as in those who present with symptoms, given the increased risk of mortality and recurrent episodes [9].
- Recurrent thrombosis: as mentioned above, oncologic patients present a higher risk for VTE recurrence. Consequently, maintenance of anticoagulation therapy must be considered taking into consideration the patient's bleeding risk and preference. Antithrombotic therapy may be continued until the cancer is considered to be cured. Recurrence in spite of antithrombotic treatment can occur. In these cases, switching to LMWH—if the patient was previously on VKA—or increasing the dose—if previously under treatment with LMWH can be considered. Placement of a vena cava filter can also be considered in these cases.
- Arterial thrombosis: arterial thrombosis is rare compared to venous events and is mainly related to metastatic cancers and therapeutic egimens involving anthracyclines, taxanes, or platines [10]. Evidence on management of these events is scarce and limits the possibility to make general recommendations. Treatment should, therefore, be based on a careful evaluation of each patient.

PROPHYLACTIC ANTICOAGULATION

Prevention of thrombotic events is frequently considered in hospitalized as well as in high-risk ambulatory cancer patients, especially in those with low bleeding risk, with LMWH as the preferred regimen. Current evidence does not support systematic primary thromboprophylaxis [11]. An individualized approach based on cancer-, patient-, and treatment-related risk factors for thrombosis seems a reasonable strategy [12]. Assessment of bleeding risk must be performed, and low-dose aspirin has been proposed as an alternative [13].

In cancer patients presenting with atrial fibrillation, CHA_2DS_2VASc score must be followed as the basis on which to indicate thromboprophylaxis. However, this does not consider the thrombotic risk intrinsically associated with cancer and anticancer therapy or the variations in predictability of response to anticoagulation [14]. Therefore an individualized assessment by a cardio-oncology team considering thrombotic/bleeding risks should be performed.

REFERENCES

[1] Rickles FR. Mechanisms of cancer-induced thrombosis in cancer. Pathophysiol Haemost Thromb 2006;35:103–10.

[2] Suter TM, Ewer MS. Cancer drugs and the heart: importance and management. Eur Heart J 2013;34(15):1102–11.

[3] Lecumberri R, Marqués M, Panizo E, Alfonso A, García-Mouriz A, Gil-Bazo I, et al. High incidence of venous thromboembolism despite electronic alerts for thromboprophylaxis in hospitalised cancer patients. Thromb Haemost 2013;110:184–90.

[4] Haddad TC, Greeno EW. Chemotherapy-induced thrombosis. Thromb Res 2006;118:555–68.

[5] Konstantinides SV, Torbicki A, Agnelli G, Danchin N, Fitzmaurice D, Galiè N, Task Force for the Diagnosis and Management of Acute Pulmonary Embolism of the European Society of Cardiology (ESC). 2014 ESC guidelines on the diagnosis and management of acute pulmonary embolism. Eur Heart J 2014;35:3033–69.

[6] Prins MH, Lensing AW, Bauersachs R, van Bellen B, Bounameaux H, Brighton TA, et al. Oral rivaroxaban versus standard therapy for the treatment of symptomatic venous thromboembolism: a pooled analysis of the EINSTEIN-DVT and PE randomized studies. Thromb J 2013;11(1):21.

[7] Schulman S, Goldhaber SZ, Kearon C, Kakkar AK, Schellong S, Eriksson H, et al. Treatment with dabigatran or warfarin in patients with venous thromboembolism and cancer. Thromb Haemost 2015;114(1):150–7.

[8] Hutten BA, Prins MH, Gent M, Ginsberg J, Tijssen JGP, Büller HR. Incidence of recurrent thromboembolic and bleeding complications among patients with venous thromboembolism in relation to both malignancy and achieved international normalized ratio: a retrospective analysis. J Clin Oncol 2000;18:3078–83.

[9] O'Connell CL, Liebman HA. Approach to the management of incidental venous thromboembolic events in patients with cancer. J Natl Compr Canc Netw 2014;12:1557–60.

[10] Di Nisio M, Ferrante N, Ferragalli B, De Tursi M, Iacobelli S, Cuccrullo F, et al. Arterial thrombosis in ambulatory cancer patients treated with chemotherapy. Thromb Res 2011;127:382–3.

[11] Carrier M, Khorana AA, Moretto P, Le Gal G, Karp R, Zwicker JI. Lack of evidence to support thromboprophylaxis in hospitalized medical patients with cancer. Am J Med 2014;127:82–6.

[12] Khorana AA, Conolly GC. Assessing risk of venous thromboembolism in the patients with cancer. J Clin Oncol 2009;27:4839–47.

[13] Larocca A, Cavallo F, Bringhen S, Di Raimondo F, Falanga A, Evangelista A, et al. Aspirin or enoxaparin thromboprophylaxis for patients with newly diagnosed multiple myeloma treated with lenalidomide. Blood 2012;119:933–9.
[14] Farmakis D, Parissis J, Filippatos G. Insights into onco-cardiology: atrial fibrillation in cancer. J Am Coll Cardiol 2014;63(10):945–53.

Chapter 34

New Drugs: The Beneficial Effects of Ranolazine

M. Galderisi

Chapter Outline

RANOLAZINE: MECHANISMS OF ACTION

Ranolazine, a piperazine derivative, was approved by the US Food & Drug Administration for the treatment of symptomatic angina pectoris. In Europe ranolazine has been approved for the treatment of stable angina pectoris in cardiac patients who do not respond adequately to standard antianginal agents such as nitrates, beta-blockers, and calcium antagonists [1]. Of note, ranolazine has been demonstrated to reduce significantly angina episodes and nitroglycerine consumption per week as well as to increase the exercise (treadmill) time without exerting any kind of hemodynamic effect, i.e., without altering double product (= systolic blood pressure × heart rate) [2]. The benefits induced by ranolazine are also balanced by only mild adverse effects (dizziness, nausea, and constipation), which are observed particularly in patients receiving the highest doses (1000 or 1500 mg bid) [2], whereas the maximal dosage recommended in Europe is 750 mg bid.

The effect of ranolazine was initially thought to be due to an inhibition of fatty acid oxidation and to a shift of metabolism toward glucose oxidation [3]. The majority of evidences now show that ranolazine exerts its action by inhibiting the late inward sodium current ($I_{\mathrm{Na,\ Late}}$) [4]. In fact, in the ischemic myocardium the delayed/incomplete inactivation of $I_{\mathrm{Na,\ Late}}$ (due to hypoxia, accumulation of ischemic metabolites, and reactive oxygen species (ROS) overproduction) induces an elevation of intracellular Na^+ which is in turn responsible for an excess of Ca^{2+} intracellular entrance such as to activate

Anticancer Treatments and Cardiotoxicity. DOI: http://dx.doi.org/10.1016/B978-0-12-802509-3.00034-0

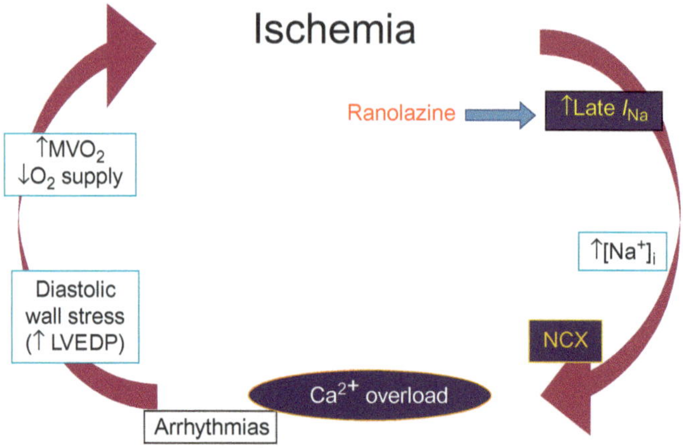

FIGURE 34.1 Schema depicting the mechanisms of action of ranolazine. *LVEDP*, left ventricular end-diastolic pressure; *MVO_2*, myocardial oxygen consumption; *NCX*, lNa(+)-Ca(2+) exchanger.

myofilaments and increase diastolic wall stress, which finally determines the reduction of coronary conductance during the diastolic phase of the cardiac cycle [5]. In such way, the ischemic heart introduces a vicious circle where ischemia begets ischemia. Ranolazine interrupts this vicious circle by activating $I_{Na, Late}$ and reducing diastolic wall stress, i.e., by improving myocardial relaxation during diastole ("*positive lusitropic effect*") (Fig. 34.1) [6,7]. It is conceivable, therefore, that this mechanism of ranolazine could be maximally exerted at the level of coronary microcirculation, where microvessels are particularly exposed to the increase of diastolic wall tension [2].

RATIONALE FOR THE USE OF RANOLAZINE TO PROTECT FROM ANTICANCER DRUGS

Anthracyclines increase the oxygen- and nitrogen-centered reactive subspecies after redox activation in cardiomyocytes and endothelial cells [8]. By favoring a continuous ROS formation, anthracyclines can also reduce the oxygen tension and set up the stage for myocardial hypoxia and metabolic ischemia [9]. In addition, the ROS activation determines cytosolic Ca^{2+} overload, mainly by an increased sarcoplasmic release [8] and also mitochondrial Ca^{2+} depletion that, in its turn, triggers a chronic vicious circle characterized by mitochondrial H_2O_2 production (increased oxidative stress), and NAD(P)H and ATP depletion (energetic stress), both sustaining ROS production [10,11]. $I_{Na, Late}$ could also be activated by anticancer drugs different from anthracycline. These drugs could induce coronary endothelial dysfunction and ischemia, whether silent or mediated by transient arrhythmias.

The rationale of using ranolazine in cancer therapy-related cardiac toxicity is therefore related to the capability of this drug in improving left ventricular (LV) diastolic function in cancer patients who also present normal LV ejection fraction (the so-called "heart failure with normal ejection fraction"), a subset of patients who may also be observed in the cancer setting.

BASIC AND CLINICAL RESEARCHERS ON THE USE OF RANOLAZINE IN THE CANCER SETTING

Some studies showed that acute intravenously administered ranolazine improves LV diastolic function in patients with previous transmural myocardial infarction [12], or in patients with type 3 long QT syndrome due to SCN5A gene mutations and slow inactivation of $I_{Na,\ Late}$ [13]. In addition, at dosages of 500 mg bid for the first week and 1000 mg bid in the following therapy, oral ranolazine improved echo indices of myocardial performance in patients with stable angina [14].

The INTERACT study, ranolazine to treat early cardiotoxicity induced by antitumor drugs (EUDRA-CT 2009-016930-29) [15], is a multicenter, phase IIb, open-label study which has been designed to show possible effectiveness of ranolazine in treating early cardiotoxicity induced by antitumor. INTERACT recruits cancer patients (nonHodgkin lymphoma and breast cancer, age 18–70 years) receiving anthracyclines and starting with normal LV function (EF >50%) and no comorbidity. It evaluates LV function by both echo-Doppler and measurements of NT-proBNP and TnI, introducing ranolazine at early post-chemotherapy.

Results from INTERACT will open a track to further studies of ranolazine in cancer patients, which is a steadily growing population at risk for cardiotoxicity.

While the beneficial effects of ranolazine can be appropriately emphasized, some limitations of its use in the oncologic setting shall also be evidenced in relation to some pharmacokinetic interactions of this drug with antitumor agents. Ranolazine is a substrate and weak inhibitor of CYP3A enzymes and also of the drug transporter P-glycoprotein, very common for drugs that are substrates of CYP3A enzymes [16]. Because metabolization and elimination of anthracyclines or other anticancer agents also depend on CYP3A enzymes and P-glycoprotein [17], concomitant administration of ranolazine might substantially modify the patient's exposure to these drugs. In this view, it is important to discourage the administration of ranolazine during chemotherapy, whereas it could be begun at the end of chemotherapy to restore early LV diastolic dysfunction and thus prevent late cardiotoxicity.

REFERENCES

[1] Task Force Members, Montalescot G, Sechtem U, Achenbach S, Andreotti F, Arden C, Budaj A, et al. ESC guidelines on chronic coronary artery disease. 2013 ESC guidelines on the management of stable coronary artery disease: the Task Force on the management of stable coronary artery disease of the European Society of Cardiology. Eur Heart J 2013;34:2949–3003.

[2] Cattaneo M, Porretta AP, Gallino A. Ranolazine: drug overview and possible role in primary microvascular angina management. Int J Cardiol 2015;181:376–81.

[3] Matsumura H, Hara A, Hashizume H, Maruyama K, Abiko Y. Protective effects of ranolazine, a novel anti-ischemic drug, on the hydrogen peroxide-induced derangements in isolated, perfused rat heart: comparison with dichloroacetate. Jpn J Pharmacol 1998;77:31–9.

[4] Belardinelli L, Shryock JC, Fraser H. Inhibition of the late sodium current as a potential cardioprotective principle: effects of the late sodium current inhibitor ranolazine. Heart 2006;92(Suppl. 4):iv6–iv14.

[5] Hale SL, Shryock JC, Belardinelli L, Sweeney M, Kloner RA. Late sodium current inhibition as a new cardioprotective approach. J Mol Cell Cardiol 2008;44:954–67.

[6] Sossalla S, Wagner S, Rasenack EC, Ruff H, Weber SL, Schöndube FA, et al. Ranolazine improves diastolic dysfunction in isolated myocardium from failing human hearts—role of late sodium current and intracellular ion accumulation. J Mol Cell Cardiol 2008;45:32–43.

[7] Hwang H, Arcidi Jr JM, Hale SL, Simkhovich BZ, Belardinelli L, Dhalla AK, et al. Ranolazine as a cardioplegia additive improves recovery of diastolic function in isolated rat hearts. Circulation 2009;120(Suppl.):S16–21.

[8] Minotti G, Menna P, Salvatorelli E, Cairo G, Gianni L. Anthracyclines: molecular advances and pharmacologic developments in antitumor activity and cardiotoxicity. Pharmacol Rev 2004;56:185–229.

[9] Ganey PE, Carter LS, Mueller RA, Thurman RG. Doxorubicin toxicity in perfused rat heart. Decreased cell death at low oxygen tension. Circ Res 1991;68:1610–13.

[10] Corradi F, Paolini L, De Caterina R. Ranolazine in the prevention of anthracycline cardiotoxicity. Pharmacol Res 2014;79:88–102.

[11] Tocchetti CG, Carpi A, Coppola C, Quintavalle C, Rea D, Campesan M, et al. Ranolazine protects from doxorubicin-induced oxidative stress and cardiac dysfunction. Eur J Heart Fail 2014;16:358–66.

[12] Hayashida W, van Eyll C, Rousseau MF, Pouleur H. Effects of ranolazine on left ventricular regional diastolic function in patients with ischemic heart disease. Cardiovasc Drugs Ther 1994;8:741–7.

[13] Moss AJ, Zareba W, Schwarz KQ, Rosero S, McNitt S, Robinson JL. Ranolazine shortens repolarization in patients with sustained inward sodium current due to type-3 long-QT syndrome. J Cardiovasc Electrophysiol 2008;19:1289–93.

[14] Jerling M. Clinical pharmacokinetics of ranolazine. Clin Pharmacokinet 2006;45:469–91.

[15] Minotti G. Pharmacology at work for cardio-oncology: ranolazine to treat early cardiotoxicity induced by anti-tumor drugs. J Pharmacol and Exper Ther 2013;346:343–9.

[16] Wilde S, Jetter A, Rietbrock S, Kasel D, Engert A, Josting A, et al. Population pharmacokinetics of the BEACOPP polychemotherapy regimen in Hodgkin's lymphoma and its effect on myelotoxicity. Clin Pharmacokinet 2007;46:319–33.

[17] Figueredo VM, Pressman GS, Romero-Corral A, Murdock E, Holderbach P, Morris DL. Improvement in left ventricular systolic and diastolic performance during ranolazine treatment in patients with stable angina. J Cardiovasc Pharmacol Ther 2011;16:168–72.

Chapter 35

Percutaneous Coronary Intervention and Cardiac Surgery in Cancer Patients

A. López López, R.A. Abellás Sequeiros and J.R. González-Juanatey

Chapter Outline

Over the last few decades to the present, cardiovascular disease and cancer have been the most frequent causes of death in developed countries [1]. Both their prevalence and incidence rates are growing, mainly due to an older population thanks to the development of new therapies, earlier diagnosis, and better life conditions. Special consideration is deserved of the relationship between cancer and coronary artery disease (CAD) [2,3]. From an etiopathogenic point of view, they share common risk factors like obesity, sedentary lifestyle, smoking, and diabetes mellitus [4]. In addition to this, cancer has been recognized as a prothrombotic state itself, mainly related to endothelial injury and high serum levels of prothrombotic agents like coagulation factor XII or tumor necrosis factor. Clotting tests are not normal in up to 50% of cancer patients and thrombocytopenia is usually present, however it is remarkable that platelets are dysfunctional and they tend to aggregate [1]. On the other hand, it is well known that cancer therapies are able to induce CAD. Radiotherapy promotes atherosclerosis and histological changes, which result in a significant reduction of luminar area of the coronary vessels. Chemotherapeutic agents like anthracyclines [5–7], 5-FU [8], or taxanes [9] can induce ischemia due to the generation of higher levels of reactive oxidant species, arterial spasm, or endothelial injury.

Anticancer Treatments and Cardiotoxicity. DOI: http://dx.doi.org/10.1016/B978-0-12-802509-3.00035-2

MANAGEMENT OF PATIENTS WITH CAD AND CANCER

Management of coronary disease in cancer patients will differ based on its form of presentation: stable disease versus acute coronary syndrome. As ESC guidelines on the management of stable coronary disease [10] propose, after demonstrating the presence of ischemia, risk stratification should guide our treatment strategy [11]. Medical therapy aims to include control of angina pectoris and limitation of atherosclerosis progression and the myocardial remodelation process. When severe myocardial ischemia is evidenced or angina is not under control, coronary revascularization should be proposed, especially if surgery is going to be performed to the patient as part of cancer treatment. However, in this context, a multidisciplinary evaluation between cardiologist and oncologist is needed in the most life-threatening situations. If cancer surgery can be delayed, percutaneous or surgical myocardial revascularization are accepted. Patients who present with acute coronary syndrome should be treated according to the ESC guidelines as cancer does not represent a significant contraindication [1]. Whereas ST segment elevation myocardial infarction (STEMI) should be considered a life-threatening situation and primary percutaneous coronary intervention (PCI) is recommended in order to restore coronary normal flow, non-STEMI (NSTEMI) and unstable angina can be managed in a conservative or an invasive way. The risks and benefits of either option should be weighed up by cardiologists and oncologists, as the revascularization process could delay cancer treatment.

Percutaneous or surgical revascularization are accepted in cancer patients. The choice of the best option should be based on individual factors like coronary anatomy, the stage of the tumor, and the overall condition of the patient. PCI is preferred in aggressive or widespread neoplasm whereas coronary artery bypass graft (CABG) seems to be a good option in potentially curable cancer [12]. Recently, Hess et al. [13] reported that PCI with stenting in patients with CAD and cancer is safe, with no differences in cardiovascular mortality, myocardial infarction, or new vessel revascularization from control patients.

PERCUTANEOUS REVASCULARIZATION

If PCI is decided on, isolated percutaneous transluminal coronary angioplasty (PTCA) or stenting with bare metal stents (BMS) or drug-eluting stents (DES) are the available options. Dual antiplatelet therapy (DAPT) is warranted after stenting as uncovered struts are highly thrombogenic. While BMS are apparently covered by neointima about 4 weeks after coronary deployment, DES however have a slower rate of endothelialization. Last-generation DES, like zotarolimus stents, are suggested to be covered about 3 months after their implantation, but first-generation ones delay this process until 1 year [14–16]. In addition to this, further delay has been described in reendothelialization in

TABLE 35.1 Advantages and Disadvantages of the Different Options for Myocardial Revascularization

Technique	Advantages	Disadvantages
PTCA	Requires only aspirin long term	Less predictable results
		Potential acute closure/dissection (1–3%)
		Restenosis 30%
BMS	Safe procedure, rare acute CABG	25% restenosis
		Requires 2–4 weeks of DAPT
DES	Safe procedure, rare acute CABG	Requires DAPT between 3–12 months
	Restenosis <10%	
CABG	2–4-week recovery	Higher risk of procedural death

Source: Adapted from Krone RJ. Managing coronary artery disease in the cancer patient. Prog Cardiovasc Dis 2010;53(2):149–56.

the presence of chemotherapeutic agents due to their antimitotic properties. Taking into account the prothrombotic environment generated by malignant disease and high prevalence of anemia and need for further surgery in cancer patients, BMS are promoted as the best stent option as they allow limiting of DAPT time [16]. In the case of bleeding tumors, isolated PTCA could be a temporary solution, although it carries a high risk of thrombosis or restenosis (Table 35.1).

Antiplatelet treatment should be based on the combination of clopidogrel and aspirin [16]. New antiplatelet agents (like ticagrelor or prasugrel) and glicoprotein IIb/IIIa receptor blockers should be avoided as there is no evidence of their use in cancer patients [1,18–20]. From a technical point of view, the radial approach should be used in order to reduce bleeding complications [16,21,22], especially in the presence of marked thrombocytopenia.

SURGICAL REVASCULARIZATION

Surgical revascularization has also been demonstrated as a safety approach for myocardial revascularization in patients with cancer [12]. Dual antiplatelet treatment is not necessary after CABG, and this is the main advantage of surgery versus percutaneous approach. However, previous exhausting tests must be done before taking the decision for a surgical revascularization. We always have to take in mind that patients who had received previous radiotherapy may suffer from radio-induced damage of their internal mammary arteries, pericardial or valvular disease, or thorax tissues changes that could lead to more difficult healing of the sternal incision [1,23,24]. Moreover, the origin, extension, and stage of the tumor must be evaluated in addition to the level of immunosuppression of the patient as the risk of mediastinitis is higher in patients with pulmonic or digestive tract neoplasm. One- or two-stage strategies are accepted for myocardial and cancer surgery [25,26]. The best option should be evaluated in an individual way. One-stage procedures are recommended when surgical oncology treatment cannot be delayed. Although they reduce cardiac or renal complications and postoperative recovery time, we have to take into account their higher rates of bleeding. The two-stage surgical approach has been demonstrated to be safer with lower morbidity and mortality rates than a combined procedure. Nevertheless, its performance includes a mandatory recovery time between the two procedures that could be unacceptable regarding cancer evolution. This resting time could vary between 7 and 60 days. From a technical point of view, available studies support the use of myocardial off-pump revascularization procedures in cancer patients [27]; however, more evidence is needed.

CONCLUSION

Although there is a strong relationship between cancer and CAD, there is a lack of evidence in the field of management of myocardial ischemia in this subgroup of patients. For decades, people with malignant diseases have been excluded from trials. Nowadays percutaneous or surgical approaches for myocardial revascularization are accepted without any preference. The cornerstone of the management decision should be the individualized evaluation of each patient under a multidisciplinary focus which must include cardiologists, oncologists, and surgeons.

REFERENCES

[1] Plana JC, López Fernández T, Gómez de Diego JJ, García Fernández MÁ. Cardio-oncology. 1st ed. Spain CTO Editorial, SL 2015.

[2] Chan AO, Jim M, Lam KF, Morris JS, Siu DC, Tong T, et al. Prevalence of colorectal neoplasm among patients with newly diagnosed coronary artery disease. JAMA 2007;298:1412–19.

[3] Yang SY, Kim Y, Chung SJ, Song JH, Choi SY, Park MJ, et al. Association between colorectal adenoma and coronary atherosclerosis detected by CT coronary angiography in Korean men; a cross-sectional study. J Gastroenterol Hepatol 2010;25:1795–9.

[4] Larsson SC, Orsini N, Wolk A. Diabetes mellitus and risk of colorectal cancer: a meta-analysis. J Natl Cancer Inst 2005;97:1679–87.

[5] Bonadonna G, Monfardini S, De Lena M, Fossati-Bellani F, Beretta G. Phase I and preliminary phase II evaluation of adriamycin (NSC 123127). Cancer Res 1970;30:2572–82.

[6] Winchester DE, Bavry A. Acute myocardial infarction during infusion of liposomal doxorubicin for recurrent breast cancer. Breast J 2010;16:313–14.

[7] Corradi F, Paolini L, De Caterina R. Ranolazine in the prevention of anthracycline cardiotoxicity. Pharmacol Res 2014;79:88–102.

[8] Kosmas C, Kallistratos M, Kopterides P, Syrios J, Skopelitis H, Mylonakis N, et al. Cardiotoxicity of fluoropyrimidines in different schedules of administration: a prospective study. J Cancer Res Clin Oncol 2008;134:75–82.

[9] Arbuck SG, Strauss H, Rowinsky E, Christian M, Suffness M, Adams J, et al. A reassessment of cardiac toxicity associated with Taxol. J Natl Cancer Inst Monogr 1993;117–30.

[10] Members TF. 2013 ESC guidelines on the management of stable coronary artery disease: the Task Force on the management of stable coronary artery disease of the European Society of Cardiology. Eur Heart J 2013;34.

[11] Chandra S, Lenihan D, Wei W, Yusuf SW, Tong AT. Myocardial perfusion imaging and cardiovascular outcomes in a cancer population. Tex Heart Inst J 2009;36:205–13.

[12] Darwazah AK, Osman M, Sharabati B. Use of off-pump coronary artery bypass surgery among patients with malignant disease. J Card Surg 2010;25:1–4.

[13] Hess CN, Roe M, Clare RM, Chiswell K, Kelly J, Tcheng JE, et al. Relationship between cancer and cardiovascular outcomes following percutaneous coronary intervention. J Am Heart Assoc 2015.

[14] Takano M, Ohba T, Inami S, Seimiya K, Sakai S, Mizuno K. Angioscopic differences in neointimal coverage and in persistence of thrombus between sirolimus-eluting stents and bare metal stents after a 6-month implantation. Eur Heart J 2006;27:2189–95.

[15] Joner M, Finn A, Farb A, Mont EK, Kolodgie FD, Ladich E, et al. Pathology of drug-eluting stents in humans: delayed healing and late thrombotic risk. J Am Coll Cardiol 2006;48:193–202.

[16] Authors/Task Force members. 2014 ESC/EACTS Guidelines on myocardial revascularization: The Task Force on Myocardial Revascularization of the European Society of Cardiology (ESC) and the European Association for Cardio-Thoracic Surgery (EACTS). Developed with the special contribution of the European Association of Percutaneous Cardiovascular Interventions (EAPCI). Eur Heart J 2014;37:2541–619.

[17] Krone RJ. Managing coronary artery disease in the cancer patient. Prog Cardiovasc Dis. 2010;53:149–56.

[18] James S, Akerblom A, Cannon CP, Emanuelsson H, Husted S, Katus H, et al. Comparison of ticagrelor, the first reversible oral P2Y(12) receptor antagonist, with clopidogrel in patients with acute coronary syndromes: Rationale, design, and baseline characteristics of the PLATelet inhibition and patient Outcomes (PLATO) trial. Am Heart J 2009;157:599–605.

[19] Steg PG, James S, Harrington RA, Ardissino D, Becker RC, Cannon CP, et al. Ticagrelor versus clopidogrel in patients with ST-elevation acute coronary syndromes intended for reperfusion with primary percutaneous coronary intervention: A Platelet Inhibition and Patient Outcomes (PLATO) trial subgroup analysis. Circulation 2010;122:2131–41.

[20] Montalescot G, Wiviott S, Braunwald E, Murphy SA, Gibson CM, McCabe CH, et al. TRITON-TIMI 38 investigators. Prasugrel compared with clopidogrel in patients undergoing percutaneous coronary intervention for ST-elevation myocardial infarction (TRITON-TIMI 38): double-blind, randomised controlled trial. Lancet 2009;373:723–31.

[21] Rao SV, Ou F, Wang TY, Roe MT, Brindis R, Rumsfeld JS, et al. Trends in the prevalence and outcomes of radial and femoral approaches to percutaneous coronary intervention: a report from the National Cardiovascular Data Registry. JACC Cardiovasc Interv 2008.

[22] Bertrand OF, Larose E, Rodés-Cabau J, Gleeton O, Taillon I, Roy L, et al. Incidence, predictors, and clinical impact of bleeding after transradial coronary stenting and maximal antiplatelet therapy. Am Heart J 2009;157:164–9.

[23] Gansera B, Schmidtler F, Angelis I, Botzenhardt F, Schuster T, Kiask T, et al. Quality of internal thoracic artery grafts after mediastinal irradiation. Ann Thorac Surg 2007.

[24] Brown ML, Schaff H, Sundt TM. Conduit choice for coronary artery bypass grafting after mediastinal radiation. J Thorac Cardiovasc Surg 2008;136:1167–71.

[25] Ozsöyler I, Yilik L, Bozok S, Emrecan B, Kestelli M, Karahan N, et al. Off-pump coronary artery bypass surgery in patients with coronary artery disease and malign neoplasia: results of ten patients and review of the literature. Heart Vessels 2006;21:365–7.

[26] Fu Q, Li Q, Liang DG, Ruan XH, Wang ZX, Wei MX. Early and long-term results of combined cardiac surgery and neoplastic resection in patients with concomitant severe heart disease and neoplasms. Chin Med J (Engl) 2011;124:1939–42.

[27] Nurözler F, Kutlu S, Kücük G. Off-pump coronary bypass for patients with concomitant malignancy. Circ J 2006;70:1048–51.

Chapter 36

Focus on the Patient With Known Cardiac Disease

R.A. Abellás-Sequeiros and J.R. González-Juanatey

Chapter Outline

PATIENTS WITH CANCER AND PREVIOUS KNOWN CARDIAC DISEASE

Nowadays, cancer has in part become a chronic disease thanks to the development of more effective cancer therapies coupled with earlier diagnosis [1]. As a result, in this population there has been an increase in the prevalence of cardiac diseases for two reasons: as in the general population, older people are at risk of developing heart diseases, such as cardiac valvular disease or heart failure and; on the other hand, we know cancer treatments can damage our cardiovascular (CV) system and favor the development of CV risk factors such as arterial hypertension [2] (Table 36.1). Moreover, it has also been suggested that cancer itself can promote CV disease as it creates a proinflammatory systemic status. This is the reason why American Heart Association (AHA) guidelines for the management of heart failure [3] state that people receiving potential cardiotoxic cancer therapies should we considered as people in stage A of heart failure classification.

In addition to this, the strong relationship between previous known cardiac disease and cancer is well known. Some CV patient series report prevalence rates between 2% and 4% for cancer [4–7] and a clear association between coronary artery disease (CAD) and colorectal neoplasm has been described [8,9]. Common risk factors like age, smoking, obesity, and diabetes mellitus (DM) have been described as the etiopathogenic basis of this association [10].

Anticancer Treatments and Cardiotoxicity. DOI: http://dx.doi.org/10.1016/B978-0-12-802509-3.00036-4

TABLE 36.1 Cancer Treatment Off-Target Cardiovascular Effects

Anthracycline	Cardiomyopathy: left ventricle diastolic and systolic dysfunction
Cyclophosphamide	Cardiomyopathy. Myocarditis. Arrhythmias. Heart failure
Ifosfamide	
Cisplatin	Cardiomyopathy: left ventricle diastolic dysfunction. Acute myocardial infarction → Vasospasm
Taxanes	Arrhythmias. Myocardial ischemia
5-Fluorouracil	Acute myocardial infarction → Vasospasm. Arrhythmias. Heart failure
Monoclonal antibodies	Cardiomyopathy: left ventricle systolic dysfunction
	Arterial hypertension
Radiotherapy	Pericardial disease. Cardiomyopathy. Valvular and coronary disease

The European Society for Medical Oncology (ESMO) and Heart Failure Association of the European Society of Cardiology (ESC) state the importance of a good stratification of cardiovascular risk (CVR) in patients who are going to receive potential cardiotoxic cancer treatments [11,12]. Special mention is reserved for patients with previous known cardiac disease. They are more vulnerable to cardiotoxicity as they have less or no cardiac reserves. For this reason, both medical associations support an exhausting CVR stratification and follow-up of these patients. Baseline and new protective cardiovascular treatments must be intensified [11,12]. The basis of this CVR stratification includes the performance of a 12-lead ECG, with QT corrected time determination and the assessment of left ventricular ejection fraction (LVEF) [11]. Although we know magnetic resonance imaging (MRI) is the gold-standard method to study LVEF or cardiac volumes, its lack of availability in most centers makes the echocardiogram the standard procedure for basal assessment of cardiac parameters. It should be noted that LVEF and volumes should be determined by modified biplane Simpson's technique. In recent years, the development of echocardiographic techniques has allowed us to assess the global longitudinal strain (GLS) of the left ventricle. Although we do not have evidence of its long-term relevance, we already know that GLS is able to detect myocardial dysfunction in its earliest phases [13]. Because of this, we should encourage strain determination in patients with previous cardiac disease who undergo cardiotoxic chemotherapy. A relative decrease in GLS >15% is considered a cancer-related myocardial dysfunction [14,15].

TABLE 36.2 Current Preventive Strategies

Cancer Treatment Adjustment	Medical Treatment	Maintenance of Hydroelectrolytic Balance
Lower doses or infusion rates	ACEI. Beta-blockers	Magnesium serum levels
More separate doses	Statins	Calcium serum levels
Discontinuation of therapy	Dexrazoxane	
	Ranolazine	

ESMO has approved some algorithms for the follow-up process of CV-naïve patients in cancer treatment with anthracyclines or with monoclonal antibodies like trastuzumab, but there is no global, evidence-based accepted algorithm for patients with prior CV disease.

Preventive therapies (Table 36.2) like the use of angiotensin-converting enzyme inhibitors (ACEI) or statins (which reduce oxidative metabolism and free radical generation) or changes in the chemotherapeutic protocol treatment (with lower doses or infusion rates, discontinuation of therapy, etc.) should be proposed in patients at high risk, not to allcomers (90% of people complete chemotherapy without developing cardiotoxicity) [16].

ACEI have risen as the most promising therapy against cardiotoxicity due to cancer treatment. Cardinale et al. [17] demonstrated that patients receiving ACEI treatment after chemotherapy developed no cardiotoxicity during a median follow-up of 12 months (43% developed cardiotoxicity in the control group versus 0% in ACEI group; $P < 0.001$).

Currently, ranolazine has also been suggested as a possible protective drug against anthracycline off-target effects [18]. These chemotherapeutic agents disturb oxidative cellular metabolism. As a result, higher levels of reactive oxygen species are warranted, with changes in the cardiomyocyte late inward sodium current. Arrhythmias or diastolic dysfunction of the myocardium due to higher cytosolic levels of calcium and sodium could be avoided with ranolazine use, as it is a selective inhibitor of this late inward sodium current. More clinical evidence is needed.

In addition to this, arterial hypertension has been described as the most frequent off-target effect of monoclonal antibodies like bevacizumab, which have antiangiogenic properties as they inhibit human VEGF (vascular endothelial growth factor). People with previous cardiac disease like hypertensive cardiomyopathy, history of heart failure, or valvular heart disease like mitral regurgitation, are especially at risk of developing complications due to refractory hypertension [2]. Because of this, ESMO guidelines support intensive treatment and follow-up of patients, and they recommend AECI or dihydropyridine calcium channel blockers as the best treatment [11].

PRE- AND PERI-OPERATIVE MANAGEMENT OF PATIENTS WITH CANCER AND KNOWN CARDIAC DISEASE

From the start of this text, we have been referring to patients with a diagnosis of cancer who are going to be treated in a medical way. However, nowadays, especially in the very early stages of neoplasic disease, surgery can be the cornerstone in cancer treatment. Preoperative risk assessment is warranted, especially in patients with previous known heart disease. According to the ESC guidelines on noncardiac surgery for CV assessment and management [19], all these patients must undergo a clinical, electro- and echocardiogram evaluation. Patients with poor functional capacity (less than 4 METS) and two of the 5 risk factors (i.e. previous CAD, heart failure, stroke, DM on insulin, and/or renal dysfunction), should be referred to a cardiologist for a test to detect myocardial ischemia. In the case of severe ischemia, guidelines recommend to balance the risk versus benefit for a previous myocardial revascularization in the context of high-risk surgery. The cardiologist and oncologist should identify together the most life-threatening situations. If previous myocardial revascularization is decided, percutaneous or surgical revascularization are accepted. Isolated percutaneous transluminal coronary angioplasty (PTCA), bare metal stents, or last-generation DES (with the suggested shortest time of mandatory double antiplatelet treatment) should be used in percutaneous coronary intervention (PCI). In the case of surgical revascularization, off-pump coronary artery bypass surgery has been demonstrated to be safe [20]. Until this moment we were talking about chronic and stable CAD. In the case that our patient suffers from a ST segment elevation myocardial infarction (STEMI), it would be considered a life-threatening condition so they can undergo primary PCI. However, patients presenting with non-STEMI (NSTEMI) and cancer should be evaluated in a multidisciplinary way to assess the emergency degree of surgery. If possible to delay it, prior myocardial revascularization should be performed [19].

Patients previously treated with aspirin (e.g., for stable CAD, prior cerebrovascular stroke, or TIA) may be considered to go on antiplatelet treatment during the perioperative period if the bleeding risk is not unacceptably high [19]. Besides, Sarkiss et al. [21] demonstrated the safety profile and CV benefit of aspirin in ACS treatment even in patients with thrombocytopenia due to cancer. Patients treated with AAS had a survival rate of 90% compared with 6% in those who did not receive it ($P < 0.0001$), without an excess in bleeding rates.

CONCLUSION

Research is needed to ameliorate our knowledge of cancer biology in order to develop new effective treatments without the off-target effects of current therapies. Besides, we need more evidence related to protective treatments, especially in patients with known previous cardiac disease, as they have been classically put out of all trials. All of this, coupled with the development of new and more specific algorithms for the surveillance of patients with previous heart disease, will allow us to give our patients the best treatment, with an increase not only in quantity, but also in quality of life.

REFERENCES

[1] DeSantis CE, Lin CC, Mariotto AB, Siegel RL, Stein KD, Kramer JL, et al. Cancer treatment and survivorship statistics, 2014. CA Cancer J Clin 2014;64:252–71.

[2] Carlos Plana JC, Teresa LF, Gomez De Diego JJ, García Fernández Miguel Angel M. Cardio-oncology. 1st ed. SL: Spain CTO Editorial; 2015.

[3] Yancy CW, Jessup M, Bozkurt B, Butler J, Casey Jr DE, Drazner MH, et al. 2013 ACCF/AHA guideline for the management of heart failure: a report of the American College of Cardiology Foundation/American Heart Association Task Force on Practice Guidelines. J Am Coll Cardiol 2013;62:147–239.

[4] Vieira RD, Pereira A, Lima EG, et al. Cancer-related deaths among different treatment options in chronic coronary artery disease: results of a 6-year follow-up of the MASS II study. Coron Artery Dis 2012;23:79–84.

[5] Mistiaen W, Van Cauwelaert PH, Muylaert PH, Wuyts FL, Harrisson F, Bortier H. Effect of prior malignancy on survival after cardiac surgery. Ann Thorac Surg 2004;77:1593–7.

[6] Carrascal Y, Gualis J, Arévalo A, et al. Cardiac surgery with extracorporeal circulation in cancer patients: influence on surgical morbidity and mortality and on survival. Rev Esp Cardiol 2008;61:369–75.

[7] Chan J, Rosenfeldt F, Chaudhuri K, Marasco S. Cardiac surgery in patients with a history of malignancy: increased complication rate but similar mortality. Heart Lung Circ 2012;21:255–9.

[8] Chan AO, Jim M, Lam KF, Morris JS, Siu DC, Tong T, et al. Prevalence of colorectal neoplasm among patients with newly diagnosed coronary artery disease. JAMA 2007;298:1412–19.

[9] Yang SY, Kim YS, Chung SJ, Song JH, Choi SY, Park MJ, et al. Association between colorectal adenoma and coronary atherosclerosis detected by CT coronary angiography in Korean men; a cross-sectional study. J Gastroenterol Hepatol 2010;25:1795–9.

[10] Larsson SC, Orsini N, Wolk A. Diabetes mellitus and risk of colorectal cancer: a meta-analysis. J Natl Cancer Inst 2005;97:1679–87.

[11] Curigliano G, Cardinale D, Suter T, Plataniotis G, de Azambuja E, Sandri MT, et al. Cardiovascular toxicity induced by chemotherapy, targeted agents and radiotherapy: ESMO Clinical Practice Guidelines. Ann Oncol 2012;23:155–66.

[12] Eschenhagen T, Force T, Ewer MS, de Keulenaer GW, Suter TM, Anker SD, et al. Cardiovascular side effects of cancer therapies: a position statement from the Heart Failure Association of the European Society of Cardiology. Eur J Heart Fail 2011;13:1–10.

[13] Sawaya H, Sebag IA, Plana JC, Januzzi JL, Ky B, Cohen V, et al. Early detection and prediction of cardiotoxicity in chemotherapy-treated patients. Am J Cardiol 2011;107:1375–80.

[14] Thavendiranathan P, Poulin F, Lim KD, Plana JC, Woo A, Marwick TH. Use of myocardial strain imaging by echocardiography for the early detection of cardiotoxicity in patients during and after cancer chemotherapy: a systematic review. J Am Coll Cardiol 2014;63:2751–68.

[15] Negishi K, Negishi T, Hare JL, Haluska BA, Plana JC, Marwick TH. Independent and incremental value of deformation indices for prediction of trastuzumab-induced cardiotoxicity. J Am Soc Echocardiogr 2013;26:493–8.

[16] Kalam K, Marwick TH. Role of cardioprotective therapy for prevention of cardiotoxicity with chemotherapy: a systematic review and meta-analysis. Eur J Cancer 2013;49: 2900–9.

[17] Cardinale D, Colombo A, Sandri MT, Lamantia G, Colombo N, Civelli M, et al. Prevention of high-dose chemotherapy-induced cardiotoxicity in high-risk patients by aniotensin-converting enzyme inhibition. Circulation 2006;114:2474–81.

[18] Corradi F, Paolini L, De Caterina R. Ranolazine in the prevention of anthracycline cardiotoxicity. Pharmacol Res 2014;79:88–102.

[19] Kristensen SD, Knuuti J, Saraste A, Anker S, Bøtker HE, Hert SD, et al. 2014 ESC/ESA Guidelines on non-cardiac surgery: cardiovascular assessment and management: The Joint Task Force on non-cardiac surgery: cardiovascular assessment and management of the European Society of Cardiology (ESC) and the European Society of Anaesthesiology (ESA). Eur Heart J 2014;35:2383–431.

[20] Darwazah AK, Osman M, Sharabati B. Use of off-pump coronary artery bypass surgery among patients with malignant disease. J Card Surg 2010;25:1–4.

[21] Sarkiss MG, Yusuf SW, Warneke CL, Botz G, Lakkis N, Hirch-Ginsburg C, et al. Impact of aspirin therapy in cancer patients with thrombocytopenia and acute coronary syndromes. Cancer 2007;109:621–7.

Chapter 37

Multidisciplinary Approach to Cardiac Disease in Cancer Patients

M. Galderisi

Chapter Outline

THE CONCEPT OF CARDIO-ONCOLOGY

Cancer and cardiac diseases are inevitably associated entities because of the sharing of common risk factors, the conjunction of both pathologies—particularly in the elderly population—and the detrimental effects exerted by cancer therapies on the cardiovascular (CV) system. This latter aspect has grown in relevant importance in the last decade, in relation with the strong reduction of morbidity and mortality of several kinds of malignancies, often converting cancer into a chronic disease [1]. At the present time, the majority of cancer patients survive and develop CV complications, which affect their quality of life and may even become the main cause of mortality of these patients [2]. The broad variety of cancer therapy-related CV complications includes not only left ventricular (LV) dysfunction and overt heart failure but also additional/alternative clinical manifestations, such as supraventricular and ventricular arrhythmias, valve heart disease, rapidly progressive atherosclerosis, and pericardial involvement (pericardial effusion and constrictive pericarditis).

Although the knowledge of these relationships is now recognized from the epidemiological point of view and the medical community is increasingly sensible to these aspects [3], the reciprocal communication between oncologists and cardiologists remains fragmentary in clinical practice. This is mainly

Anticancer Treatments and Cardiotoxicity. DOI: http://dx.doi.org/10.1016/B978-0-12-802509-3.00037-6

due to the fact that cardiologists have limited training or disclosure to the main advances in cancer therapy and their side effects, whereas oncologists are strongly anchored to a traditional approach of CV complications in cancer patients. In this view, a continuous and effective interaction between oncologists and cardiologists should be encouraged in order to increase adherence to cancer therapy, reduce the burden of cardiac toxicity, and improve both the quality of life and survival of cancer patients. Prospectively, this mainly corresponds to the realization of a multidisciplinary approach to cardiac diseases, where the work of a cardiologist could be inextricably linked to that of a clinical oncologist in daily practice. The term "cardio-oncology" has been created to define the kind of activity that could be defined as a medical subspeciality aimed at the diagnosis and management of cardiac diseases in cancer patients. In particular, it should include the sequence of CV risk definition, as well as the comprehension, prevention, and therapy of cardiac toxicity [4,5]. This subspeciality should not be limited to cardiologists and clinical oncologists but also involve radiotherapists, surgeons, and all medical doctors who are charged in caring for cancer patients with heart diseases.

Nowadays, some cardio-oncology units have been created and operate around the world. They are entitled to create several activities which include translational research programs from molecular studies to clinical programs aiming at the prediction of CV complications, epidemiological observations on the weight of these complications and, possibly, interventional strategies capable of reducing their burden in the clinical setting. Samples of this kind of coordinated activities (e.g., the Department of Cardiology at MD Anderson Cancer Center) are actually reported in particular in the United States, including diagnostic laboratories, electrophysiology units, and interventional and advanced heart failure services [6]. In general, however, these activities are performed solitarily, without true coordination of CV services for cancer patients. At the present time, most cancer patients and survivors are managed not in specialized centers but in community-based outpatient clinics, which have low or even minimal experience in CV complications of cancer therapy. Some observations point to the fact that cancer patients and survivors are treated inadequately in relation to their CV risk and in comparison with cancer-free cardiac patients [7,8].

Fig. 37.1 illustrates a multidisciplinary proposal to different clinical stages of cancer patients.

THE IMPORTANCE OF A PRELIMINARY CV RISK ASSESSMENT IN CANCER PATIENTS

Only a subset of cancer patients undergoing chemotherapy, targeted therapy, and/or radiotherapy meets CV complications. The predisposition to cardiac toxicity is individual and has a multifactorial basis which is determined by

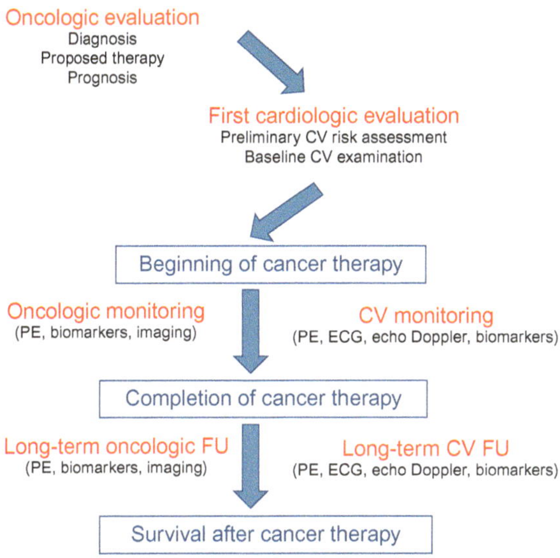

FIGURE 37.1 Proposal of an algorithm of cooperation between cardiologist and oncologist before, during, and after cancer therapy. *CV*, cardiovascular; *FU*, follow-up; *PE*, physical examination.

the concurrence of genetic and environmental factors. The genetic susceptibility of cancer patients toward cardiac toxicity has been particularly investigated in those treated with anthracyclines [9–11]. Also, the familial risk for CV diseases has been demonstrated to increase the rate of developing cancer therapy-related cardiac complications [12]. Additional individual factors such as age, sex, and concomitant CV risk factors should be taken into account. The likelihood of developing cardiac toxicity is in fact lower in premenopausal women than in men of the same age, but the possibility of atherosclerosis increases in women after menopause [13]. Arterial systemic hypertension is the most frequent CV risk factor observed in cancer registries [3]. Also, so-called "radiation-induced heart disease" (RIHD), which encompasses all CV complications consequent to radiotherapy, may be accelerated by the contribution of the common CV risk factors such as obesity, cigarette smoking, and physical inactivity [14]. Accordingly, an accurate familial and personal clinical history will allow early identification of patients with an effectively increased CV risk and also a personalization of cancer treatment. Data previously published on CV screening before the beginning of cancer therapy [15,16] demonstrate that the prevalence of CV disease is substantially underestimated but also open a track for appropriate CV monitoring and management of these patients, after their careful and appropriate baseline identification.

THE ROLE OF A BASELINE CV EXAMINATION

A baseline comprehensive CV examination, i.e., before starting cancer therapy, shall be promoted by clinical oncologists in order to prevent cardiac side effects of anticancer drugs and also to exclude the use of some of these drugs in patients with high CV risk. For instance, the use of antiangiogenic agents (bevacizumab, sorafenib, and sunitinib) should be avoided in patients who present with high blood pressure despite the use of antihypertensive drugs.

The baseline CV examination should be combined at least with an ECG at rest, which can detect signs of overt or even silent myocardial ischemia and both supraventricular and ventricular arrhythmias. It could be particularly useful in cancer patients who refer previous episodes of paroxysmal atrial fibrillation, eventually in combination with a 24-h holter ECG. The occurrence of atrial fibrillation in cancer patients may be due to comorbidities, to direct tumor action, or even represent a complication of surgical or medical cancer treatment, whereas inflammation may be a common denominator for both conditions [17].

This baseline CV examination should also be enriched by a complete echo Doppler evaluation [18], able to explore LV and right ventricular (systolic and diastolic) function, heart valves, pulmonary arterial pressure, and pericardium. The baseline assessment of cardiac function has a key role to identify patients at risk of developing heart failure under the effects of anticancer drugs such as anthracyclines and adjuvant drugs. Patients with evidence of baseline valvular heart disease should be addressed carefully toward radiotherapy which is needed in certain kinds of malignancies but increases the risk of valvular deterioration. Patients with increased pulmonary arterial pressure should be avoided, or started with great care on anticancer therapies including tyrosine kinase inhibitors (e.g., imatinib), which can increase or even provoke the onset of pulmonary arterial hypertension. In all these preexisting CV conditions, a strict link between cardiologists and oncologists should be established, after a careful baseline physical and instrumental cardiac examination, in order to evaluate the risk/benefit ratio and achieve the most appropriate choice for the safety of the individual cancer patient.

THE ROLE OF A CARDIOLOGIC FOLLOW-UP DURING CANCER THERAPY

Currently, oncologists ask for cardiologic consultation during cancer therapy when the patient complains of cardiac symptoms, such as shortness of breath, palpitations, and angina, or presents with signs of liver congestion and peripheral edema. In these situations, cancer patients should undergo periodical (at regular intervals) cardiologic check-up, including physical examination, ECG, complete echo Doppler, and/or control of some biohumoral markers (troponin I and, to a lesser extent, B-type natriuretic peptide (BNP) or pro-BNP) [4,18,19]. This could allow detection of subclinical signs of cardiac toxicity but also identification of pericardial and/or pleural effusion, as well as the onset of valve heart disease and vessel (coronary and/or carotid) involvement. This cardiologic follow-up could have a key role not only for planning and performing an early pharmacologic intervention by cardiac drugs (ACE inhibitors, beta-blockers, and diuretics) but also for modulating the same cancer treatment. Choice of therapeutic management and even prognosis depends strictly on the delicate balance between cancer treatment and CV complications. This choice should be individualized to each patient. For instance, the subclinical alteration of echocardiographic indices of cardiac function and/or the increase of biomarkers during cancer therapy should induce the oncologist to reduce the doses of some anticancer drugs or to change the type of treatment in order to prevent subsequent therapeutic withdrawal. Even some side effects of the anticancer therapy could be monitored by searching their possible CV effects: e.g., hypokalemia induced by vomiting and diarrhea, often associated with the use of anthracycline, could induce typical ECG signs (QT interval prolongation, T-wave flattening, and inversion, ST-segment depression, first degree atrioventricular block), which could be successfully used to prevent the onset of life-threatening arrhythmias by the simple recovery of potassium blood levels.

This kind of cardiologic follow-up should obviously be repeated at the end of cancer therapy.

CARDIOLOGIC FOLLOW-UP OF CANCER SURVIVORS AFTER THERAPY COMPLETION

It is well known that some cancer treatments, mainly anthracyclines and radiotherapy (RIHD) and their interactions, can induce very late signs and/or symptoms of cardiac toxicity, even several years after therapy completion. Of note, the late manifestations of RIHD are, for the most part, indistinguishable from those presented in cardiac patients with other etiologies. Globally, this phenomenon is defined as "late cardiac toxicity" and is often underestimated, in particular in pediatric cancer patients, who can present with sudden but not unexpected cardiac damage during adulthood. It is reasonable, therefore, to prolong the cardiologic follow-up of patients who, despite being asymptomatic for cardiac symptoms/signs, have undergone anthracycline chemotherapy and/or radiotherapy even 10 years after treatment, given the high likelihood of detecting very late CV complications. This cardiologic follow-up should obviously include instrumental examination, such as ECG at rest and echocardiography [14,18,19]. In patients who have undergone radiotherapy (in particular those with breast cancer, lymphoma, or esophageal cancer), the cardiologic follow-up should be extended to the performance of repeated stress testing (echocardiographic or nuclear) of inducible ischemia (at least every 5 years), because of their increased risk of coronary events.

REFERENCES

[1] Todaro MC, Oreto L, Qamar R, Paterick TE, Carerj S, Khandheria BK. Cardioncology: state of the heart. Int J Cardiol 2013;168:680–7.

[2] Lenihan DK, Olive S, Chow EJ, Cardinale D. Cardiac toxicity in cancer survivors. Cancer 2013;119(Suppl. 11):2131–42.

[3] Yeh ET, Bickford C. Cardiovascular complications of cancer therapy: incidence, pathogenesis, diagnosis, and management. J Am Coll Cardiol 2009;53:2231–47.

[4] Albini A, Pennesi G, Donatelli F, Cammarota R, De Flora S, Noonan DM. Cardiotoxicity of anticancer drugs: the need for cardio-oncology and cardio-oncological prevention. J Natl Cancer Inst 2010;102:14–25.

[5] Yeh ET. Onco-cardiology: the time has come. Tex Heart Inst 2011;38:246–7.

[6] Barac A, Murtagh G, Carver JR, Chen MH, Freeman AM, Herrmann J, et al. Cardiovascular health of patients with cancer and cancer survivors: a roadmap to the next level. J Am Coll Cardiol 2015;65:2739–94.

[7] Yoon GJ, Telli ML, Kao DP, Matsuda KY, Carlson RW, Witteles RM. Left ventricular dysfunction in patients receiving cardiotoxic cancer therapies are clinicians responding optimally. J Am Coll Cardiol 2010;56:1644–50.

[8] Ammon M, Arenja N, Leibundgut G, Buechel RR, Kuster GM, Kaufmann BA, et al. Cardiovascular management of cancer patients with chemotherapy-associated left ventricular systolic dysfunction in real-world clinical practice. J Card Fail 2013;19:629–34.

[9] Deng S, Wojnowski L. Genotyping the risk of anthracycline-induced cardiotoxicity. Cardiovasc Toxicol 2007;7:129–34.

[10] Duan S, Bleibel WK, Huang RS, Shukla SJ, Wu X, Badner JA, et al. Mapping genes that contribute to daunorubicin-induced cytotoxicity. Cancer Res 2007;67:5425–33.

[11] Huang RS, Duan S, Kistner EO, Bleibel WK, Delaney SM, Fackenthal DL, et al. Genetic variants contributing to daunorubicin-induced cytotoxicity. Cancer Res 2008;68:3161–8.

[12] Andersson A, Näslund U, Tavelin B, Enblad G, Gustavsson A, Malmer B. Long-term risk of cardiovascular disease in Hodgkin lymphoma survivors—retrospective cohort analyses and a concept for prospective intervention. Int J Cancer 2009;124:1914–17.

[13] Mendelsohn M, Karas R. Molecular and cellular basis of cardiovascular gender differences. Science 2005;308:1583–7.

[14] Lancellotti P, Nkomo VT, Badano LP, Bergler-Klein J, Bogaert J, Davin L, et al. European Society of Cardiology Working Groups on Nuclear Cardiology and Cardiac Computed Tomography and Cardiovascular Magnetic Resonance; American Society of Nuclear Cardiology; Society for Cardiovascular Magnetic Resonance; Society of Cardiovascular Computed Tomography. Expert consensus for multi-modality imaging evaluation of cardiovascular complications of radiotherapy in adults: a report from the European Association of Cardiovascular Imaging and the American Society of Echocardiography. Eur Heart J Cardiovasc Imaging 2013;14(8):721–40.

[15] Schmidinger M, Zielinski CC, Vogl UM, Bojic A, Bojic M, Schukro C, et al. Cardiac toxicity of sunitinib and sorafenib in patients with metastatic renal cell carcinoma. J Clin Oncol 2008;26:5204–12.

[16] Zell JA, Pelot D, Chen WP, McLaren CE, Gerner EW, Meyskens FL. Risk of cardiovascular events in a randomized placebo-controlled, double-blind trial of difluoromethylornithine plus sulindac for the prevention of sporadic colorectal adenomas. Cancer Prev Res 2009;2:209–12.

[17] Farmakis D, Parissis J, Filippatos G. Insights into onco-cardiology: atrial fibrillation in cancer. J Am Coll Cardiol 2014;63:945–53.

[18] Plana JC, Galderisi M, Barac A, Ewer MS, Ky B, Scherrer-Crosbie M, et al. Expert consensus for multimodality imaging evaluation of adult patients during and after cancer therapy: a report from the American Society of Echocardiography and the European Association of Cardiovascular Imaging. Eur Heart J Cardiovasc Imaging 2014;15:1063–93.

[19] Galderisi M, Marra F, Esposito R, Lomoriello VS, Pardo M, de Divitiis O. Cancer therapy and cardiotoxicity: the need of serial Doppler echocardiography. Cadiovasc Ultrasound 2007;5:4.

Section VIII

Future Research Priorities

Chapter 38

Pharmacogenomics Screening

C. Oury and V. Bours

Chapter Outline

PHARMACOGENOMICS: BACKGROUND

The first comprehensive picture of the human genome emerged a decade after the start of the Human Genome Project in 1990. Since its first draft, the latest human genome assembly GRCh38.p2 has dramatically improved our information about gene architecture through more accurate functional annotations of expressed elements. The GENCODE project provides a vast encyclopedia of genes and gene variants built of complete Ensembl gene models and the latest Havana gene annotation (http://www.gencodegenes.org/).

Single-nucleotide polymorphisms (SNPs) are heritable single-nucleotide variants. Common SNPs are arbitrarily defined as having a minor allele frequency (MAF) >5% in the targeted population. Homozygosity for an allele with a MAF of 5% means that only 2.5 homozygous individuals will be identified in a sample of 1000. Common variants account for approximately 90% of the genetic difference between individuals [1], The HapMap project gives a list of tag SNPs that captured most of the common genomic variation in a number of human populations [2]. While most common variants are function-neutral, some modify the risk of diseases, or can impact on drug efficacy or toxicity.

The goals of pharmacogenomics are to prevent adverse drug reactions and maximize drug effectiveness for individual patients. In other words, pharmacogenomic studies are performed in populations of subjects treated with a specific drug to identify genetic variants that predict drug response and the

Anticancer Treatments and Cardiotoxicity. DOI: http://dx.doi.org/10.1016/B978-0-12-802509-3.00038-8

occurrence of adverse reactions. Pharmacogenomics can improve the benefits and reduce the risks of medications by determining which patients are most likely to respond favorably to a specific medication and by predicting which individuals are at greater risk for an adverse drug reaction. This information can be used to adjust an individual's dosage according to their likely response to treatment.

Much research is underway to understand how genomic information can be used to develop more personalized and cost-effective strategies for using drugs to improve human health. Pharmacogenomics research has led to several genetic tests that provide clinical dosing recommendations. For instance, the FDA is considering genetic testing for drugs like clopidogrel bisulfate, an antiplatelet drug commonly used in cardiovascular disease patients to prevent myocardial infarction and stroke [3]. Cancer is another very active area of pharmacogenomic research. Studies have found that the chemotherapy drugs, gefitinib and erlotinib, work much better in lung cancer patients whose tumors have a certain genetic change [4].

In a general manner, pharmacogenetic association of a particular drug may concern either pharmacokinetic pathways (what the body does to the drug; absorption, distribution, metabolism, elimination) or pharmacodynamic pathways (what the drug does to the body; target, mechanism of action, drug response, efficacy, toxicity) [5].

A pharmacogenomics knowledge resource is available to clinicians and researchers at the PharmGKB website (www.pharmgkb.org). This resource encompasses clinical information including dosing guidelines and drug labels, potentially actionable gene–drug associations and genotype–phenotype relationships. Users have access to integrated information from gene–drug knowledge to implementation of pharmacogenomics in the clinic. Pharmacogenomics of chemotherapy-induced cardiotoxicity is still at its infancy. According to PharmGKB, there are currently no clinical variants that meet a high level of criteria. However, some genetic information reaching lower levels of criteria is included in the database.

Considering breast cancer, a recent systematic review reports on the findings of existing genetic association studies that have examined the genetic variants underlying chronic and late toxicities, specifically cardiotoxicity, cognitive dysfunction, fatigue, and peripheral neuropathy, in patients treated with different chemotherapy modalities [6]. In this review, the quality of the studies was assessed with the Strengthening the Reporting of Genetic Association Studies (STREGA) reporting guidelines. According to these guidelines, only four studies reached the STREGA quality criteria for cardiotoxicity [7–10].

This chapter provides an overview of the major findings in this area of research. Data are available for patients treated for breast cancer, nonHodgkin's lymphoma, acute lymphoblastic leukemia (ALL), and acute myeloid leukemia (AML).

GENETIC DETERMINANTS OF ANTHRACYCLINE-INDUCED CARDIOTOXICITY

Although clinical and demographic factors may predispose certain individuals to greater risk and severity of cardiotoxicity, the vast interindividual variation in their manifestation accentuates the idiosyncratic nature of these toxicities.

Some patients experience cardiotoxicity with doses as low as 200 mg/m^2, while others tolerate doses as high as 1000 mg/m^2 [11]. While some patients with little exposure have considerable cardiac damage, others with higher exposure do not develop heart problems. A genetic contribution to the variability in sensitivity is supported by the relatively high heritability of anthracycline cytotoxicity ($h^2 = 0.18-0.63$) [12].

Up to now, there have been very limited large-scale efforts to interrogate the human genome for markers of risk for chemotherapy-induced cardiotoxicity. Investigators have tested the association of common genetic variants with cardiotoxicity using a candidate-gene approach. The selection of SNPs has been guided by the presumed mechanism of myocardial injury highlighted in animal studies and cellular models, or by knowledge of the pathways responsible for drug trafficking and elimination [13]. This approach inherently has been limited by the incomplete understanding of the mechanisms underlying the myocardial insult, which is insufficient to inform effective candidate-gene efforts. Animal studies have suggested critical roles for genes involved in oxidative stress (*Nox2, MnSOD, PTGS2, MT, TRX1*), drug transport and metabolism (*CBR1, CBR3, ABCB1*), or transcriptional regulation (*GATA4, STAT3*) [14,15]. However, although such studies may provide some insight regarding the effect of dramatic alterations in the abundance or function of a given protein, they rarely predict a response in the human system. This is part of the reason why candidate-gene approaches to identify determinants of cardiotoxicity have not been particularly fruitful.

Early studies suggest that inherited SNPs in one of the carbonyl reductase genes (*CBR1* and *CBR3*) that catalyze the metabolism of anthracyclines to highly cardiotoxic C-13 alcohol metabolites may be involved in anthracycline-induced cardiotoxicity [16,17]. The *CBR1* gene variant increased the risk of heart problems more than fivefold, and the *CBR3* gene variant increased the risk more than threefold. By using the ITMAT/Broad CARe cardiovascular SNP array to profile common SNPs in 2100 genes considered relevant to de novo cardiovascular disease (93 cases, 194 controls), Wang et al. identified a common SNP, rs2232228, in the hyaluronan synthase 3 (HAS3) gene that exerts a modifying effect on anthracycline dose-dependent cardiomyopathy risk [18]. In individuals exposed to high-dose ($>$250 mg/m^2) anthracyclines, the rs2232228 AA genotype conferred an 8.9-fold increased cardiomyopathy risk compared with the GG genotype. Mechanistically, since HAS3 produces hyaluronan, a ubiquitous component of the extracellular that also reduces reactive oxygen species (ROS)-induced cardiac injury, the authors proposed that high cardiomyopathy risk associated with AA genotype could be due to inadequate remodeling and/or inadequate protection of the heart from ROS-mediated injury on high anthracycline exposure.

In a study of adults with nonHodgkin's lymphoma (1697 participants of the German High-Grade nonHodgkin Lymphoma Study Group who developed either chronic or acute cardiotoxicity after a cumulative doxorubicin dose of 300 mg/m^2), genetic variants in 82 candidate genes were examined. The authors identified five SNPs of the NADPH oxidase (*NCF4, RAC2, CYBA*) and doxorubicin efflux transporters (*MRP1/ABCC1* and *MRP2/ABCC2*) that conveyed up to a 2.5-fold increased risk for cardiotoxicity [19]. They proposed that genetic variants in doxorubicin transport and free radical metabolism may modulate the individual risk to develop antracycline-induced cardiotoxicity. A subsequent study from a separate group confirmed an increased susceptibility to doxorubicin-induced cardiotoxicity in patients with the c.212A>G missense variant of the gene encoding the NCF4 subunit of NADPH oxidase [20]. Pediatric studies were undertaken showing an intronic variant (rs10836235) in the catalase gene (CAT) associated with cardiotoxicity in 76 children with ALL, a variant in the ABCC1 gene was associated with lower left ventricular fractional shortening in 235 ALL children [21]. The Canadian Pharmacogenomics Network for Drug Safety (CPNDS) consortium analyzed 2977 variants in 220 key drug biotransformation genes. The subjects were children who received anthracyclines for the treatment of various malignancies and developed cardiotoxicity during at least 5 years of follow-up. The authors identified a highly significant association of cardiotoxicity with a synonymous coding variant within the solute carrier family 28 (*SCL28A3*) gene in three independent cohorts (156 children in British Columbia, 188 Canadians, 96 from Amsterdam) [22]. This consortium also identified highly associated variants in genes, including drug transporters (*SCL28A1, ABCB1, ABCB4, ABCC1*) and an enzyme of the glucuronidation pathway, UDP-glucuronosyltransferase (*UTG1A6*) [23]. They proposed that combining multiple genetic variants with clinical risk factors may predict anthracyclin-induced cardiotoxicity and might thus be used to identify high-risk patients who can then be provided with safer treatment options.

Using a multi-SNP-based approach, Lubieneicka et al. examined 60 genes coding for proteins involved in drug metabolism and efflux and identified the *P450 oxidoreductase* (POR) gene to be most strongly associated with daunorubicin-induced cardiotoxicity in a population of 286 AML patients [24]. Variation in the POR gene was estimated to account for some 11.6% of the variability in the drop of left ventricular ejection fraction (LVEF) after daunorubicin treatment, compared to the estimated 13.2% accounted for by the cumulative dose and ethnicity.

Vivenza et al. conducted a study on 48 early breast cancer patients treated with adjuvant anthracycline chemotherapy with the aim to determine whether SNPs in the renin–angiotensin–aldosterone system and in the glutathione S-transferase family of phase 2 detoxification enzymes might be useful predictors of chemotherapy-induced cardiotoxicity [7]. Whereas *RAAS* gene SNPs were not significantly associated with the development of cardiotoxicity, this study suggested that SNPs in *GSTM1* may be useful as a biomarker of higher risk of cardiotoxicity.

In a recent preliminary study by Triggiani et al. [25] on 66 early breast cancer patients treated with epirubicin (90 mg/m^2 for three or four cycles every 21 days) with or without radiation and hormone therapy, three variants, rs4148808 [C/T] for ABCB4 transporter, rs7853758 [A/G], and rs885004 [A/G] for SLC28A3, combined with serial measurements of plasma cardiac troponin I levels had predictive value for individual anthracycline cardiotoxicity.

Anthracycline-induced cardiotoxicity is a complex phenotype with many genes, environmental factors, and gene–environment interactions contributing to its development [26]. For such complex traits, several genetic determinants underly the final phenotype and variants at each of the genetic loci will generally have a modest effect. Therefore, they will often be missed by the standard single-variant-based association tests [27]. In this respect, genome-wide association studies (GWASs) enable to interrogate more than one million SNPs. GWASs are powered to detect association with causal variants that are relatively common in the population. In contrast to the candidate-gene approach, GWASs are unbiased with respect to prior biological knowledge and with respect to genome location. In the last decade, GWASs have been successfully used to dissect the genetic basis of complex diseases and quantitative traits [28]. To date, more than 2000 disease-associated common variants have been identified through GWASs. The latest technological advances together with biobanks of population cohorts or case-control samples greatly facilitate the ability to conduct these studies.

GWASs of anthracycline-induced cardiotoxicity have been initiated. An abstract by Wells et al. [29] reports on the identification of a new locus for anthracycline cardiotoxicity on chromosome 1p32.1 encompassing the genes *Clorf87*, *CYP2J2,* and *HOOK1*. This study included 385 subjects with anthracycline exposure and measures of LVEF before and after drug exposure. The most common malignancies were nonHodgkin's lymphoma (28.3%), breast (20.3%), acute myelogenous leukemia (15.3%), sarcoma (10.3%), and Hodgkin's lymphoma (7.3%). Median anthracycline dose (converted to doxorubicin equivalents) was 240 mg/m^2. Interestingly, overexpression of CYP2J2 in mouse has previously been shown to be protective from anthracycline cardiotoxicity, and thus represents a biologically plausible candidate gene.

A clinical trial (ClinicalTrials.gov identifier: NCT02078388) is ongoing with the aim to identify genetic variants that are associated with a higher risk of doxorubicin-induced cardiotoxicity in breast cancer patients, toward developing a predictive algorithm comprising both clinical and genetic factors to select patients who should avoid treatment with anthracyclines.

GENETIC DETERMINANTS OF CARDIOTOXICITY OF TARGETED THERAPIES

Knowledge of the genetic determinants of susceptibility to the cardiotoxicity of trastuzumab and other targeted therapies is limited. Candidate-gene approaches naturally have focused on variants in the molecular targets for these drugs, although this approach clearly underestimates their mechanistic complexity. One small study (61 advanced breast cancer patients) suggested that a HER2 SNP (I655V) conferred both increased growth potential in tumor cells and an increased propensity for cardiotoxicity in patients treated with trastuzumab [10]. The association of HER2 I655V with trastuzumab-induced cardiotoxicity (decline in LVEF) was also found in a retrospective cohort study of 237 women with nonmetastatic HER2-positive breast cancer [9].

Another study investigated the predictive value of HER2 I655V, FCGR2A H131R, and FCGR3A V158F variants for cardiac toxicity and efficacy of trastuzumab in 132 HER2-positive breast cancer patients (participants of the prospective node-positive-breast cancer trial HER2 containing-regimen UNICANCER-PACS 04 trial) [8]. The HER2 I655V genotype was found to be significantly associated with cardiac toxicity, whereas the FCGR2A 131 H/H genotype was significantly correlated with a shorter event-free survival. It was concluded that these genetic variants might be useful in making a treatment choice of HER2 blockers in an adjuvant setting with an increase in efficacy and decrease in toxicity.

As stated above, it is unlikely that a single, common variant is sufficient to explain the risk of trastuzumab-induced cardiotoxicity and further large-scale, genome-wide studies are awaited.

There are currently no data on genetic variants that would affect patient risk for cardiotoxicity induced by tyrosine kinase inhibitors.

CONCLUSIONS

Predicting and preventing chemotherapy-induced cardiotoxicity, in addition to understanding its underlying pathophysiology, may significantly improve outcomes in survivors of cancer.

Results from candidate-gene-based studies strongly suggest that genetic markers may be useful to mitigate individual risk for chemotherapy-induced cardiotoxicity. There is still a long way to go before clinical application. Future unbiased genome-wide association and/or exome sequencing in large patient cohorts holds the promise for identifying a broader spectrum of candidate genes that might determine the susceptibility to chemotherapy-induced cardiotoxicity and improve patient care. Indeed, the discovery of genetic biomarkers and their combination with clinical or demographic risk factors may identify patients at risk prior to treatment, thereby guiding suitable therapeutic measures to prevent or limit cardiotoxicity.

The mechanisms underlying chemotherapy-induced cardiotoxicity are still poorly understood. Genome-wide data may provide greater insights into the development of these cancer treatment-induced toxicities. The identification of functional genetic variants associated with these toxicities may improve our understanding of the underlying mechanistic pathways, in order to path the way for development of novel therapies targeting these toxicities.

In addition, the use of genomic tools to better identify chemotherapy-sensitive tumors could also help improve the risk/benefit ratio for related toxicity by reducing chemotherapy exposure in patients unlikely to receive anticancer benefit. Besides improving the ways in which existing drugs are used, genome research will lead to the development of better drugs. The goal is to produce new drugs that are highly effective and do not cause serious side effects.

REFERENCES

[1] Sachidanandam R, Weissman D, Schmidt SC, et al. A map of human genome sequence variation containing 1.42 million single nucleotide polymorphisms. Nature 2001;409(6822):928–33.

[2] Frazer KA, Ballinger DG, Cox DR, et al. A second generation human haplotype map of over 3.1 million SNPs. Nature 2007;449(7164):851–61.

[3] Pare G, Mehta SR, Yusuf S, et al. Effects of CYP2C19 genotype on outcomes of clopidogrel treatment. N Engl J Med 2010;363(18):1704–14.

[4] Mayo C, Bertran-Alamillo J, Molina-Vila MA, Gimenez-Capitan A, Costa C, Rosell R. Pharmacogenetics of EGFR in lung cancer: perspectives and clinical applications. Pharmacogenomics 2012;13(7):789–802.

[5] Whirl-Carrillo M, McDonagh EM, Hebert JM, et al. Pharmacogenomics knowledge for personalized medicine. Clin Pharmacol Ther 2012;92(4):414–17.

[6] Ng T, Chan M, Khor CC, Ho HK, Chan A. The genetic variants underlying breast cancer treatment-induced chronic and late toxicities: a systematic review. Cancer Treat Rev 2014;40(10):1199–214.

[7] Vivenza D, Feola M, Garrone O, Monteverde M, Merlano M, Lo Nigro C. Role of the renin-angiotensin-aldosterone system and the glutathione S-transferase Mu, Pi and Theta gene polymorphisms in cardiotoxicity after anthracycline chemotherapy for breast carcinoma. Int J Biol Markers 2013;28(4):e336–347.

[8] Roca L, Dieras V, Roche H, et al. Correlation of HER2, FCGR2A, and FCGR3A gene polymorphisms with trastuzumab related cardiac toxicity and efficacy in a subgroup of patients from UNICANCER-PACS 04 trial. Breast Cancer Res Treat 2013;139(3):789–800.

[9] Lemieux J, Diorio C, Cote MA, et al. Alcohol and HER2 polymorphisms as risk factor for cardiotoxicity in breast cancer treated with trastuzumab. Anticancer Res 2013;33(6):2569–76.

[10] Beauclair S, Formento P, Fischel JL, et al. Role of the HER2 [Ile655Val] genetic polymorphism in tumorogenesis and in the risk of trastuzumab-related cardiotoxicity. Ann Oncol 2007;18(8):1335–41.

[11] Yeh ET, Bickford CL. Cardiovascular complications of cancer therapy: incidence, pathogenesis, diagnosis, and management. J Am Coll Cardiol 2009;53(24):2231–47.

[12] Peters EJ, Motsinger-Reif A, Havener TM, et al. Pharmacogenomic characterization of US FDA-approved cytotoxic drugs. Pharmacogenomics 2011;12(10):1407–15.

[13] Jensen BC, McLeod HL. Pharmacogenomics as a risk mitigation strategy for chemotherapeutic cardiotoxicity. Pharmacogenomics 2013;14(2):205–13.

[14] Menna P, Paz OG, Chello M, Covino E, Salvatorelli E, Minotti G. Anthracycline cardiotoxicity. Expert Opin Drug Saf 2012;11(Suppl. 1):S21–36.

[15] Sawyer DB, Peng X, Chen B, Pentassuglia L, Lim CC. Mechanisms of anthracycline cardiac injury: can we identify strategies for cardioprotection? Prog Cardiovasc Dis 2010;53(2):105–13.

[16] Blanco JG, Leisenring WM, Gonzalez-Covarrubias VM, et al. Genetic polymorphisms in the carbonyl reductase 3 gene CBR3 and the NAD(P)H:quinone oxidoreductase 1 gene NQO1 in patients who developed anthracycline-related congestive heart failure after childhood cancer. Cancer 2008;112(12):2789–95.

[17] Jamieson D, Boddy AV. Pharmacogenetics of genes across the doxorubicin pathway. Expert Opin Drug Metab Toxicol 2011;7(10):1201–10.

[18] Wang X, Liu W, Sun CL, et al. Hyaluronan synthase 3 variant and anthracycline-related cardiomyopathy: a report from the children's oncology group. J Clin Oncol 2014;32(7): 647–53.

[19] Wojnowski L, Kulle B, Schirmer M, et al. NAD(P)H oxidase and multidrug resistance protein genetic polymorphisms are associated with doxorubicin-induced cardiotoxicity. Circulation 2005;112(24):3754–62.

[20] Rossi D, Rasi S, Franceschetti S, et al. Analysis of the host pharmacogenetic background for prediction of outcome and toxicity in diffuse large B-cell lymphoma treated with R-CHOP21. Leukemia 2009;23(6):1118–26.

[21] Semsei AF, Erdelyi DJ, Ungvari I, et al. ABCC1 polymorphisms in anthracycline-induced cardiotoxicity in childhood acute lymphoblastic leukaemia. Cell Biol Int 2012;36(1): 79–86.

[22] Visscher H, Ross CJ, Rassekh SR, et al. Pharmacogenomic prediction of anthracycline-induced cardiotoxicity in children. J Clin Oncol 2012;30(13):1422–8.

[23] Visscher H, Ross CJ, Rassekh SR, et al. Validation of variants in SLC28A3 and UGT1A6 as genetic markers predictive of anthracycline-induced cardiotoxicity in children. Pediatr Blood Cancer 2013;60(8):1375–81.

[24] Lubieniecka JM, Graham J, Heffner D, et al. A discovery study of daunorubicin induced cardiotoxicity in a sample of acute myeloid leukemia patients prioritizes P450 oxidoreductase polymorphisms as a potential risk factor. Front Genet 2013;4:231.

[25] Triggiani M, Fragni M, Bonetti G, Pizzuto A, Papa I, Capellini S, et al. Abstract P3644. Genetic variants in antracicline biotransformation genes and risk of cardiotoxicity. Eur Heart J 2014;35:A665.

[26] Duan S, Bleibel WK, Huang RS, et al. Mapping genes that contribute to daunorubicin-induced cytotoxicity. Cancer Res 2007;67(11):5425–33.

[27] Kraft P, Hunter DJ. Genetic risk prediction—are we there yet? N Engl J Med 2009; 360(17):1701–3.

[28] Visscher PM, Brown MA, McCarthy MI, Yang J. Five years of GWAS discovery. Am J Hum Genet 2012;90(1):7–24.

[29] Wells QS, Mosley JD, Van Driest SL, Weeke P, Karnes JH, Shaffer CM, et al. Abstract 15509: genomwide-association identifies a novel locus for anthracycline cardiotoxicity. Circulation 2013;128:A15509.

Chapter 39

Cardiac Monitoring During Clinical Trials

M. Moonen, P. Frere, P. Lancellotti and G. Jerusalem

Chapter Outline

INTRODUCTION

Systematic cardiac monitoring during clinical trials, particularly in trials investigating anticancer therapeutics, emerged as a field in cardiology about 15 years ago. Indeed, anticancer agent-related cardiac dysfunction has been a nonanticipated adverse event in a phase 3 trial published in 2001, comparing standard chemotherapy plus a monoclonal antibody against HER2 (trastuzumab) for metastatic breast cancer that overexpresses HER2 [1]. The trial randomized 234 patients to receive standard chemotherapy alone (doxorubicin 60 mg/m^2 or epirubicin 75 mg/m^2 plus cyclophosphamide 600 mg/m^2, or paclitaxel 175 mg/m^2 for patients who had already received adjuvant anthracyclines) and 235 patients to receive standard chemotherapy concurrently with trastuzumab. The addition of trastuzumab to chemotherapy was effective in that it reduced the relative risk of death by 20% at a median follow-up of 30 months. Only very few studies of metastatic breast cancer had until then demonstrated a survival advantage of that magnitude in association with the addition of a single agent. However, 25 patients stopped taking trastuzumab because of adverse events, mainly including 20 cases of cardiac events attributable to trastuzumab, which had not been anticipated on the basis of the preclinical or early clinical studies data. These adverse cardiac events

Anticancer Treatments and Cardiotoxicity. DOI: http://dx.doi.org/10.1016/B978-0-12-802509-3.00039-X

commissioned a retrospective analysis by an independent cardiac review and evaluation committee. A total of 63 patients were retrospectively identified with symptomatic or asymptomatic cardiac dysfunction. The 27% incidence of cardiac dysfunction among patients who were given an anthracycline, cyclophosphamide, and trastuzumab and the 13% incidence among those who were given paclitaxel and trastuzumab largely exceeded the expected incidence of 8% associated with corresponding cumulative doses of anthracyclines. The incidence of cardiac dysfunction of New York Heart Association (NYHA) class III and IV was highest among patients treated with an anthracycline, cyclophosphamide, and trastuzumab. Of these 63 patients, 44 had received standard heart failure treatment, with improvement of the condition in 33 (five did not change, four worsened, two died), suggesting the potential reversibility of the trastuzumab-associated cardiac dysfunction. The mechanism of the cardiotoxicity of trastuzumab is explained by the expression of HER2/erbB2 in adult myocardium. Trastuzumab alters the expression of genes for DNA repair, which is associated with cardiomyocyte lesions promoting apoptosis.

In these circumstances, the intrinsic or potentiating cardiac toxicity of trastuzumab, or of other new anticancer agents, must be weighed against their clinical benefit, considering the extremely poor prognosis of patients with HER2-positive metastatic breast cancer, and introduced the need for precautions with extended indications. Particularly, the adjuvant (postoperative) setting is an important concern both in clinical trials and in real-life situations, when considering concomitant or sequential treatment with agents with cardiotoxic effects, since many patients with early-stage breast cancer can be cured by surgery and radiotherapy. The benefits should outweigh the risks of short-term and long-term toxicity. In this chapter, dedicated to "cardiac monitoring during clinical trials," we propose a description of the different strategies worked out to prevent cardiac dysfunction attributable to trastuzumab when it was evaluated in the adjuvant setting.

PHASED STUDY DESIGN

The first reaction of study designers was to work out studies including prospective evaluation of cardiotoxicity with several stages.

For example, the National Surgical Adjuvant Breast and Bowel Project (NSABP) trial B-31, comparing doxorubicin and cyclophosphamide followed by paclitaxel with the same scheme plus 52 weeks of trastuzumab beginning concurrently with paclitaxel, included two stages, with assessment of cardiac dysfunction as the primary aim of the first stage [2]. The stage 1 included approximately one-third of patients (the first 1000 patients in 2700 planned patients) and required a favorable review of the cardiac data by an independent data-monitoring committee before extending accrual to the stage 2. This strategy was used subsequently in other trials.

CAREFUL PATIENT SELECTION

After the result of the pivotal trial demonstrating for the first time the significant rate of cardiac dysfunction associated with trastuzumab administration [1], all the following trials included specific cardiac eligibility and exclusion criteria (Table 39.1). However, different eligibility criteria were used, complicating comparison between trials. In the case of regimens with sequential administration of anticancer agents, the study design included an evaluation of the left ventricular ejection fraction (LVEF) baseline but also particularly after the completion of anthracycline-based chemotherapy. The LVEF at that time should remain above the lower limit of normal and not be decreased by more than 15 percentage points from the preentry level. Indeed, the mean cumulative dose of anthracyclines appears as an important parameter predicting the occurrence of congestive heart failure associated with trastuzumab infusion. In the HERA trial, the mean cumulative dose among patients with a cardiac event was significantly higher for doxorubicin (287 vs 257 mg/m^2) or epirubicin (480 vs 422 mg/m^2). The mean cumulative dose of paclitaxel showed a trend to a higher dose among patients with a cardiac event that was not significant, possibly because of the small sample size of patients receiving paclitaxel in this trial [3].

It must also be pointed out that some risks factors not considered at baseline as cardiac exclusion criteria should be evaluated before starting trastuzumab as they have been demonstrated to significantly increase the risk of cancer therapeutics-related cardiac dysfunction:

- Lower screening LVEF or a lower postanthracycline LVEF [2,4];
- High (>25) BMI [4];
- Older patients [2].

Other parameters such as hypertension, being a current smoker, diabetes, hypothyroidism, age ≥ 60 showed a trend to a higher incidence of cardiac events that was not significant, possibly due to the limited number of patients presenting those characteristics [4]. The large underrepresentation of patients with diabetes or metabolic syndrome included in trials suggests great caution considering treating them with potential cardiotoxic agents in real-life situations.

Left-sided lesions receiving radiotherapy did not appear associated with an increase in congestive heart failure [2].

CAUTIOUS CARDIAC MONITORING

Close cardiac monitoring is assumed most of the time combining clinical evaluation, 12-lead electrocardiogram, and LVEF monitoring (Table 39.2).

The NYHA functional class is classically used for the evaluation of symptoms. Severe cardiac heart failure symptoms are generally defined as NYHA class III or IV. A cardiologist usually confirms the symptomatic evaluation.

TABLE 39.1 Cardiac Eligibility and General and Cardiac-Specific Exclusion Criteria

	Cardiac Eligibility Criteria	General Exclusion Criteria	Cardiac-Specific Exclusion Criteria
HERA trial [3,4]	Normal LVEF (≥55% measured by echocardiography or multiple gated acquisition scanning) after completion of all chemotherapy and radiotherapy	Prior mediastinal irradiation (except internal mammary-node irradiation for the present breast cancer) Cumulative doses of anthracycline exceeding 360 mg per square meter of body-surface area for doxorubicin or 720 mg per square meter for epirubicin	History of documented congestive heart failure Coronary artery disease with previous Q-wave myocardial infarction Angina pectoris requiring medication Uncontrolled hypertension (systolic blood pressure >180 mmHg or diastolic blood pressure >100 mmHg) Clinically significant valvular disease High-risk arrhythmias
NSABP B-31 [2]	LVEF on multiple gated acquisition scan ≥the lower limit of normal (which was more often an LVEF >49%) or LVEF drop after anthracycline and cyclophosphamide <15% compared to baseline LVEF		Prior myocardial infarction, chronic heart failure, or other cardiomyopathy Active cardiac disease: • angina pectoris • cardiac arrhythmia requiring medication • severe conduction abnormalities • clinically significant valvular disease • cardiomegaly • ventricular hypertrophy • poorly controlled hypertension
Trial N9831 [6]	LVEF within the institutional normal range	Prior anthracycline or taxane therapy for any malignancy	Myocardial infarction Documented congestive heart failure Clinically significant arrhythmia Valvular heart disease requiring medication Uncontrolled hypertension (diastolic pressure >100 mmHg or systolic pressure >200 mmHg) Clinically significant pericardial effusion

FinHer study [13]			Severe hypertension Cardiac disease (cardiac failure of any degree, arrhythmia requiring regular medication and any myocardial infarction within the previous 12 months)

LVEF, left ventricular ejection fraction.

TABLE 39.2 Cardiac Monitoring in Clinical Trials

	Clinical Evaluation		LVEF Monitoring	
HERA trial [3,4]	Cardiac questionnaire, physical examination, 12-lead electrocardiogram	Baseline and 3, 6, 12, 18, 24, 30, 36, and 60 months after randomization	Echocardiography or MUGA scanning	Baseline and 3, 6, 12, 18, 24, 30, 36, and 60 months after randomization
NSABP B-31 [2]	Cardiac history forms	Entry, every 6 months for the first 5 years and yearly thereafter	MUGA scans	Before entry, after anthracyclines, and at 6, 9, and 18 months
Trial N9831 [6]			Echocardiography or MUGA scanning	Baseline, 3 weeks after the end of anthracycline therapy, 6 months after registration (3 weeks after completing paclitaxel with or without trastuzumab), 9 months after registration, and 3 months after study completion

Echocardiography or MUGA scanning is used for the assessment of LVEF. It is now strongly recommended to monitor the LVEF using the same method and radiology facility throughout the study [5]. LVEF drop has to be systematically confirmed by repeated cardiac imaging performed 2–4 weeks after the first cardiac study showing a decrease in LVEF.

In regimens including sequential administration of new agents following anthracycline administration, patients should also be evaluated for cardiac symptoms and LVEF measurement 3 weeks postanthracyclines to exclude cardiac toxicity of anthracyclines and to permit the administration of the tested agent. In N9831, trastuzumab was not administered if a patient showed significant cardiac symptoms related to left ventricular (LV) dysfunction, cardiac ischemia, or arrhythmia or if the 3-week postanthracycline LVEF relative to pretreatment LVEF levels decreased by more than 15% or by $\leq$5% to a level below the radiology facility's lower limit of normal [6].

The generally applied timing of LVEF evaluation is baseline evaluation and then every 3–6 months for the first year and then every 6–12 months. The total duration of the cardiac monitoring is most of the time limited to the study follow-up and regrettably does not provide long-term monitoring. In the NSABP B-31 trial, three of the 31 congestive heart failures observed in the trastuzumab arm occurred more than 1 year after initiation of trastuzumab [2]. In the Herceptin, Cyclophosphamide and Epirubicin (HERCULES) trial, all cardiac events were recorded after completion of chemotherapy [7].

A core laboratory or science staff has generally been in charge of reviewing the echocardiograms and the MUGA scan results.

The study design should also include timely prespecified interim cardiac safety analyses by independent cardiac review panel blinded to treatment arm. An absolute difference of more than a prefixed percentage point level (in general 4%) in the incidence of severe congestive heart failure or cardiac death between the treatment group and the observation group should trigger a recommendation by the independent data-monitoring committee to stop or modify the trial.

CLEAR STOPPING RULES (INTERRUPTION AND DISCONTINUATION)

The cardiac safety and tolerability of agents should be assessed based on prespecified cardiac endpoints, e.g., cardiac death (death definitely due to heart failure, myocardial infarction, or documented arrhythmia or probable cardiac death within 24 h of a cardiac event), severe congestive heart failure (NYHA class III or IV and significant LVEF drop), or confirmed significant LVEF drop (confirmation requires a repeat LVEF assessment 3 weeks after the first documented significant LVEF drop).

The HERA trial was the first to apply an algorithm for discontinuation of trastuzumab in patients based on periodic LVEF assessment and careful symptom monitoring (http://jco.ascopubs.org/content/25/25/3859/F2.expansion.html). The NSABP trial B-31 also proposed a similar algorithm although not identical (http://jco.ascopubs.org/content/23/31/7811/T2.expansion.html). In the HERA trial, trastuzumab was stopped if symptomatic congestive heart failure and LVEF ≤44% developed or if an LVEF <50% with confirmed absolute reduction of ≥10% from baseline developed. In patients without signs of congestive heart failure, the same criteria for left ventricular function were used to withhold treatment. Trastuzumab was discontinued if, in asymptomatic patients, left ventricular function did not return to a level above the criteria for withholding treatment after the therapy was stopped for 3 weeks [4]. The NSABP trial B-31 criteria for trastuzumab suspension included NYHA class III or IV symptoms with either a decrease from baseline in LVEF of more than 10 percentage points to less than 55% or a decrease of more than 5 percentage points to less than the lower limit of normal. Discontinuation was considered after 4 weeks if LVEF remains below the criteria for withholding treatment [2]. The National Cancer Institute Common Toxicity Criteria (version 2.0) was used to grade cardiac toxicity in the N9831 trial [6].

Cardiac follow-up forms that summarized ongoing symptoms, LVEF values, and cardiac medications should monitor the patients for whom cardiac dysfunction has been reported.

It should also be noted that in some clinical trials, not only symptoms of congestive heart failure or LVEF drop motivated trastuzumab discontinuation but other cardiac manifestations, such as coronary heart disease, tachyarrthymias, and pericardial effusion [3].

The definition of the recovery after a cardiac event should also be prespecified. The following definition has been especially used: a patient's LVEF is considered to be recovered from a cardiac endpoint if the patient has a LVEF ≥55% at any time after the cardiac event [3].

SEQUENTIAL SCHEMES OF ANTHRACYCLINE–TRASTUZUMAB ADMINISTRATION

Cardiotoxicity of trastuzumab has been reported in 1.4% of women who received the drug as a single agent for metastatic disease [8,9]. A 27% incidence of cardiac dysfunction is reached in patients receiving concurrently an anthracycline, cyclophosphamide, and trastuzumab [1] and to a lesser extent to 13–17% incidence in case of concomitant administration of taxanes and trastuzumab [1,10], exceeding anyway the expected incidence of cardiotoxicity associated with corresponding cumulative doses of anthracyclines. This damaging interaction between trastuzumab and anthracyclines on the heart, and to a lesser magnitude between trastuzumab and taxanes, has been a concern in the design of studies in the adjuvant setting, since the established efficacy of anthracyclines and taxanes currently keeps them as preferred first-line treatment options in the management of breast cancer.

The HERA study was the first trial designed of sequential chemotherapy and trastuzumab. It is important to note that adjuvant chemotherapy, neoadjuvant chemotherapy, or both (consisting of at least four cycles) should be completed before the beginning of trastuzumab administration and only patients who after completion of (neo)adjuvant chemotherapy had LVEF $\geq 55\%$ were eligible. The study confirmed the favorable expected effects on disease-free survival (approximately 50% reduction in the rate of recurrence, particularly distant recurrence) and demonstrated a lower incidence of symptomatic congestive heart failure (1.7% of patients in the trastuzumab group and 0.06% of patients in the observation group) [4].

The NSABP B-31 trial went further and proposed to compare doxorubicin and cyclophosphamide followed by paclitaxel with doxorubicin and cyclophosphamide followed by paclitaxel plus 52 weeks of trastuzumab beginning concurrently with paclitaxel. As mentioned above, the study was designed in two stages with assessment of cardiac dysfunction as the primary aim of the first stage. The cardiotoxicity interim analysis found a difference in cardiac events of less than 4%, so accrual was continued. Cumulative incidence of cardiac events 3 years after day 1 of cycle 5 was 0.8% in the control arm and 4.1% in the trastuzumab-treated patients (3.3% difference between both arms). Interestingly three of the 31 cases of congestive heart failure occurred more than 1 year after initiation of trastuzumab. The joint efficacy analysis of the N9831 and NSABP B-31 trials demonstrated that adding trastuzumab to chemotherapy reduced disease recurrence by 52% and risk of death by 33% compared with chemotherapy. In the N9831 trial, the 3-year cumulative incidence of class III or IV congestive heart failure or death from cardiac causes was 2.9% in the trastuzumab group [11]. So, in both studies, the cumulative 3-year incidence of congestive heart failure increased by about 3 percentage points with the concomitant administration of paclitaxel and trastuzumab.

It is noteworthy that, in the case of sequential anthracycline–trastuzumab chemotherapy, acute decreases in LVEF have been frequently observed when measured 3 weeks after the fourth cycle of treatment [6].

Finally, the N9831 trial was also designed to address the efficacy of trastuzumab initiated sequentially to an anthracycline but concurrently with paclitaxel as opposed to sequentially. The comparison suggests that delayed administration of trastuzumab (i.e., after completion of paclitaxel) is less effective than concurrent administration and the 3-year cumulative incidence of cardiac events is 3.3% and 2.8%, respectively [12].

ALTERNATIVE SCHEMES

The FinHer (Finland Herceptin) study is a trial of concurrent chemotherapy and trastuzumab. The patients were randomized to receive three cycles of docetaxel or vinorelbine, administered with or without 9-weekly infusion of trastuzumab, followed in both groups by three cycles of fluorouracil, epirubicin, and cyclophosphamide (FEC) [13]. The study design specified no trastuzumab administration during administration of FEC. The hypothesis was that such a schedule would limit cardiotoxicity and maintain efficacy. The study design has cardiac exclusion criteria (Table 39.1). The cardiac monitoring is not described in the study report. This short course of trastuzumab given concomitantly with the chemotherapy resulted in no significant increase in the frequency of adverse events related to vinorelbine or docetaxel and the LVEF in women who received trastuzumab was even slightly better than those who did not receive the antibody [14]. The authors suggested that the administration of trastuzumab before FEC and radiotherapy, as well as the small cumulative dose of epirubicin given, might be alternative schemes to preserve cardiac function. The main limitation of the study is the small sample size, and the relatively young age of the study participants.

The BCRIG 0006 trial, also addressing the adjuvant use of trastuzumab, was conducted to evaluate the efficacy and safety of a nonanthracycline regimen in a sequential chemotherapy and trastuzumab scheme [15]. This nonanthracycline regimen consisted of docetaxel, carboplatin, and trastuzumab. The trial was designed for a comparison of each of two different chemotherapy–trastuzumab combinations, doxorubicin–cyclophosphamide followed by docetaxel every 3 weeks plus 52 weeks of trastuzumab or docetaxel–carboplatin plus 52 weeks of trastuzumab, against a chemotherapy control (doxorubicin–cyclophosphamide followed by docetaxel every 3 weeks). The authors confirmed that the addition of 1 year of adjuvant trastuzumab significantly improved disease-free and overall survival among women with HER2-positive breast cancer. They observed at a median follow-up of 65 months no significant differences in efficacy between the two trastuzumab regimens. The rates of congestive heart failure and cardiac dysfunction were significantly higher in the group receiving anthracycline plus trastuzumab than in the nonanthracycline regimen. Therefore the postulate of the higher risk–benefit ratio, favoring the nonanthracycline regimen, has been stated. However, some authors have emphasized that the trial was not designed to compare the two trastuzumab-based arms and, for different reasons, extreme caution should at this stage be taken before systematically privileging a nonanthracycline regimen [16].

The HERCULES trial proposed to test epirubicin instead of doxorubicin [7]. Epirubicin has been shown as equally effective and less toxic than doxorubicin. HER2-positive metastatic breast cancer patients received first-line trastuzumab plus cyclophosphamide and one of two dosages of epirubicin (60 mg/m^2 or 90 mg/m^2) for six cycles, followed by trastuzumab monotherapy until progression. HER2-negative disease received epirubicin (90 mg/m^2) and cyclophosphamide alone. So the trial was not a comparison of epirubicin and doxorubicin. The primary endpoint was dose-limiting cardiotoxicity. The results demonstrated that the low dosage of epirubicin (60 mg/m^2) was associated with similar safety findings as a nonanthracycline regimen (1.7% incidence of cardiotoxicity) with efficacy similar to trastuzumab/docetaxel in patients with HER2-positive metastatic breast cancer [10] and superior to outcomes with trastuzumab/doxorubicin in the pivotal H0648g trial [1].

Compared with conventional anthracyclines, pegylated liposomal doxorubicin has been observed to be significantly less cardiotoxic. Based on these findings, it has been hypothesized that substituting pegylated liposomal doxorubicin for doxorubicin may permit concurrent administration of trastuzumab with anthracycline. A phase II study (BACH trial) was therefore conducted. In the arm receiving pegylated liposomal doxorubicin, trastuzumab therapy was initiated concurrently, compared with the arm receiving doxorubicin in which trastuzumab was administered after completion of the anthracycline. Cardiac assessment included clinical evaluation and LVEF measurements (MUGA or ECHO) with one method used consistently throughout the study. The cardiac safety analysis suggested that administering trastuzumab concurrently with pegylated liposomal doxorubicin is feasible and resulted in lower rates of early cardiotoxicity and premature cessation of trastuzumab due to cardiotoxicity. The protocol failed to evaluate relapse-free survival. The possible clinical benefit of this strategy therefore requires a comparison of the current strategy to an optimal nonanthracycline trastuzumab-based regimen, but as mentioned above no agreement has been reached until now.

CONCLUSION AND PERSPECTIVES FOR CARDIAC MONITORING AND MANAGEMENT

Breast cancer is the most frequent malignancy among women and HER2-positive tumors have been associated with the worst prognosis. Current adjuvant treatment for HER2-positive tumors now includes an anti-HER2 monoclonal antibody, trastuzumab, either concurrent with or sequential to chemotherapy with up to 50% reduction in 3-year breast cancer recurrence and death rate. Given these positive results, trastuzumab has been approved since 2006 by the FDA for adjuvant treatment of HER2-positive breast cancer. However, an adverse effect of trastuzumab that has not been anticipated is symptomatic LV dysfunction that can lead to overt heart failure and death. The conception of adjuvant regimens limiting the risk of cardiotoxicity has therefore been an important area of research. Different precautions and strategies have been proposed for minimizing the risks of cardiac damages. They have been developed in the chapter.

However, it is noteworthy that the rate of cardiac dysfunction reported in clinical trials seems to underestimate the extent of the problem in real clinical practice [17]. Trastuzumab cardiotoxicity has also been considered reversible based on follow-up of patients included in trials. However, real-life data seem to be less optimistic [18]. An explanation of these observations comes from the fact that standard practice concerns patients not strictly sticking to the stringent cardiac exclusion criteria applied in clinical trials. Moreover, older women represent a fast-growing group of patients, unavoidably at higher cardiovascular risk. These over-60 patients have been shown to be at higher risk of (a) symptomatic heart failure and treatment discontinuation [19]. Currently, we are unfortunately not able to accurately predict which patients receiving anticancer therapy are at increased risk of cardiac toxicity based on pretreatment patient characteristics or the changes in LVEF during treatment.

These observations gave rise to a new development of aspects of cardiac monitoring in trials.

The LV lesions that precede severe symptomatic congestive heart failure can now technically be analyzed thanks to the progress of noninvasive cardiac imaging. Cardiovascular magnetic resonance (CMR) imaging has emerged as the reference method for quantification of ventricular volumes and ejection fraction. Higher cost, lesser accessibility, and not uncommon contraindications (cardiac device, claustrophobia, etc.) represent however important limitations of the technique. Two-dimensional echocardiography and recent three-dimensional echocardiography and speckle tracking technology remain serious alternatives. The increased accuracy of all these tools allows the detection of subclinical changes in left ventricular function that precedes overt heart failure. These at-risk patients could therefore benefit from preventive interventions, i.e., early pharmacological treatment with beta-blockers and angiotensin-converting enzyme inhibitors. The MANTICORE 101—Breast (Multidisciplinary Approach to Novel Therapies in Cardiology Oncology Research) is a currently monocentric-randomized trial to determine whether conventional heart failure pharmacological treatment can prevent trastuzumab-mediated LV remodeling [20].

Moreover, cardiac monitoring, by routinely measuring LVEF before, during, and after adjuvant therapy, is only a standard of care for trastuzumab-based anticancer therapy. The EACVI/HFA Cardiac Oncology Toxicity (COT) registry in breast cancer patients is a EURObservational research program of the European Society of Cardiology designed for comprehensive data collection and evaluation of the current European practice in terms of diagnosis and management of anticancer drug-related cardiotoxicity in breast cancer patients [21]. Several critical missing pieces of information should become available thanks to the COT registry: predisposing factors, rate of subclinical LV dysfunction, and its transition to overt heart failure, clinical impact, and outcome of anticancer drug-related cardiotoxicity.

In addition to imaging, cardiac biomarker monitoring is now included in trial design in some studies. It has implications on early detection of cardiotoxicity, physiopathology assessment, and predictive value. Troponin and brain natriuretic peptide are the most studied biomarkers, but the area of cardiac biomarkers is quickly moving and new promising cardiac biomarkers with high physiopathological value are emerging.

Until more data are available, it is important to remind clinicians and patients that the highly studied and highly effective adjuvant regimen remains the mainstay of therapy for higher-risk HER2 breast cancer patients, even if the concern about cardiomyopathies justifies the development of regimens that minimize cardiac toxicity [16].

REFERENCES

[1] Slamon DJ, Leyland-Jones B, Shak S, Fuchs H, Paton V, Bajamonde A, et al. Use of chemotherapy plus a monoclonal antibody against HER2 for metastatic breast cancer that overexpresses HER2. N Engl J Med 2001;344(11):783–92.

[2] Tan-Chiu E, Yothers G, Romond E, Geyer Jr. CE, Ewer M, Keefe D, et al. Assessment of cardiac dysfunction in a randomized trial comparing doxorubicin and cyclophosphamide followed by paclitaxel, with or without trastuzumab as adjuvant therapy in node-positive, human epidermal growth factor receptor 2-overexpressing breast cancer: NSABP B-31. J Clin Oncol 2005;23(31):7811–19.

[3] Suter TM, Procter M, van Veldhuisen DJ, Muscholl M, Bergh J, Carlomagno C, et al. Trastuzumab-associated cardiac adverse effects in the herceptin adjuvant trial. J Clin Oncol 2007;25(25):3859–65.

[4] Piccart-Gebhart MJ, Procter M, Leyland-Jones B, Goldhirsch A, Untch M, Smith I, et al. Trastuzumab after adjuvant chemotherapy in HER2-positive breast cancer. N Engl J Med 2005;353(16):1659–72.

[5] Plana JC, Galderisi M, Barac A, Ewer MS, Ky B, Scherrer-Crosbie M, et al. Expert consensus for multimodality imaging evaluation of adult patients during and after cancer therapy: a report from the American Society of Echocardiography and the European Association of Cardiovascular Imaging. Eur Heart J Cardiovascu Imaging 2014;15(10):1063–93.

[6] Perez EA, Suman VJ, Davidson NE, Kaufman PA, Martino S, Dakhil SR, et al. Effect of doxorubicin plus cyclophosphamide on left ventricular ejection fraction in patients with breast cancer in the North Central Cancer Treatment Group N9831 Intergroup Adjuvant Trial. J Clin Oncol 2004;22(18):3700–4.

[7] Untch M, Muscholl M, Tjulandin S, Jonat W, Meerpohl HG, Lichinitser M, et al. First-line trastuzumab plus epirubicin and cyclophosphamide therapy in patients with human epidermal growth factor receptor 2-positive metastatic breast cancer: cardiac safety and efficacy data from the Herceptin, Cyclophosphamide, and Epirubicin (HERCULES) trial. J Clin Oncol 2010;28(9):1473–80.

[8] Vogel CL, Cobleigh MA, Tripathy D, Gutheil JC, Harris LN, Fehrenbacher L, et al. Efficacy and safety of trastuzumab as a single agent in first-line treatment of HER2-overexpressing metastatic breast cancer. J Clin Oncol 2002;20(3):719–26.

[9] Baselga J, Carbonell X, Castaneda-Soto NJ, Clemens M, Green M, Harvey V, et al. Phase II study of efficacy, safety, and pharmacokinetics of trastuzumab monotherapy administered on a 3-weekly schedule. J Clin Oncol 2005;23(10):2162–71.

[10] Marty M, Cognetti F, Maraninchi D, Snyder R, Mauriac L, Tubiana-Hulin M, et al. Randomized phase II trial of the efficacy and safety of trastuzumab combined with docetaxel in patients with human epidermal growth factor receptor 2-positive metastatic breast cancer administered as first-line treatment: the M77001 study group. J Clin Oncol 2005;23(19):4265–74.

[11] Romond EH, Perez EA, Bryant J, Suman VJ, Geyer Jr. CE, Davidson NE, et al. Trastuzumab plus adjuvant chemotherapy for operable HER2-positive breast cancer. N Engl J Med 2005;353(16):1673–84.

[12] Perez EA, Suman VJ, Davidson NE, Sledge GW, Kaufman PA, Hudis CA, et al. Cardiac safety analysis of doxorubicin and cyclophosphamide followed by paclitaxel with or without trastuzumab in the North Central Cancer Treatment Group N9831 adjuvant breast cancer trial. J Clin Oncol 2008;26(8):1231–8.

[13] Joensuu H, Kellokumpu-Lehtinen PL, Bono P, Alanko T, Kataja V, Asola R, et al. Adjuvant docetaxel or vinorelbine with or without trastuzumab for breast cancer. N Engl J Med 2006;354(8):809–20.

[14] Joensuu H, Bono P, Kataja V, Alanko T, Kokko R, Asola R, et al. Fluorouracil, epirubicin, and cyclophosphamide with either docetaxel or vinorelbine, with or without trastuzumab, as adjuvant treatments of breast cancer: final results of the FinHer Trial. J Clin Oncol 2009;27(34):5685–92.

[15] Slamon D, Eiermann W, Robert N, Pienkowski T, Martin M, Press M, et al. Adjuvant trastuzumab in HER2-positive breast cancer. N Engl J Med 2011;365(14):1273–83.

[16] Burstein HJ, Piccart-Gebhart MJ, Perez EA, Hortobagyi GN, Wolmark N, Albain KS, et al. Choosing the best trastuzumab based adjuvant chemotherapy regimen: should we abandon anthracyclines? J Clin Oncol 2012;30(18):2179–82.

[17] McArthur HL, Chia S. Cardiotoxicity of trastuzumab in clinical practice. N Engl J Med 2007;357(1):94–5.

[18] Wadhwa D, Fallah-Rad N, Grenier D, Krahn M, Fang T, Ahmadie R, et al. Trastuzumab mediated cardiotoxicity in the setting of adjuvant chemotherapy for breast cancer: a retrospective study. Breast Cancer Res Treat 2009;117(2):357–64.

[19] Tarantini L, Gori S, Faggiano P, Pulignano G, Simoncini E, Tuccia F, et al. Adjuvant trastuzumab cardiotoxicity in patients over 60 years of age with early breast cancer: a multicenter cohort analysis. Ann Oncol 2012;23(12):3058–63.

[20] Pituskin E, Haykowsky M, Mackey JR, Thompson RB, Ezekowitz J, Koshman S, et al. Rationale and design of the Multidisciplinary Approach to Novel Therapies in Cardiology Oncology Research Trial (MANTICORE 101--Breast): a randomized, placebo-controlled trial to determine if conventional heart failure pharmacotherapy can prevent trastuzumab-mediated left ventricular remodeling among patients with HER2+ early breast cancer using cardiac MRI. BMC Cancer 2011;11:318.

[21] Lancellotti P, Anker SD, Donal E, Edvardsen T, Popescu BA, Farmakis D, et al. EACVI/HFA Cardiac Oncology Toxicity Registry in breast cancer patients: rationale, study design, and methodology (EACVI/HFA COT Registry)-EURObservational Research Program of the European Society of Cardiology. Eur Heart J Cardiovascu Imaging 2015;16(5):466–70.

Chapter 40

Preventive Therapy

M. Scherrer-Crosbie

Chapter Outline

DEXRAZOXANE

Dexrazoxane (also called ICRF-187 or ADR-589), a molecule that belongs to the bisdioxopiperazine agents, was initially developed as a potential anticancer drug [1]. Despite abundant research, the mechanism by which dexrazoxane prevents anthracycline cardiotoxicity remains incompletely understood. The prevailing theory is that when dexrazoxane becomes hydrolyzed, it produces ADR-925 and some intermediate products that are able to chelate iron [2]. As ADR-925 is a stronger iron chelator than anthracyclines, it displaces Fe^{3+} from the complex with this drug. As detailed in the mechanistic section of the book, the production of reactive oxidant species (ROS) by anthracyclines is considerably augmented by the presence of iron. Iron binds to anthracyclines to create anthracycline–Fe^{3+}complexes; when these complexes are reduced to anthracycline-Fe^{2+}, they can react with oxygen to form the oxidant, O_2^-. Additionally, iron catalyzes the reactions of H_2O_2 and O_2^- to produce the oxidant, OH.

Dexrazoxane was shown to protect rat neonatal cardiomyocytes from apoptosis induced by daunorubicin [3]. Interestingly, it did not protect cardiomyocytes from necrosis induced by higher doses of daunorubicin. There is a large body of evidence that dexrazoxane protects from apoptosis and left ventricular (LV) dysfunction in small and large animal models of doxorubicin-induced cardiotoxicity (for a review, see [4]). Similarly, in patients with a variety of cancers, dexrazoxane has shown its efficiency in decreasing cardiotoxicity [5–9]. In humans, dexrazoxane is given in a short (approximately 15 min) infusion immediately prior to anthracycline treatment. Lipshultz et al. measured troponin T before, during, and after

Anticancer Treatments and Cardiotoxicity. DOI: http://dx.doi.org/10.1016/B978-0-12-802509-3.00040-6

treatment in a population of children with acute lymphoblastic leukemia treated by doxorubicin, with or without dexrazoxane, and demonstrated that 300 mg/m^2 dexrazoxane decreased the proportion of patients with elevated troponin T from 50% to 21% [6]. A follow-up study 5 years after the completion of doxorubicin revealed that children who had received doxorubicin alone had significantly worse shortening fraction than their healthy counterparts, however, the shortening fraction was not decreased in children who had received dexrazoxane. The decrease in wall thickness and the increase in the ratio of LV diameter/wall thickness were also limited in children who had received dexrazoxane [5]. Three additional studies were conducted in patients with breast cancer. An early randomized study in 150 anthracycline-naïve women with breast cancer reported that women receiving dexrazoxane were able to be treated with higher doses of anthracyclines, yet developed less cardiac events than untreated women [8]. Thirty-seven patients on the placebo group had to discontinue anthracyclines due to cardiac toxicity as compared to only six in the dexrazoxane arm, and the left ventricular ejection fraction (LVEF) was lower in the untreated women group for all subcategories of anthracycline doses. Marty et al. randomized 164 women with recurrent breast cancer who had previously been treated with anthracyclines to further anthracyclines with or without dexrazoxane [7]. The group treated with dexrazoxane experienced less cardiac events (defined as a significant reduction in LVEF or symptomatic heart failure, 13% vs 39%, $P<0.001$) than the placebo-treated group. Another study [9], grouping two randomized trials in anthracycline-naïve women with breast cancer confirmed the earlier results, however, it raised the concern that dexrazoxane interfered with the anticancer effect of anthracyclines. Specifically, in one of the two trials (293 women), a significant difference in the tumor response to treatment was noted (47% in patients treated with dexrazoxane vs 61% in patients treated with placebo, $P=0.019$). Of note, there was no difference noted in the other trial (tumor response was 54% in patients treated with dexrazoxane vs 49% in patients treated with placebo, $P=0.63$), and there was no difference in the time to progression or the overall survival between groups in either trial. There had been no difference in tumor response noted in any of the other reported trials. These isolated results regarding the impairment of the anticancer effect of the anthracyclines by dexrazoxane were extensively analyzed, including by an expert panel directed by the first author reporting the incriminating study [10]. Their conclusion was that the deleterious effect of dexrazoxane on the anticancer effect of anthracyclines was an isolated finding, possibly due to the unusually high tumor response of the placebo group. Furthermore, two meta-analyses of all existing randomized trials using dexrazoxane [11,12] did not confirm this finding. The most recent meta-analysis in 2011, including 1619 patients from 10 randomized studies found that dexrazoxane provided a benefit on heart failure with a risk ratio of 0.29 and no deleterious effect on overall survival [11]. Nevertheless, the stain has remained, and the guidelines of oncological societies recommend the use of dexrazoxane only in metastatic breast cancer and when the cumulative dose of doxorubicin exceeds 300 mg/m^2 [13].

The side effects of dexrazoxane appear to be rare, however, leukopenia and myelotoxicity have been noted. Leukopenia in particular appears to be more frequent in dexrazoxane-treated patients [9], maybe due to an inhibition of topoisomerase 2. One study in pediatric patients suggested that the incidence of secondary malignancy was higher in pediatric Hodgkin patients treated with dexrazoxane [14]. An analysis of studies in pediatric patients with T-cell lymphoblastic leukemias reported 4.2% secondary cancers in the group treated with dexrazoxane and 1.3% secondary cancers in the placebo-treated group at 10 years ($P = 0.15$) [15]. This additional concern led the European Medicine Agency (EMA) to discontinue the use of dexrazoxane in children in Europe for the prevention of cardiotoxicity in 2011; both the FDA and the EMA recommendations are now similar and restrict the use of dexrazoxane to women with advanced or metastatic breast cancer who receive more than 300 mg/m^2 doxorubicin or 540 mg/m^2 epirubicin [16].

STATINS

There are significant experimental data suggesting statin therapy given during cardiac injury decreases the development of systolic dysfunction [17,18]. In mice treated with anthracyclines, statins reduced oxidative stress, apoptosis, and inflammation, and preserved cardiac function [19,20]. These effects and an additional decrease in fibrosis were confirmed in a rat chronic model of doxorubicin-induced cardiotoxicity [21].

In a retrospective study of 201 patients treated with anthracyclines (67 treated with statins and 134 matched by propensity score), statins were associated with a reduction in heart failure (6% in the statin group and 18% in the control group, over a period of 2.6 years) [22]. A small randomized study (20 patients per group) demonstrated that atorvastatin pretreatment preserved the LVEF [23]. The use of statins, while not free of side effects, is not limited by the adverse hemodynamic changes associated with ACE inhibition or beta-blockade, nor by the concerns of increased risk of secondary malignancies, and represent a potentially promising therapy that needs to be confirmed in larger studies.

THALIDOMIDE

Thalidomide (α-*N*-phtalimido-glutarimide) was initially marketed in the 1950s as a sedative and antiemetic drug. It became popular to treat morning sickness in pregnancy but was discovered to result in major limb deformities; it is thought that between 8000 and 12,000 children were affected in utero. Interest was revived in 1965 when it was shown that thalidomide had antiinflammatory and immunomodulatory properties in erythema nodosum leprosum, a complication of leprosy. More recently, thalidomide was shown to inhibit basic fibroblast growth factor-induced angiogenesis [24] and is now indicated in the treatment of newly diagnosed multiple myeloma [25]. However, work by Fischer et al. [26] on the mechanism of action of thalidomide recently showed that the molecule can both upregulate or downregulate the ubiquitination (a process that can affect many properties of the protein, including its activity and degradation) of proteins, depending on the cell type and on the proteins expressed. It is important to note that thalidomide appears to have antiangiogenic properties at high doses but proangiogenic properties at low doses, and that at these lower doses it also increases vessel maturation and pericyte proliferation in microvessels through a platelet-derived growth factor [27].

Sunitinib, a tyrosine-kinase inhibitor used in renal cell carcinoma and gastrointestinal stromal tumors, and sorafenib, used in advanced renal cell or liver carcinoma, mainly target the vascular endothelial growth factor receptor (VEGFR) and the platelet-derived growth factor receptor (PDGFR) families. It is well known that both the VEGF and PDGFR pathways are cardioprotective and proangiogenic (see [28]). In a recent study, Chintalgattu et al. [29] also reported a novel effect of sunitinib-induced PDGFR inhibition, namely a depletion of coronary microvascular pericytes. Pericytes are cells that are closely associated with certain microvessels and that promote microvascular function. Of note, they did not find a similar pericyte depletion in doxorubicin-induced cardiotoxicity. Thalidomide prevented sunitinib-induced pericyte cell death in vitro and reversed both the microvascular dysfunction and the decrease in cardiac function in vivo, suggesting potential novel therapeutic applications of the drug.

METFORMIN

Metformin, an antihyperglycemic drug from the biguanide family, is widely used for the treatment of type II diabetes mellitus. Beyond its glucose-lowering properties, metformin has been reported to display direct antioxidant effects that may be advantageous in anthracycline-induced cardiotoxicity. Several mechanisms have been described, including increases in the antioxidant systems properties [30], decreases in lipid peroxidation [31], decreases in the generation of ROS through inhibition of protein kinase C [32], and also reduces apoptosis in heart failure by activation of 5′-adenosine monophosphate-activated protein kinase (AMPK) [33]. Three studies including one published very recently, have documented that metformin decreases the production of ROS, decreases apoptosis and the impairment of antioxidant defenses in isolated cardiomyocytes or cardiomyoblasts exposed to doxorubicin [34–36]. Mechanisms involved may include an upregulation of adiponectin pathways [35], increasing the expression of an iron-storage protein [34] and an AMPK-PDGFR pathway [36]. Whether these in vitro effects translate in vivo is currently unknown.

Metformin has also been tested in the setting of sunitinib-induced cardiotoxicity. Indeed, sunitinib is known to decrease AMPK in cardiomyocytes and in mice [37,38], and in cardiomyocytes, restoring AMPK by introducing a constitutively active AMPK decreases sunitinib-induced cell death [38]. This improvement has not been reproduced by pretreatment with metformin [37], warranting further studies.

REFERENCES

[1] Creighton AM, Birnie GD. The effect of bisdioxopiperazines on the synthesis of deoxyribonucleic acid, ribonucleic acid and protein in growing mouse-embryo fibroblasts. Biochem J 1969;114:58P.

[2] Diop NK, Vitellaro LK, Arnold P, Shang M, Marusak RA. Iron complexes of the cardioprotective agent dexrazoxane (ICRF-187) and its desmethyl derivative, ICRF-154: solid state structure, solution thermodynamics, and DNA cleavage activity. J Inorg Biochem 2000;78:209–16.

[3] Sawyer DB, Fukazawa R, Arstall MA, Kelly RA. Daunorubicin-induced apoptosis in rat cardiac myocytes is inhibited by dexrazoxane. Circ Res 1999;84:257–65.

[4] Herman EH, Ferrans VJ. Preclinical animal models of cardiac protection from anthracycline-induced cardiotoxicity. Semin Oncol 1998;25:15–21.

[5] Lipshultz SE, Scully RE, Lipsitz SR, Sallan SE, Silverman LB, Miller TL, et al. Assessment of dexrazoxane as a cardioprotectant in doxorubicin-treated children with high-risk acute lymphoblastic leukaemia: long-term follow-up of a prospective, randomised, multicentre trial. Lancet Oncol 2010;11:950–61.

[6] Lipshultz SE, Rifai N, Dalton VM, Levy DE, Silverman LB, Lipsitz SR, et al. The effect of dexrazoxane on myocardial injury in doxorubicin-treated children with acute lymphoblastic leukemia. N Engl J Med 2004;351:145–53.

[7] Marty M, Espié M, Llombart A, Monnier A, Rapoport BL, Stahalova V, Dexrazoxane Study Group. Multicenter randomized phase III study of the cardioprotective effect of dexrazoxane (Cardioxane) in advanced/metastatic breast cancer patients treated with anthracycline-based chemotherapy. Ann Oncol 2006;17:614–22.

[8] Speyer JL, Green MD, Zeleniuch-Jacquotte A, Wernz JC, Rey M, Sanger J, et al. ICRF-187 permits longer treatment with doxorubicin in women with breast cancer. J Clin Oncol 1992;10:117–27.

[9] Swain SM, Whaley FS, Gerber MC, Weisberg S, York M, Spicer D, et al. Cardioprotection with dexrazoxane for doxorubicin-containing therapy in advanced breast cancer. J Clin Oncol 1997;15:1318–32.

[10] Swain SM, Vici P. The current and future role of dexrazoxane as a cardioprotectant in anthracycline treatment: expert panel review. J Cancer Res Clin Oncol 2004;130:1–7.

[11] van Dalen EC, Caron HN, Dickinson HO, Kremer LC. Cardioprotective interventions for cancer patients receiving anthracyclines. Cochrane Database Syst Rev 2011;CD003917. Available from: http://dx.doi.org/10.1002/14651858.CD003917.pub4.

[12] Seymour L, Bramwell V, Moran LA. Use of dexrazoxane as a cardioprotectant in patients receiving doxorubicin or epirubicin chemotherapy for the treatment of cancer. The Provincial Systemic Treatment Disease Site Group. Cancer Prev Control 1999;3:145–59.

[13] Hensley ML, Schuchter LM, Lindley C, Meropol NJ, Cohen GI, Broder G, et al. American Society of Clinical Oncology clinical practice guidelines for the use of chemotherapy and radiotherapy protectants. J. Clin. Oncol 1999;17:3333–55.

[14] Tebbi CK, London WB, Friedman D, Villaluna D, De Alarcon PA, Constine LS, et al. Dexrazoxane-associated risk for acute myeloid leukemia/myelodysplastic syndrome and other secondary malignancies in pediatric Hodgkin's disease. J Clin Oncol 2007;25:493–500.

[15] Salzer WL, Devidas M, Carroll WL, Winick N, Pullen J, Hunger SP, et al. Long-term results of the pediatric oncology group studies for childhood acute lymphoblastic leukemia 1984-2001: a report from the children's oncology group. Leukemia 2010;24:355–70.

[16] FDA. Recommendations of the FDA regarding dexrazoxane. [Internet]. 2011 [cited 2015 Feb 10]; Available from: http://www.fda.gov/Drugs/DrugSafety/ucm263729.htm.

[17] Hayashidani S, Tsutsui H, Shiomi T, Suematsu N, Kinugawa S, Ide T, et al. Takeshita A. Fluvastatin, a 3-hydroxy-3-methylglutaryl coenzyme a reductase inhibitor, attenuates left ventricular remodeling and failure after experimental myocardial infarction. Circulation 2002;105:868–73.

[18] Landmesser U, Engberding N, Bahlmann FH, Schaefer A, Wiencke A, Heineke A, et al. Statin-induced improvement of endothelial progenitor cell mobilization, myocardial neovascularization, left ventricular function, and survival after experimental myocardial infarction requires endothelial nitric oxide synthase. Circulation 2004;110:1933–9.

[19] Ramanjaneyulu SVVS, Trivedi PP, Kushwaha S, Vikram A, Jena GB. Protective role of atorvastatin against doxorubicin-induced cardiotoxicity and testicular toxicity in mice. J Physiol Biochem 2013;69:513–25.

[20] Riad A, Bien S, Westermann D, Becher PM, Loya K, Landmesser U, et al. Pretreatment with statin attenuates the cardiotoxicity of Doxorubicin in mice. Cancer Res 2009;69: 695–9.

[21] Kim Y-H, Park S-M, Kim M, Kim SH, Lim S-Y, Ahn J-C, et al. Cardioprotective effects of rosuvastatin and carvedilol on delayed cardiotoxicity of doxorubicin in rats. Toxicol Mech Meth 2012;22:488–98.

[22] Seicean S, Seicean A, Plana JC, Budd GT, Marwick TH. Effect of statin therapy on the risk for incident heart failure in patients with breast cancer receiving anthracycline chemotherapy: an observational clinical cohort study. J Am Coll Cardiol 2012;60:2384–90.

[23] Acar Z, Kale A, Turgut M, Demircan S, Durna K, Demir S, et al. Efficiency of atorvastatin in the protection of anthracycline-induced cardiomyopathy. J Am Coll Cardiol 2011; 58:988–9.

[24] D'Amato RJ, Loughnan MS, Flynn E, Folkman J. Thalidomide is an inhibitor of angiogenesis. Proc Nat Acad Sci 1994;91:4082–5.

[25] Singhal S, Mehta J, Desikan R, Ayers D, Roberson P, Eddlemon P, et al. Antitumor activity of thalidomide in refractory multiple myeloma. N Engl J Med. 1999;341:1565–71.

[26] Fischer ES, Böhm K, Lydeard JR, Yang H, Stadler MB, Cavadini S, et al. Structure of the DDB1-CRBN E3 ubiquitin ligase in complex with thalidomide. Nature 2015;512:49–53.

[27] Lebrin F, Srun S, Raymond K, Martin S, van den Brink S, Freitas C, et al. Thalidomide stimulates vessel maturation and reduces epistaxis in individuals with hereditary hemorrhagic telangiectasia. Nat Med 2010;16:420–8.

[28] Hahn VS, Lenihan DJ, Ky B. Cancer therapy-induced cardiotoxicity: basic mechanisms and potential cardioprotective therapies. J Am Heart Assoc 2014;3:e000665.

[29] Chintalgattu V, Rees ML, Culver JC, Goel A, Jiffar T, Zhang J, et al. Coronary microvascular pericytes are the cellular target of sunitinib malate-induced cardiotoxicity. Sci Transl Med 2013;5:187ra69-187ra69.

[30] Faure P, Rossini E, Wiernsperger N, Richard MJ, Favier A, Halimi S. An insulin sensitizer improves the free radical defense system potential and insulin sensitivity in high fructose-fed rats. Diabetes 1999;48:353–7.
[31] Kanigür-Sultuybek G, Güven M, Onaran I, Tezcan V, Cenani A, Hatemi H. The effect of metformin on insulin receptors and lipid peroxidation in alloxan and streptozotocin induced diabetes. J Basic Clin Physiol Pharmacol 1995;6:271–80.
[32] Mahrouf M, Ouslimani N, Peynet J, Djelidi R, Couturier M, Therond P, et al. Metformin reduces angiotensin-mediated intracellular production of reactive oxygen species in endothelial cells through the inhibition of protein kinase C. Biochem Pharmacol 2006;72:176–83.
[33] Sasaki H, Asanuma H, Fujita M, Takahama H, Wakeno M, Ito S, et al. Metformin prevents progression of heart failure in dogs: role of AMP-activated protein kinase. Circulation 2009;119:2568–77.
[34] Asensio-López MC, Sánchez-Más J, Pascual-Figal DA, Abenza S, Pérez-Martínez MT, Valdés M, et al. Involvement of ferritin heavy chain in the preventive effect of metformin against doxorubicin-induced cardiotoxicity. Free Radic Biol Med 2012.
[35] Asensio-López MC, Lax A, Pascual-Figal DA, Valdés M, Sánchez-Más J. Metformin protects against doxorubicin-induced cardiotoxicity: involvement of the adiponectin cardiac system. Free Radic Biol Med 2011;51:1861–71.
[36] Kobashigawa LC, Xu YC, Padbury JF, Tseng Y-T, Yano N. Metformin protects cardiomyocyte from doxorubicin induced cytotoxicity through an AMP-activated protein kinase dependent signaling pathway: an in vitro study. PLoS One 2014;9:e104888.
[37] Hasinoff BB, Patel D, O'Hara KA. Mechanisms of myocyte cytotoxicity induced by the multiple receptor tyrosine kinase inhibitor sunitinib. Mol Pharmacol 2008;74:1722–8.
[38] Kerkelä R, Woulfe KC, Durand J-B, Vagnozzi R, Kramer D, Chu TF, et al. Sunitinib-induced cardiotoxicity is mediated by off-target inhibition of AMP-activated protein kinase. Clin Transl Sci 2009;2:15–25.

Chapter 41

Cardiotoxicity: Future Research Directions

T. López Fernández and J. López Sendón

Chapter Outline

Cardiovascular toxicity is a reality that impacts the quality of life and the overall survival of cancer patients. Careful analysis of the needs of these patients is mandatory to develop preventive strategies focused on the early detection and treatment of cardiovascular toxicities. Two major dilemmas are facing both the cardiologist and the hematologist/oncologist: the first is how to predict the risk of cancer therapeutics-related cardiac disease (CTRCD) [1,2], and the second how to improve therapeutic strategies to reduce cardiotoxicity without losing antitumor activity [3]. The quality of cancer care requires a cultural transformation. We need cardio-oncology multidisciplinary teams to integrate skills and abilities and to standardize the care process [4]. All the diagnostic and therapeutic specialties involved in the multidisciplinary team must unify their clinical criteria in standardized protocols, to reduce the risk of cardiac diseases and the risk of discontinuation of cancer therapy. Multidisciplinary teams must agree quality standards and must also be involved in research and educational projects [5,6].

HOW TO PREDICT THE RISK OF CTRCD

The expansion of cancer therapies to individuals with preexisting cardiovascular (CV) diseases, and the improvements in cancer survival, have increased the need for a thorough risk assessment of patients that will undergo active therapy. Moving toward a protective chemoprevention approach, we need as soon as possible a prospective risk score to optimize patient daily care from

Anticancer Treatments and Cardiotoxicity. DOI: http://dx.doi.org/10.1016/B978-0-12-802509-3.00041-8

both the medical and economical perspectives. Multiple definitions of CTRCD exist and are predominantly based on a change in left ventricular ejection fraction (LVEF). However, even a precise LVEF detects myocardial damage only when a functional impairment has already occurred, not allowing for early preventive strategies. Identification of cardiotoxicity with specific cardiac biomarkers and new imaging techniques may be more suitable to identify early asymptomatic and potentially reversible cardiac injury. Repeated measures of specific biomarkers show excellent promise for cancer treatment monitoring. To date, the largest body of literature has focused upon the assessment of troponins during anthracycline and trastuzumab treatments. Additional studies are necessary to clarify the optimal timing of biomarker assessment, the optimal level to improve the negative predictive value and the potential of new cardiac biomarkers in this field. CTRCD surveillance with myocardial strain [7], or cardiovascular magnetic resonance (CMR) tissue characterization [8], requires expensive technology and specific staff training, which makes it difficult to implement in all centers. Furthermore, in the best scenario, if all these techniques are available, prospective information is needed to standardize monitoring protocols and to explore their real predictive value in daily practice. The complexity of antitumoral agents, different dosing, and changes in treatment further challenge the appropriate identification of patients at risk.

HOW TO IMPROVE THERAPEUTIC STRATEGIES TO REDUCE CARDIOTOXICITY

Much research needs to be done to identify the most appropriate protective strategies against the development of CTRCD in cancer patients. We must focus on a tailored cancer therapy based on a cardiotoxicity risk evaluation. Patients with a low CTRCD risk profile need few clinical controls, whereas moderate- to high-risk patients will benefit from close follow-up or a primary CTRCD prevention therapy. The most common CV toxicity, or at least the better recognized, is left ventricular dysfunction, mainly associated with the use of anthracyclines and trastuzumab. On the basis of observational studies, it appears that a number of agents may be effective in primary CTRCD prevention. Statins, beta-blockers, and ACE inhibitors have been shown to reduce the risk of left ventricular dysfunction in high-risk populations treated with anthracyclines [9]. However, there is limited evidence to support the use of a widespread intervention strategy. The development of new cancer treatments increases the number of open questions in this field. The most effective means of delivering protective strategies remains to be defined. Are new cancer treatments as cardiotoxic as anthracyclines? Must we ask for a change in the preclinical development of new anticancer drugs, in terms of cardiovascular safety?

REFERENCES

[1] Plana JC, Galderisi M, Barac A, et al. Expert consensus for multimodality imaging evaluation of adult patients during and after cancer therapy: a report from the american society of echocardiography and the european association of cardiovascular imaging. J Am Soc Echocardiogr 2014;27:911−39.

[2] Lancellotti P, Nkomo VT, Badano L. Expert consensus for multi-modality imaging evaluation of cardiovascular complications of radiotherapy in adults: a report from the european association of cardiovascular imaging and the american society of echocardiography. J Am Soc Echocardiogr 2013;26:1013−32.

[3] Berardi R, Caramanti M, Savini A, et al. State of the art for cardiotoxicity due to chemotherapy and to targeted therapies: a literature review. Rev Oncol/Hematol 2013;88:75−86.

[4] Albini A, Pennesi G, Donatelli F, et al. Cardiotoxicity of anticancer drugs: the need for cardio-oncology and cardio-oncological prevention. J Natl Cancer Inst 2010;102:14−25.

[5] Holmes D, Rich JB, Zoghbi WA, et al. The heart team of cardiovascular care. J Am Coll Cardiol 2013;61:903−7.

[6] Prades J., van Hoof E., Remue E., Borras J.M. Multidisciplinary teams in cancer care: a systematic review of the evidence. Deliverable 1, specific objective 1.1; Work Package 7 of the European Partnership for Action Against Cancer (EPAAC). Available from: www.epaac.eu.

[7] Thavendiranathan P, et al. Use of myocardial strain imaging by echocardiography for the early detection of cardiotoxicity in patients during and after cancer chemotherapy: a systematic review. J Am Coll Cardiol 2014;63(25 Pt A):2751−68.

[8] Tham EB, Haykowsky MJ, Chow K, Spavor M, Kaneko S, Khoo NS, et al. Diffuse myocardial fibrosis by T1-mapping in children with subclinical anthracycline cardiotoxicity: relationship to exercise capacity, cumulative dose and remodeling. J Cardiovasc Magn Reson 2013;15(1):48.

[9] Bosch X, Rovira M, Sitges M, Domenech A, Ortiz-Perez JT, de Caralt TM, et al. Enalapril and carvedilol for preventing chemotherapy-induced left ventricular systolic dysfunction in patients with malignant hemopathies: the OVERCOME trial (preventiOn of left Ventricular dysfunction with Enalapril and caRvedilol in patients submitted to intensive ChemOtherapy for the treatment of Malignant hEmopathies). J Am Coll Cardiol 2013;61(23):2355−62.

Multiple Choice Questions

Italicized the correct answer

How Big Is the Problem? The Oncologist's View?

1. **One important challenge concerning cardiotoxicity from the oncologist point of view**
   a. Toxicity is not a concern if the patient is cured
   b. *Cardiotoxicity is frequently seen only many years after systemic therapy*
   c. No effective treatments are available even if toxicity is detected early
   d. All anticancer treatment options are associated with the same cardiac risk

2. **Cardiac toxicity in the real world**
   a. Younger age is an important risk factor for developing cardiac problems after chemotherapy
   b. *Cardiotoxicity is higher in the real world compared to clinical trials as patients are less selected (older patients presenting more comorbidities in the real world)*
   c. Cardiotoxicity is not a concern as most patients are not cured after adjuvant therapy
   d. Cardiotoxicity is not a concern as preventive therapies allow today the elimination of long-term cardiac side effects

3. **Perspectives of cardio-oncology**
   a. *Close collaboration of cardiologists and oncologists is needed for early identification and optimal management of cardiotoxicity*
   b. Cardiologists should not interfere with oncological treatments
   c. Biomarkers and new imaging techniques should not be developed because current results are disappointing
   d. Preventive therapies with cardioprotective agents are contraindicated from the oncological point of view

General Considerations

1. **Increased intima medial thickness and higher grade of abnormality in the bulb wall were observed at doses higher than**
   a. 20 Gy
   b. 30 Gy
   c. *35 Gy*
   d. 50 Gy

2. **Postradiation effects are due to**
   a. Fibrosis of vasa vasorum
   b. Adventia fibrosis
   c. Accelerated atherosclerosis
   d. *All the above answers*

3. **Which ECG abnormality is more frequent after radiation therapy?**
   a. *Right bundle branch block*
   b. Left bundle branch block
   c. A-V block
   d. Premature ventricular beats

Detrimental Effects of Anticancer Drugs and Radiotherapy on the Heart

1. **Regarding anthracycline cardiotoxicity, which of these statements is wrong**
   a. It is involved in an excess of ROS
   b. One of the mechanisms is the topoisomerase inhibition
   c. *None of the above*
   d. All previous

2. **Strategies for reducing anthracycline cardiotoxicity include**
   a. Using lower doses of anthracycline
   b. Using liposomal formulations
   c. Use of dexrazoxane
   d. *All of the above*

3. **Which of these drugs is the founder of ErbB2 inhibitors**
   a. Lapatinib
   b. TDM1
   c. *Trastuzumab*
   d. None of the above

4. **Regarding the cardiotoxicity induced by trastuzumab which is incorrect**
   a. It is not dose-dependent
   b. It is frequently reversible after suspension of therapy

c. *It is not possible to restart the therapy when the EF is completely restored*
d. This type of cardiomyopathy is defined as type II

5. **Mechanisms of radiation-induced valvular disease (RIVD) include**
   a. Microvascular damage
   b. Macrovascular damage
   c. Accelerated development of age-related atherosclerosis
   d. *All of the above*

6. **Risk factors for the onset of RIVD are**
   a. Total radiation dose
   b. The irradiated volume
   c. Use of chemotherapy
   d. *All of the above*

7. **Which of these statements concerning the anthracyclines is incorrect**
   a. *They do not produce negative effects additional to ionizing radiation*
   b. Safe doses can also produce negative effects additional to ionizing radiation
   c. They produce negative effects regardless of the timing of the injection in relation to radiation
   d. Anthracyclines produce negative effects on the heart additional to ionizing radiation

8. **Which of these statements is incorrect**
   a. The incidence of RIVD appears to be higher on the left side of the heart
   b. The reported median interval from radiation to symptomatic RIVD is 22 years
   c. *The incidence of RIVD appears to be higher on the right side of the heart*
   d. The left chambers are subjected to a greater hemodynamic stress

Cardiovascular Complications of Cancer Treatments

1. **A 58-year-old man with known promyelocytic leukemia is diagnosed with a relapse. Treatment with arsenic trioxide was started 6 weeks ago given the refractory nature of the disease. He has been undergoing weekly EKGs to assess for QT prolongation. ECG performed in the office today shows QT interval of 520 ms. Patient is currently asymptomatic. What should be the most appropriate next step in management?**
   a. Send the patient home and advise him to return if he experiences palpitations or syncope
   b. Perform a stat echocardiogram
   c. Initiate amiodarone to prevent fatal ventricular arrhythmias
   d. *Admit the patient under telemetry, check serum electrolytes, and administer IV magnesium sulfate*

Note: Arsenic trioxide causes QT prolongation. If a patient develops QT of >500 ms or reports symptoms such as palpitations or syncope, he/she should be promptly hospitalized under cardiac telemetry and the offending agent should be temporarily held while reassessing the QT. Administration of intravenous magnesium sulfate with prompt correction of electrolyte abnormalities should be done.

2. **A 74-year-old female with ovarian cancer now being treated with paclitaxel infusion starts complaining of sweating, flushing, dizziness. ECG showed sinus bradycardia with HR 44. Which of the following step could have prevented this**
   a. Prophylactic temporary transvenous pacer
   b. *Pretreatment with antihistamines and corticosteroids*
   c. Evaluation for carcinoid syndrome
   d. IV hydration before chemotherapy infusion

   Note: Cremophor EL, the vehicle used for paclitaxel formulation, causes histamine release which produces bradycardia. Pretreatment with antihistamines and corticosteroids to avoid the release of histamine may prevent bradycardia due to this mechanism.

3. **A 59-year-old female is admitted to the hospital for intractable nausea and vomiting which began after receiving cisplatin for non small-cell lung cancer 2 days ago. She is started on ondansetron for chemotherapy-induced nausea and vomiting. Her EKG on day 3 of admission is significant for prolonged QT interval of 503 ms. Patient reports no symptoms and has no known cardiovascular comorbidities. What is the most likely cause of the QT interval prolongation?**
   a. Hypovolemia secondary to nausea and vomiting
   b. Cisplatin
   c. *Ondansetron*
   d. Coronary artery disease

4. **A 50-year-old male with prior history of mediastinal mantle radiation for Hodgkin's lymphoma 18 years ago, now comes with palpitations, dizziness and two episodes of syncope. ECG showed complete heart block. What is the most likely explanation?**
   a. *Progressive fibrosis of conduction system of the heart*
   b. Hypothyroid
   c. Medication-induced
   d. Age-related calcification of conduction system of heart

   Note: Complete heart block, syncope, and sudden death can occur even 10 years after mediastinal radiotherapy. Age-related calcification is seen usually beyond 70 years of age. Permanent pacemaker implantation is indicated for high-degree AV blocks.

5. **A 65-year-old male with history of lung cancer who underwent lung resection. The patient is now evaluated due to intractable pain, hence placed on methadone 120 mg po once daily and amitriptyline. His EKG in clinic showed atrial tachycardia. Which medication should be avoided for rate control in this patient?**
   a. Metoprolol
   b. Diltiazem
   c. *Amiodarone*
   d. Adenosine

   Note: Both methadone and amitriptyline cause QT prolongation. Adding amiodarone may further prolong the QT and will increase the risk of life-threatening Torsades de pointes and sudden death.

6. **A 65-year old male with non small-cell lung cancer who underwent video-assisted thoracoscopic surgery (VATS) 8 h ago. Cardiology evaluation was requested due to new episode of atrial fibrillation. Baseline electrocardiogram showed normal sinus rhythm with left ventricular hyperthrophy. What is the best statement regarding the current arrhythmia**
   a. It increases the risk of bleeding during early postoperative time
   b. It is associated with an increased risk of hospital-acquired pneumonia
   c. Calcium channel blockers are contraindicated
   d. *Patient has an increased risk of cardiovascular events*

   Note: Atrial fibrillation during POP time has been associated with increased postoperative mortality, critical care unit admission rates, longer hospitalization, and higher rates of death from cardiovascular diseases.

7. **A 66-year-old man with medical history of hypertension, and esophageal cancer who underwent surgical resection and chemotherapy. Patient has chronic renal disease with a creatinine clearance of 29 mL/min. A recent Holter monitoring reported episodes of paroxysmal atrial fibrillation without associated symptoms. What is the best choice for this patient regarding stroke prevention?**
   a. ASA 81 mg/day
   b. *Warfarin to keep INR between 2 and 3*
   c. Rivaroxaban 15 mg daily with the evening meal (reduced dose due to renal function)
   d. Dabigatran 75 mg po every 12 h

   Note: ASA is no longer recommended for stroke prevention. Warfarin is recommended in all guidelines from cardiology societies. There is no experience/evidence of NOACs in cancer patients.

8. **A 52-year-old woman who is seen in the cardiology clinic due to new onset of atrial fibrillation. She has a history of breast cancer treated with trastuzumab. No prior surgical interventions. She has**

normal renal function. Her CHA2Ds2-Vasc is 3. Patient denies any cardiovascular symptoms including chest pain, palpitations, or shortness of breath. Her daughter has recently noticed minor memory problems and frequent mood changes. Twelve-lead ECG showed atrial fibrillation with a ventricular rate of 100. What is the most appropriate next step for stroke prevention?

a. ASA
b. Warfarin for INR 2–3
c. Dabigatran
d. *MRI of the brain*
e. Transesophageal echocardiogram

Note: MRI of the brain for screening of brain metastasis, which it is considered a contraindication for systemic AC. The initiation of anticoagulation must be weighed against the risk of hemorrhage in certain cases.

9. **A 29-year old woman with history of diabetes mellitus, chronic kidney disease, and claudication, is seen in the oncology unit due to new-onset atrial fibrillation with rapid ventricular response. Patient was admitted due to fever and malaise. She has a history of acute promyelocytic leukemia treated with chemotherapy (all-trans retinoic acid [ATRA] and arsenic trioxide). Coagulation times are normal with slightly elevated plasma fibrinogen and elevated D-dimer. Platelet count is 35,000. Chronic DIC is suspected. There is no evidence of active bleeding at this time. What is the best step regarding management and stroke prevention?**

a. ASA for stroke prevention and rate control with calcium channel blockers
b. Warfarin for stroke prevention and rate control with calcium channel blockers
c. ASA for stroke prevention and rate control with amiodarone
d. *Avoid systemic anticoagulation until improvement of platelet count. Consider rate control*
e. Warfarin for stroke prevention and rate control with β-blockers

Note: Severe thrombocytopenia is usually a contraindication for systemic AC. Risk versus benefits of anticoagulation must be weighed against the risk of hemorrhage versus thrombosis in certain cases.

10. **A 69-year old man with history of hypertension, diabetes mellitus, paroxysmal atrial fibrillation on metoprolol succinate 100 mg/day, amiodarone 200 mg/day and systemic anticoagulation for stroke prevention, and metastatic pancreatic cancer on chemotherapy with 5-FU (fluorouracil), leucovorin, oxaliplatin, and irinotecan (FOLFIRINOX). Twelve-lead ECG showed sinus tachycardia with a ventricular rate of 106, and a QT interval of 499 ms. Successful**

chemotherapy infusion was administered. What medication should be given with caution to avoid cardiovascular events?

a. Metoprolol succinate
b. Warfarin
c. Acetaminophen
d. *Ondansetron*
e. Diphenhydramine

Note: Ondansetron has to be avoided to prevent further prolongation of the QT interval.

11. **What percentage of patients with metastatic disease who experience STEMI and NSTEMI received PCI?**

a. 100% and 50%
b. 75% and 25%
c. 50% and 25%
d. *25% and 10%*
e. 10% and 5%

Note: 25% and 10% of patients receive PCI for STEMI and NSTEMI, respectively.

12. **What type or radiation carries the highest risk of coronary artery disease?**

a. *Hodgkin's lymphoma*
b. Left-sided breast cancer radiation
c. Thyroid radiation
d. Left lung cancer radiation
e. Hepatic cancer radiation

Note: Hodgkin's lymphoma, with an average of >30 Gy radiation, carries the highest risk of coronary artery disease.

13. **Fluorouracil (5-FU) toxicity may present clinically as**

a. NSTEMI
b. STEMI
c. Unstable angina
d. *All of the above*

Note: 5-FU toxicity may present as unstable angina, NSTEMI, or STEMI.

14. **Fluorouracil (5-FU) cardiotoxicity is likely to present within**

a. *12–48 h*
b. 48 h–7 days
c. 7–30 days
d. >30 days
e. Month to years

Note: 5-FU cardiotoxicity usually presents within 12–48 h.

15. How do you treat 5-FU vasospasm?

a. *Nitrates*
b. Angioplasty
c. CABG
d. TNK—thrombolytics
e. PCI with stenting.

Note: 5-FU vasospasm is initially treated with nitrates.

16. Subclinical LV dysfunction is defined as

a. GLS <16%
b. GLS <18%
c. 15% reduction when compared to reference value from JUSTICE study
d. *15% reduction in GLS when compared to baseline value*

Note: Subclinical LV dysfunction is defined as a 15% reduction in GLS when compared to baseline value.

17. When using GLS, it is important to take into consideration

a. BP
b. Loading conditions
c. Age
d. Gender
e. *All of the above*

Note: When using GLS it is important to take into consideration the age and gender of the patient as well as the BP and loading conditions in the moment of the interrogation.

18. In the treatment of atrial fibrillation in patients under anticancer treatment

a. Amiodarone is not considered a treatment option due to its potential interaction with other QT-prolonging drugs
b. Sotalol is not considered a treatment option due to its potential interaction with other QT-prolonging drugs
c. Digoxin should be considered the first choice for rate control since it does not impact systolic function negatively
d. *Amiodarone should be considered for rate control in patients with severely depressed ejection fraction or in a situation of severe heart failure*
e. Class IC antiarrhythmic agents such as flecainide should be considered for rate control in patients with severely depressed ejection fraction or in a situation of severe heart failure

19. Anticoagulation therapy in patients under anticancer treatment who develop atrial fibrillation

a. Should be initiated immediately after diagnosis given the increased thrombogenic risk in cancer patients

b. Should only be considered in patients with previous ischemic stroke given the increased bleeding risk in cancer patients
c. The use of CHA_2DS_2-VASc and HAS-BLED scores should guide decision-making also considering the type of cancer and its influence on bleeding or thrombogenic risk
d. *In cancer patients, other factors such as the presence of left atrial dilatation must be taken into consideration in the indication for anticoagulant therapy*
e. Low-dose aspirin is an effective alternative to antithrombotic therapy in cancer patients with atrial fibrillation

20. **Bradycardia and conduction disturbances in cancer patients**
   a. Are rare complications of cancer treatment
   b. Require permanent pacemaker implantation since the damage to the conduction system due to cancer treatment is permanent
   c. Are seldom related to correctable factors
   d. Are the most frequent cause of syncope and loss of physical capacity
   e. *Can be related to the development of ventricular arrhythmias such as Torsade de Pointes*

21. **Regarding the use of diuretics in patients under anticancer treatment, one of the following statements is FALSE**
   a. Spironolactone is useful in preserving left ventricular systolic function in patients under treatment with anthracyclines
   b. Spironolactone may have a cardioprotective effect in patients under treatment with trastuzumab
   c. *Treatment with spironolactone should be titrated to the maximum tolerated dose*
   d. Loop diuretics should not be considered on a systematic basis, but indicated depending on the patient's symptomatic status
   e. Combining different diuretics should be considered in patients with resistance to loop diuretics

Imaging Evaluation of Cardiac Structure and Function in Cancer Patients

1. **Find the correct answer**
   a. Left ventricular ejection fraction (EF) by 2D echocardiography is more accurate and reproducible than EF by 3D, and better suited to discover cardiotoxicity
   b. *Left ventricular EF by 3D echocardiography is more accurate and reproducible than EF by 2D, and better suited to discover cardiotoxicity*

c. Left ventricular ejection fraction (EF) by 3D echocardiography needs less training than EF by 3D
d. EF by 2D echocardiography is generally more dependent on image quality than EF by 3D echocardiography

2. **Find the correct answer**
   a. Speckle tracking echocardiography (STE) is a volume-based measure of myocardial function
   b. The speckles followed by the STE software are natural speckles found in the myocardium
   c. *EF and global longitudinal strain are both dependent on left ventricular load*
   d. STE cannot be used for assessment of right ventricle

3. **Find the correct answer**
   a. *A relative percentage reduction of GLS of 15% from baseline is very likely to be abnormal*
   b. A relative reduction of GLS of 15% from baseline should urge the cardiologist to stop further cancer treatment
   c. There is no need to use the same vendor-specific ultrasound machine when applying STE for the longitudinal follow-up of cancer patients
   d. A drop of GLS occurs in all patients treated for cancer

4. **Has stress echocardiography any role in the risk stratification of cancer patients?**
   a. No
   b. Only in CAD patients
   c. *Unsettled*

5. **Which is the preferred stressor in these patients?**
   a. Exercise
   b. *Pharmacologic*
   c. Handgrip

6. **An elicitable contractile reserve in patients with evidence of posttherapy cardiomyopathy**
   a. Is related to worse outcome
   b. *Is related to better outcome*
   c. Is not related to outcome

7. **According to the 2014 joint ASE/EACVI expert consensus document for multimodality imaging evaluation of adult patients during and after cancer therapy, when is CMR recommended?**
   a. In all patients
   b. In patients with LV dysfunction before chemotherapy

c. *In patients with LV dysfunction during chemotherapy in whom discontinuation of chemotherapy is considered*
d. In patients with ferromagnetic implants

8. **Which of the following LGE pattern has not been described in anthracycline cardiomyopathy**
   a. *Subendocardial*
   b. Epicardial
   c. Mid-wall
   d. Insertion points of the RV into the LV

9. **Which of the following statements is false**
   a. LGE identifies focal myocardial fibrosis
   b. Native T1 mapping identifies myocardial and interstitial fibrosis
   c. ECV identifies interstitial myocardial fibrosis
   d. *LGE identifies diffuse myocardial fibrosis*

Detection of Cardiac Dysfunction and Predictors of Cardiotoxicity

1. **Which variable is not included in the Lee index or "revised cardiac risk" index**
   a. History of ischemic heart disease
   b. *Disseminated cancer*
   c. History of cerebrovascular disease
   d. Preoperative treatment with insulin
   e. Preoperative creatinine >2 mg/dL

2. **Echocardiography in the preoperative setting**
   a. Echocardiography is the cornerstone in the cardiac evaluation and is mandatory in all patients before surgery
   b. Appropriate use criteria for echocardiography state that it is "appropriate" to assess ventricular function in patients without signs or symptoms of cardiovascular disease in the preoperative setting
   c. *Appropriate use criteria for echocardiography state that it is "inappropriate" to assess ventricular function in patients without signs or symptoms of cardiovascular disease in the preoperative setting*
   d. Left ventricular ejection decrease doesn't modify preoperative risk evaluation
   e. Left ventricular ejection fraction is a variable of the NSQIP risk calculator

3. **In patients with previous history of heart failure**
   a. If patients are asymptomatic, the risk for perioperative complications doesn't increase

b. *Left ventricular ejection fraction dysfunction (<30%) is an independent contributor to preoperative outcome*
c. LV dysfunction (<30%) itself is not a risk factor for death in patients undergoing intermediate- or high-risk noncardiac surgery
d. The risk of postoperative death is the same as patients with coronary artery disease
e. Heart failure is not included in cardiac risk calculator models

4. **Natriuretic peptides in perioperative risk of HF**
a. Measurement of biomarkers, especially natriuretic peptides, is not helpful in assessing patients with HF
b. Increases in cardiac troponin I or BNP concentrations have not been related to risk of cardiotoxicity
c. *Preoperative natriuretic peptide levels independently predict cardiovascular events in the first 30 days after vascular surgery*
d. Baseline assessment of biomarker concentrations is not useful in patients with left ventricular dysfunction
e. Prospective randomized studies have demonstrated the utility of baseline assessment of biomarker concentration

5. **On preoperative evaluation of patients treated with anticancer drugs, which is false**
a. The majority of risk calculator models don't include cancer or previous chemotherapy as a variable
b. Evaluation of left ventricular function should be considered in preoperative evaluation, especially in patients treated with anthracycline and high risk of development cardiotoxicity
c. Determination of preoperative natriuretic peptide levels at baseline could be a useful approach, especially in patients with left ventricular dysfunction
d. *The effect of asymptomatic left ventricular dysfunction on perioperative outcomes is well known*
e. Risk index models provide complementary prognostic perspectives and can help the clinician in the decision-making process

Cardiotoxicity in Childhood

1. **Which are the most common cancers in childhood**
a. Leukemia and lymphoma
b. Solid tumors of the central nervous system
c. Neuroblastomas
d. *All of the above*

2. **In which proportion of childhood cancer are anthracycline used**
a. *50%*
b. 70%

c. 30%
d. 40%

3. **In which proportion of childhood cancer is radiotherapy used**
   a. *50%*
   b. 25%
   c. 10%
   d. 60%

Management of Anticancer Drugs Related Cardiotoxicity

1. **What is the most recommended drug for the treatment of arterial hypertension induced by monoclonal antibodies, especially those who have antiangiogenic properties**
   a. Calcium channel blockers
   b. β-Blockers
   c. *Angiotensin-converting enzyme inhibitors*
   d. Diuretics
   e. α-Blockers

2. **What is the relative decrease in the global longitudinal strain of the left ventricle that is considered as a marker of cardiotoxicity related to cancer treatments**
   a. >20%
   b. *>15%*
   c. >30%
   d. 53%
   e. Longitudinal strain of the left ventricle is not an important factor in the follow-up process of these patients

3. **All of these following drugs have been suggested as protective drugs against the adverse effects of cardiotoxic chemotherapy except one. Which is this one**
   a. Statins
   b. Angiotensin-converting enzyme inhibitors
   c. Dexrazoxane
   d. Ranolazine
   e. *Trimetazidine*

4. **Which one between these sentences is the false one**
   a. During an acute coronary syndrome people on cancer treatments should receive complete antithrombotic therapy
   b. *Isolated ACTP is the best option, as it has no risk of restenosis*
   c. Percutaneous or surgical revascularization is accepted in cancer patients

d. Thrombocytopenia is not a contraindication for treatment with aspirin
e. Second or one-stage procedures are accepted for surgical myocardial revascularization

5. **One patient on anticancer treatment arrives at an emergency department presenting an STEMI. Time of ischemia: 60 min. Which is the best treatment option for him**
   a. Isolated medical treatment is the best option as he is at high risk of bleeding
   b. Surgical myocardial revascularization is the best option as it avoids double antiplatelet treatment
   c. *Primary PCI is the best option for treatment*
   d. STEMI is not a life-threatening situation as cancer is the real one
   e. He should be treated only with aspirin as he is at high risk of bleeding

Multidisciplinary Approach to Cardiac Disease in Cancer Patients

1. **An ideal cardio-oncology team should involve**
   a. Oncologists and cardiologists
   b. Oncologists, radiotherapists, and cardiologists
   c. Oncologists, surgeons, and cardiologists
   d. *Oncologists, radiotherapists, surgeons, and cardiologists*

2. **A cardiovascular evaluation during cancer therapy should include**
   a. Physical exam
   b. Physical exam and ECG
   c. Physical exam and echocardiogram
   d. *Physical exam, ECG, and echocardiogram (or control of biomarkers)*

3. **It is reasonable to prolong the cardiologic follow-up of patients who have undergone anthracycline chemotherapy and/or radiotherapy for**
   a. *10 years*
   b. 20 years
   c. 15 years
   d. 1 year

Future Research Priorities

1. **Pharmacogenomics identifies genetic variants that predict drug response and the occurrence of adverse reactions. These variants are common SNPs (heritable single-nucleotide polymorphisms) accounting for approximately**
   a. *90% of the genetic difference between individuals*
   b. 50% of the genetic difference between individuals
   c. 10% of the genetic difference between individuals

2. **Common SNPs are arbitrarily defined as having a minor allele frequency (MAF) >5% in the targeted population. Homozygosity for an allele with an MAF of 5% means that**
   a. Only five homozygous individuals will be identified in a sample of 1000
   b. *Only five homozygous individuals will be identified in a sample of 2000*
   c. Only five homozygous individuals will be identified in a sample of 100

3. **A pharmacogenomics knowledge resource is**
   a. *Freely available to clinicians*
   b. Not yet available
   c. Available but does not include clinical dosing guidelines yet

4. **Extensive research is underway to understand how genomic information can be used to develop more personalized and cost-effective strategies for using drugs to improve human health**
   a. Genetic markers are useful to mitigate individual risk for chemotherapy-induced cardiotoxicity, and genetic testing is already approved by the FDA for anthracyclines
   b. *Genetic markers may be useful to mitigate individual risk for chemotherapy-induced cardiotoxicity, but there is still a long way to go before clinical application*
   c. Genetic markers are not useful to mitigate individual risk for chemotherapy-induced cardiotoxicity

5. **Up to now, there have been very limited large-scale efforts to interrogate the human genome for markers of risk for chemotherapy-induced cardiotoxicity**
   a. *Most of the studies focused on anthracyclines, and therefore knowledge of the genetic determinants of susceptibility to the cardiotoxicity of trastuzumab and other targeted therapies is limited*
   b. Most of the studies focused on trastuzumab and other targeted therapies, and therefore knowledge of the genetic determinants of susceptibility to the cardiotoxicity of anthracyclines is limited
   c. Most of the studies focused on tyrosine kinase inhibitors, and therefore knowledge of the genetic determinants of susceptibility to the cardiotoxicity of anthracyclines and HER2 inhibitors is limited

6. **While some patients with little exposure to anthracyclins have considerable cardiac damage, others with higher exposure do not develop heart problems**
   a. *Although clinical and demographic factors may predispose certain individuals to greater risk and severity of cardiotoxicity, the relatively high heritability of anthracycline cytotoxicity supports a genetic contribution to the variability of sensitivity*

b. Clinical and demographic factors predispose certain individuals to greater risk and severity of anthracyclin-induced cardiotoxicity, a genetic contribution to the variability of sensitivity is unlikely
c. Clinical and demographic factors predispose certain individuals to greater risk and severity of cardiotoxicity, the relatively low heritability of anthracycline cytotoxicity does not support a genetic contribution to the variability of sensitivity

Index

Note: Page numbers followed by "*f*" and "*t*" refer to figures and tables, respectively.

B

F

P

S

W

FSC
www.fsc.org
MIX
Papier | Fördert gute Waldnutzung
FSC® C083411

Kolibri 360 GmbH
Ferdinand-Jühlke-Straße 7
99095 Erfurt, Deutschland
produktsicherheit@kolibri360.de